Postcards of Nursing

A WORLDWIDE TRIBUTE

Postcards of Nursing

A WORLDWIDE TRIBUTE

Michael Zwerdling, RN

Providence Hospital

Washington, D.C.

◆ LIPPINCOTT WILLIAMS & WILKINS
A **Wolters Kluwer** Company

Philadelphia • Baltimore • New York • London
Buenos Aires • Hong Kong • Sydney • Tokyo

Acquisitions Editor: Patricia Casey
Editorial Assistant: Megan Klim/Dana Irwin
Senior Project Editor: Tom Gibbons
Senior Production Manager: Helen Ewan
Managing Editor/Production: Erika Kors
Art Director: Carolyn O'Brien
Illustration Coordinator: Brett MacNaughton
Manufacturing Manager: William Alberti
Indexer: Manjit Sahai
Compositor: Circle Graphics
Printer: R. R. Donnelley
Prepress/scans: Steven Edson Photography

9 8 7 6 5 4 3 2 1

Library of Congress Cataloging-in Publication Data

Zwerdling, Michael.
    Postcards of Nursing : a worldwide tribute / Michael Zwerdling.
        p. cm.
    Includes bibliographical references and index.
    ISBN 0-7817-4050-9 (cloth : alk. paper)
        1. Nursing—Miscellanea. 2. Postcards. I. Title.

RT55.Z94 2003
610.73—dc21

                                                2003054093

Care has been taken to confirm the accuracy of the information presented and to describe generally accepted practices. However, the authors, editors, and publisher are not responsible for errors or omissions or for any consequences from application of the information in this book and make no warranty, express or implied, with respect to the content of the publication.

The authors, editors, and publisher have exerted every effort to ensure that drug selection and dosage set forth in this text are in accordance with the current recommendations and practice at the time of publication. However, in view of ongoing research, changes in government regulations, and the constant flow of information relating to drug therapy and drug reactions, the reader is urged to check the package insert for each drug for any change in indications and dosage and for added warnings and precautions. This is particularly important when the recommended agent is a new or infrequently employed drug.

Some drugs and medical devices presented in this publication have Food and Drug Administration (FDA) clearance for limited use in restricted research settings. It is the responsibility of the health care provider to ascertain the FDA status of each drug or device planned for use in his or her clinical practice.

This book is dedicated to
The Company of the Daughters of Charity

and to

The Providence Hospital Emergency Department
Washington, D.C.

Reviewers

Dean Krimmel
Director
University of Maryland School of
    Nursing Museum
University of Maryland
Baltimore, Maryland

Philip Maples, BS, MA
Curator/Director
Baker-Cederberg Museum and Archives
Rochester General Hospital
Rochester, New York

Mary May, RN, BSN
Staff Nurse
Oncology
Alegent Health Immanuel Medical Center
Omaha, Nebraska

ool of Nursing

Susan Brown Nicholson
Author, postcard expert
Lisle, Illinois

N, MSN

cology
norial Hospital
alifornia

Contents

Introduction

The most beautiful and informative images of nursing are found on picture postcards. No other format, including the photograph, the book, the magazine, or the postage stamp, has depicted 20th-century nursing with such scope and diversity.

The postcards in this book date from 1893 to 2002. Many are taken from the period of 1907 through World War I, known as the Golden Age of postcards. During that time, according to International Postal Union figures, approximately 140 billion postcards were mailed worldwide. Great as it is, that number represents only a fraction of the total production because vast numbers of postcards were kept or exchanged without mailing.

During the same period, in both the United States and in Europe, the industrial revolution had created dire conditions. Immigrants' rush to the cities, and the subsequent widespread unsanitary living conditions, had resulted in epidemic-level diseases. Machines at factories, construction sites, farms, and mines were complex, had fast-moving parts or operated under pressure, and were often unstable. Corrosive and flammable chemicals created their own hazards. Labor laws were few, and safety measures were primitive at best. The situation created a desperate need for health care reform.

Thousands of nurses were needed to work with the increasing numbers of patients in both urban and rural settings. Then came World War I, creating an emergent need for thousands more to staff the hospitals in Europe (while not depleting the number of nurses available at home). Finally, coinciding with the peak of the major Allied offensive, the 1918 flu pandemic struck, killing tens of millions of victims worldwide, putting a further strain on health care resources. The critical need for nurses, then, overlapped with the Golden Age of postcards. Postcards reflected and, in turn, fueled the public's awareness of the importance of the nurse.

This book is offered as a tribute to all nurses—past, present and future. Filled with images of rare and beautiful postcards, it is primarily an art book. It documents not the history of nursing per se, but rather nursing's relationship to the significant forces in 20th-century society and culture.

I hope that, in addition to finding the social history informative and interesting, you are refreshed by the therapeutic quality of the images themselves. And, for those of you who are not nurses, I hope that you become inspired to investigate nursing as a career path. Nursing is experiencing the most critical shortage in its history. Literally hundreds of thousands of additional nurses are needed now, and the need grows daily. There is no better profession, and we most certainly can use your help.

Although there are many ways to approach this book, I want to tell you what I had in mind when I designed it. The idea was for the reader to approach each chapter as if it were a museum or gallery exhibit, each double-page spread representing one wall. If you wish, you can read the introduction to each exhibit (chapter) or simply walk right in and wander around, so to speak. Whenever you come to an image about which you would like to know more, the notes are available. The notes are intended to be unpredictable; that is, they are not uniform in degree of detail and may not even relate to nursing, though each note does relate directly, in some way, to the postcard. For those who prefer a more guided tour, the postcards do follow a sequence based mostly on chronology and geography, but visual compatibility was the prime consideration in placement.

I hope you'll enjoy perusing this book as much as I enjoyed putting it together.

Michael Zwerdling, R.N.
Burtonsville, Maryland
www.nursepostcard.com
November 18, 2002

Note: The original dimensions of most postcards printed before 1930 were a uniform $3\frac{1}{2}$ inches by $5\frac{1}{2}$ inches. Most of the postcards printed after 1930 were 4 inches by 6 inches.

Postcards of Nursing

A WORLDWIDE TRIBUTE

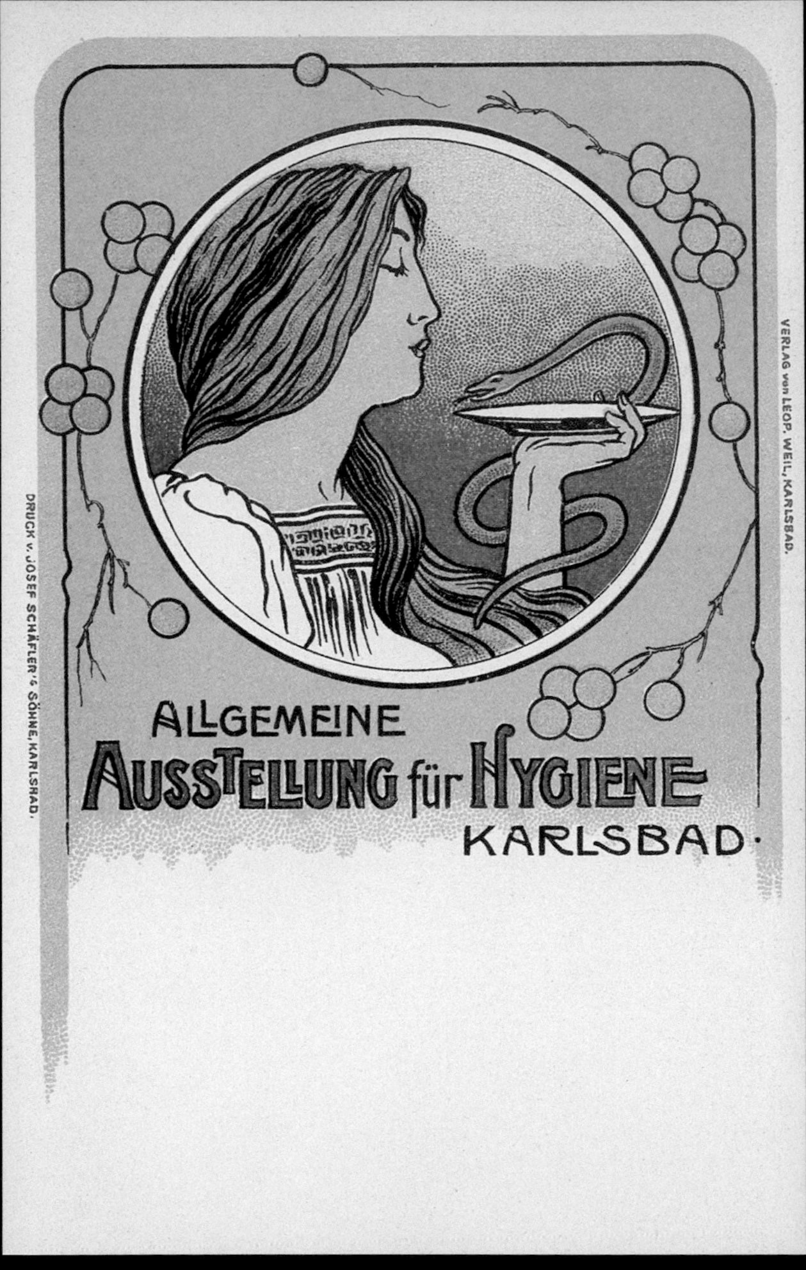
ALLGEMEINE
AUSSTELLUNG für HYGIENE
KARLSBAD·
VERLAG von LEOP. WEIL, KARLSBAD.
DRUCK v. JOSEF SCHÄFLER's SÖHNE, KARLSBAD.

Figure 1.1. German Hygiene Exposition.
Karlsbad, Germany. 1900. *(See note.)*

Symbols of Care

*M*ost of us, at one time or another, get so caught up in the urgencies and details of our lives that we are unable to view things from a more panoramic perspective. We forget who we really are and the extent to which imagination and spirit shape our identity. We become less resilient to stress, more prone to illness and accident. Fortunately, however, we left some things along the way to remind ourselves who we truly are. We created, and continue to create, images that recall truths beyond routine perceptions. Whenever we come upon one of these images, we wake a bit, step outside (or perhaps inside) ourselves, and see more clearly, becoming more mindful of our greater selves.

Some conditions are universal; we are all subject to birth, pain, and death. The profession of nursing is connected intimately to all three states. The nurse assists at the first breath and the final breath, and, in the interim, serves the patient during times of pain and debility. This service, bound intimately to universal truths, gives nursing the privilege of a mythical heritage as well as a historic one. Its practitioners draw inspiration from both. Few other professions have such a resource.

No single image of a nurse can demonstrate the entire range of professional qualities, but specific qualities or roles can be artistically isolated, emphasized in an image, and even personified. The personification of specific attributes fundamental to all nurses is known as a *nursing archetype*. The artist can convey specific attributes by using symbolic devices, such as implements, insignia, and so forth. Some roles lend themselves to representation better than others. For example, the image of a nurse interposing a shield between a patient and a snake (representing disease) is unmistakably the archetype of the Nurse Guardian. The role—to protect and defend against harm—is represented by the nurse holding the shield. The position of the nurse with respect to the menace illustrates the qualities of courage and dedication to the patient.

Recognizing archetypes and symbols in nursing art is like recognizing the constellations while stargazing. Knowing the forms of the constellations and the names of the stars is simply another way to enjoy the night skies. However, the stars do not need names for a single one of them, or the vast expanse of them, to affect us. Good renditions of archetypes, especially ones that are alive in our culture, also affect us without explanation. They are our own reflections: as nurses we *are* guardians, we *are* servants, we *are* keepers of the flame of knowledge and compassion.

Although the power of nursing archetypes and symbols affects us without explanation, to heighten our enjoyment and understanding of them, this chapter explores their origins and development and the uses to which they have been put over time. The nurse archetypes most often found on postcards are the Nurse Healer (Figs. 1.1 to 1.5), the Nurse Angel (Figs. 1.6 to 1.12), the Nurse Servant (Figs. 1.13 to 1.23), the Nurse Guardian (Figs. 1.24 to 1.33), the Lady with the Lamp (Figs. 1.34 to 1.37), and the Nurse Mother (Figs. 1.38 to 1.41).

The Healer

Asclepius (or Aesculapius, as the Romans called him) was the son of Apollo (the Greek god of health, prophecy, and light) and Coronis. Some say Coronis was simply an ordinary young woman; some say she was a nymph (also mortal but not fully human, a spirit of the rivers, woods, and meadows). Apollo took her as a lover. He later found out that she had been unfaithful and had her slain with arrows, only to discover that she was pregnant with his child. As Coronis lay on her funeral pyre, Apollo sent Hermes to deliver the infant Asclepius from her womb.

Because his father was the god of health, Asclepius trained to become a healer. His teacher was Chiron, a renowned physician who was also a centaur. At one point Asclepius obtained a drop of blood, which had magical properties, from the Gorgon's head. Zeus punished him for this act, in which Asclepius had attempted to bring mortals the promise of eternal life. Apollo again intervened, and Asclepius was placed among the heavens with the other gods. Over time, he became known as the god of medicine. In ancient Greece, a cult sprang up around him. Hippocrates, regarded as the father of Western medicine, was a 20th-generation member of this following (Fenkl, 2000).

Early images of Asclepius show his left hand resting on the head of a snake, his right hand holding a staff. The staff represents strength and authority. The snake was originally a symbol of renewal, dating back to the Egyptian cultures. Ancient people interpreted the snake's shedding of skin as a return to youth and thus believed snakes had discovered the secret of eternal life. Eventually, images depicted the snake on the staff, forming one symbol, known as the Staff of Asclepius. It appears today in emblems of the American Medical Association and the Emergency Services Association.

Another staff-and-snake motif depicts a second snake twined around the staff and a pair of wings at the top of the staff. The two-winged staff, originally the wand of the Greek messenger god Hermes, was a symbol of speed and inviolability. (A messenger was not permitted to be attacked by either warring party.) It is properly termed a caduceus from the Latin *caduceum*, derived from the Greek, meaning "herald's staff." Around 1500, printers began using the winged caduceus as an emblem of their craft because they felt it signified their roles as messengers. Publishers of medical texts began prominently displaying the caduceus on their books. The image appeared on most medical texts, so physicians and students using those books gradually came to take the symbol as representing medicine. In 1902, the U.S. Army Medical Department made the two-snake image its emblem, in part because it was already associated with medicine and in part due to the neutrality accorded the Department's noncombatant status. Today, the Staff of Asclepius and the Staff of Hermes are both symbols of the health sciences and are both commonly referred to as the caduceus.

Asclepius had eight children, of whom the best known is Hygeia (Roman Hygea, without the "i"). Hygeia is the nurse goddess, the goddess of health and healing. Although she is now usually represented as the daughter of Asclepius, originally she had no special relation to him, except that she was worshiped together with him. At one point, she was even regarded as his wife, a marriage of medicine and health. The oldest traces of Hygeia are from Corinth, around 800 BC.

Hygeia had two brothers and five sisters, all healers. One of her sisters, Panacea, still lives, but only in our language. In previous times, a panacea was taken literally as a healing power applicable to any misfortune and actively prayed for and sought after as a real possibility. Today the word has negative connotations, as a panacea has yet to be found.

Hygeia, on the other hand, is active in art as well as language. Her devices include the sacred snake, the same serpent associated with Asclepius, and the *patera*, a shallow bowl or libation dish. The dish, sometimes replaced by a chalice or a deeper bowl, is a symbol of nourishment. It is also a symbol of potency. Because the patera contains highly toxic venom, the wisdom of the goddess is necessary to dispense the medicine correctly; it can kill as easily as cure. The snake is often shown wound around Hygeia's wrist, which represents Hygeia's intimate bond to nature and to power.

Sometimes Hygeia is seen without the serpent, but with the bowl. Because the bowl is also a symbol of the Samaritan, the two archetypes overlap. The Samaritan, a symbol of charity, is often portrayed as a man or woman offering water to a thirsty stranger. Water can be seen as the most basic form of medicine and so, especially when the recipient of this bowl is obviously in dire need, the Samaritan can be seen as an aspect of Hygeia, and vice versa.

With the advent of Christianity, and specifically the Serpent of Eden, the snake changed in art from a positive to a negative symbol. In Western post-classical iconography, the snake almost always represents menace. In nursing postcards, the menace is most often disease, death, or preventable injury.

Jesus and the Angels

All nurse images have a symbolic component, because the nurse is a symbol of compassion. In fact, compassion is so associated with the nursing profession that the nurse is the only widespread secular symbol of it. Compassion, as activity or state of mind, is embraced and taught by all major religions. In this section, we focus principally on Judeo-Christian biblical expressions because nursing postcard art stems primarily from Judeo-Christian culture. From the Judeo-Christian point of view, all compassion flows from God.

From a specifically Christian point of view, Jesus, being an aspect of divinity, manifested on earth as a being of perfect compassion. He tended the sick, restored health and life, and gave comfort and instruction. Because nurses perform some of these activities as well, albeit in a limited human way, Jesus can serve as a nurse role model. He is viewed as such especially in the hospitals and nursing schools run by or descended from Christian nursing orders. In some nurse postcards, Jesus appears standing by the bedside, ministering to the patient, or, more often, watching over the fallen or receiving the souls of the deceased. On some postcards, a human nurse is given a deliberately and unmistakably Christlike appearance.

Jesus, however, does not appear on many nurse postcards. The most prevalent symbol of divine intervention in that venue belongs to the angel. Angels are closely connected with nursing in the broad range of art in general. In artistic renditions of angels, representatives of only six earthly professions appear with any regularity: the religious, the gatekeeper, the messenger, the musician, the warrior (usually depicted with a sword raised against the forces of Satan), and the nurse. Nurses are now so associated with angels that they, along with guardian angels, form the basis for the current acceptance that angels are feminine. (Until the middle of the 19th century, angels were seen as sexless or male.)

Although the Nurse Angel is an artistic metaphor, she is often literally real in the minds of patients, especially in extreme situations. A nurse on any battlefield, or in any situation where, without intervention, pain and death are inevitable, is most definitely a manifestation of salvation. Who can say, in such situations, that salvation is not divine in origin?

Old Testament angels were sometimes given the role of agents of death. They ended all suffering (or initiated an everlasting torment, depending on the state of grace of the departed). These angels of death usually bear a scythe, an instrument or symbol of reaping. Not all angels present at the time of death are reapers. Some simply witness death, guide the soul through it, and often show the saved or innocent souls to their heavenly abode. They are known as angels of the final moments.

Death, whether represented by a snake, a grim reaper, or even an angel, is usually vilified in nurse postcards. Although some acknowledgment is given to Death as the end of suffering, it is rarely represented as being kind. Death personified is either indifferent or inimical, and invariably something to be avoided if not feared. The nurse is always seen in opposition to death.

The time of our death is unpredictable and is often closer than people would like to think. Therefore, Death as a companion may be as useful a metaphor as Death as an enemy. As a companion, Death becomes more familiar to us, and we lose our fear of it. Also, being reminded that our lives are short affects the way we live, enabling us to set priorities in a more meaningful order. Hospices originally were places where pilgrims on the road and dying patients shared rooms because they were in one sense equals, both travelers on life's road.

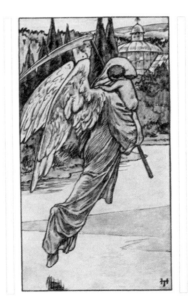

Hans Tegner (1853–1932). Story of a Mother.
Germany, c. 1910.

The Servant

The Christian religious orders from which modern nursing evolved have as their mandate the care of the sick and the poor. Monks and nuns in these orders place themselves in service to God, and therefore in service to all God's unfortunates. Nurses and healthcare workers who work in hospitals that are run by such orders also participate in this type of service. However, there are also secular servants, members of service-oriented trades or professions with specific obligations and rules.

Is the nurse a type of secular servant? It depends on how servant is defined. A servant can be someone who voluntarily makes someone else's welfare a prime concern, even to the extent of risking his or her own life. Soldiers, firefighters, and police all represent this type of servant. Also, a servant can be someone who is hired to do for an individual what they cannot easily do, or do not wish to do, on their own. In that respect, the nurse is a servant whenever she washes, feeds, or ambulates a patient, or simply makes him more comfortable.

Health and healing depend on favorable states of mind; the nurse contributes to the patient's well being in many ways, some of which are beyond the scope of clinical technique, to generate a therapeutic atmosphere. Nurses may read to their patients or write letters for them. Pediatric nurses may play with their charges. Home-bound patients often look forward to the nurse's visit as the most social part of their day.

During the two world wars, rehabilitation hospitals often organized social functions, such as picnics, fairs, and concerts, and patients and nurses attended them together. Sometimes a patient would be well enough to go off the hospital grounds, accompanied by his nurse. Shared experiences such as these have the potential for generating affectionate feelings. Because the patient's well being had priority, the relationship remained therapeutic and within professional boundaries. There may have been some hopeful flirting on the part of the patient, which may even have been returned by the nurse, but with rare exception the relationship remained strictly platonic. This type of companionable Nurse Servant is depicted as the Sister. In the United Kingdom, charge nurses are referred to as Sister (a holdover from nursing's religious origins), so the word "sister" became the basis of a double entendre sometimes found on captions of English postcards (see Fig. 2.30).

Another type of nurse servant evolved from the nursery maid of the 17th century. Called a nursemaid, originally she had no formal training as a professional nurse, but was employed to take care of the children. Later, a distinction was made between a professionally trained nanny, who took care of the children beyond the nursery, and a professional private nurse, whose duties included taking care of the children but could extend to adults as well. At the turn of the 20th century, many upper class families in Europe had private nurses and physicians to care for them at home, because the hospital experience was still unpleasant, if not outright revolting. Moreover, families preferred to keep their illnesses private.

The nanny and private nurse often lived in the house and were treated as high-level house servants. Their uniforms were similar to—sometimes indistinguishable from—maids' outfits. In some households, the nanny assisted the mother; however, more often the nanny, not the mother, was the primary caretaker. The nanny woke, dressed, bathed, and fed the children, supervised their play, presented them to the parents at certain times of the day, and put them to bed. She also took care of them when they were sick. There are two theories of the origin of the word "nanny." One is that "nanny" comes from "nanna," which is what young children called their grandmother or aunt. Another is that "nanny" was simply easier for a child to pronounce than "nurse."

An American counterpart to the nanny was the mammy, an African American woman, usually a mother, owned or, later, employed by southern white families to take care of their children. However, the mammy's origin was through slavery; and even after the abolition of slavery, she was subjected to the highly discriminatory social mores and laws of the Jim Crow era. Some mammies, just as adept at their jobs as their European counterparts, voluntarily stayed with families over several generations, out of mutual respect and love (see Fig. 6.25).

At the beginning of the 20th century, the nurse was perceived as being completely dependent on and subservient to the physician. She was someone who followed orders, waited on the patient, and was permitted no independent decision-making in the plan of the patient's care. For example, in the 1890s, if a doctor left a chair in the middle of a hospital room, a nurse might not move it without permission from her superior. This inferior relationship began to erode dramatically during World War I, and today is as outdated as bloodletting to cure yellow fever. Unfortunately, the "physician's handmaid" stereotype still persists, although weakly supported, in the minds of the woefully uninformed.

The Guardian

The Nurse Guardian is a defender and a warrior. (A warrior's path, regardless of cultural origin, requires commitment, patience, and unbroken attention. There arises a certain nonduality of self and other. As it happens, the nurse mind and the warrior mind have a good deal in common; however, the artists did not express that aspect of Nurse Guardian.) The Nurse Guardian's primary devices are the shield and the cross. The cross, in its various varieties, was worn on the breast and was the common badge of every order of Christian knighthood. The Cross of Lorraine and the Cross of St. George are the two versions that appear most often on nurse postcards.

The Cross of Lorraine

The Cross of Lorraine.

The concept of hygiene as warfare arose toward the end of the 19th century, following the establishment of germ theory of disease. Until then, no one knew the direction of the "enemy" because infection seemed to spring from everywhere. It could appear out of the air with no apparent cause, it could seep up from the ground, lie in wait in water, and so forth. Once microorganisms were identified as the causative agents and once it became known how they proliferated, the forces of science could be brought to bear.

When a disease reaches the level of universal or critical concern, the war waged against it may take the form of a crusade. The most publicly embraced anti-disease crusade of the 20th century was the crusade against tuberculosis (TB). Tuberculosis has been with humankind since antiquity, found in bones of people as far back as 2400 BC. In ancient Greece, it was labeled phthisis (pronounced "thy-sis") from the word meaning "a wasting away." Hippocrates identified phthisis as the most widespread disease of the times, and noted that it was almost always fatal. There were outbreaks of the disease in Europe in plague proportions throughout the Middle Ages. From the progressive wasting of the body, it appeared that the disease consumed its victims, and so it became known as consumption.

With the onset of the industrial revolution, the population crowded into the cities and lived packed together in poorly ventilated, unsanitary tenements. Conditions were perfect for the spread of tuberculosis. In 1800, tuberculosis was the most common cause of death in Western Europe, accounting for 25% of all deaths (Eyenet, 2000). From the 1860s to the 1940s, tuberculosis killed more people each year in the United States than any other contagious disease, with most of its victims young people in the prime of their lives (Keiger, 1998).

The introduction of the sanatorium cure (although it was not called that at the time) provided the first important step against TB. It was demonstrated as early as 1854 that tuberculosis could be controlled and even cured with proper nutrition and exposure to a fresh air climate. However, the etiology of the disease was still unknown. The real campaign against the disease began in 1882, the year Robert Koch first saw and identified *Mycobacterium tuberculosis* under the microscope. The campaign lasted until 1943, with the discovery of streptomycin.

At the outset, some imaginative strategy was definitely needed. It was known how the disease propagated, but there was still no way to kill it. The existence of little creatures, invisible to the eye, as the cause of TB was still considered dubious by many. Most of the public believed that the disease was hopeless, neither preventable nor alterable in its usually fatal course. It was a fact of life and nothing could be done about it. If tuberculosis were to be controlled at all, habits would have to change, living quarters would have to be designed differently, and recuperative institutions would have to be established. Because all of this would take massive public support and significant funding, something was needed that would engage the uninformed and somewhat uninterested public on a wide scale.

At the time, there was a European infatuation with all things medieval. The relentless changes wrought by the new technologies had created in many a profound yearning for an idealized medieval past, with its chivalry, pageantry, and simplicity. It was a natural step, therefore, to associate a modern crusade with a medieval crusade.

In fact, the fight against tuberculosis was deliberately modeled after the first Christian Crusade, the only crusade in which the Christians were ultimately victorious. The First Crusade began in 1095 with a proclamation from Pope Urban II concerning an appeal for help from the Byzantine Emperor, who was being threatened by attacks from Turks and Arabs. It ended in 1099 with the Christians capturing Jerusalem. Godefroy de Boullion, the Duke of Lorraine, was given credit for the victory. The device on Lorraine's standard was a double-barred Latin cross. (The second bar is a representation of the sign "INRI" added to the cross of Jesus on Pilate's order.) This device was designated the Cross of Lorraine by the Patriarch of Jerusalem and proclaimed a symbol of Christ Victorious.

Eight hundred years later, on October 23, 1902, at an international conference in Berlin, the Cross of Lorraine was chosen as the symbol of the anti-tuberculosis crusade. Just as in the first Christian Crusade, thousands surged forth in support. Supporters and volunteers were the army victorious. Children, by raising funds, could become pages, squires, and knights. Bacteriologists and physicians were seen as "heroes engaged in a sanctified struggle against the overwhelming beast of infection" (Keiger, 1998). The nurses became the guardians and defenders, standing between the evil and its intended victims.

The Cross of Lorraine appeared in 1907 on American Christmas Seals, which were part of a fund-raising effort to keep open an early tuberculosis sanitarium. Soon, all across the Western world, contributors to TB fund-raising efforts were given banners, certificates, and other awards bearing the Cross of Lorraine. The campaign was successful, and TB, the enemy, was driven back and subdued, if not outright vanquished.

Today, TB has returned in force. According to the World Health Organization (WHO), it infects over one third of the world's population, arising as a complication of AIDS and improperly taken antibiotics. In 1997, the WHO predicted that 30 million people would die from TB over the next 10 years (Keiger, 1998). The Cross of Lorraine is now the registered trademark of the American Lung Association.

The Cross of St. George

The Cross of St. George. The Cross of St. George, red on a white background, is the most ubiquitous symbol in nursing. Known in the crusades as the Greek Cross, it was one of the most prominent Christian emblems. It was also the device worn by St. George, an early Christian martyr who became inextricably entwined with the myth of a medieval dragon-slayer knight. St. George the Dragon Slayer became the patron saint of England, and appears, wearing his cross, on innumerable British documents, edifices, statuary, art, and coinage.

The red cross associated with nursing, however, originated at a convention held in Geneva, Switzerland in 1863. There, the red cross on a white ground was adopted as the emblem of the International Committee for the Relief of the Wounded, now known as the International Committee of the Red Cross (ICRC). In 1864, the first Geneva Convention stipulated that the emblem would guarantee safe passage and exemption from attack by all parties signatory to the treaty. The exact circumstances under which the device can be displayed, and by whom, are still part of international law.

There is some speculation that the emblem may have been designed simply as a reversal of the Swiss flag colors. However, there is no question that the emblem has religious connotations. As early as 1876, during one of the Russo-Turkish Wars, the Ottoman Empire claimed that the cross "offended the sensibilities of Muslim soldiers (IRC, 2000)." They elected to use a red crescent instead. Today, 145 countries use the red cross, and 30 countries have adopted the red crescent as the symbol of the International Red Cross (IRC).

The Maltese Cross

The Maltese Cross. The Maltese Cross or Cross of St. John was another prominent cross of the crusades. It was the device of the Knights Hospitallers of the Order of St. John, one of the first and most important of the Christian nursing orders. The order originated in Jerusalem in 1042 and later established its headquarters at Malta (from 1530 until 1798). It is from the later period that the emblem acquired the name by which it is most commonly known today.

The Maltese Cross is seen on nurse postcards as the symbol of the St. John Ambulance Association, which traces its origins to the Knights Hospitallers. St. John Ambulance is one of the United Kingdom's leading charities; its volunteers treat more than 130,000 casualties a year. St. John Ambulance has trained and placed nurses in hospitals and in the field since 1887.

The Maltese Cross is also incorporated in firefighters' emblems. Its use stems from the fact that the Hospitallers are recognized as the first firemen. When their fellow knights approached Saracen fortresses, they were exposed to a new weapon: naphtha. Naphtha would be poured over the attackers from above and then lighted with flaming arrows. Knights of the order risked their own lives to pull their brethren from the flames. The firefighters' first duty was, and still is, rescuing victims, not saving property. Since both nurses and firefighters were originally Knights Hospitallers, the two professions have a common origin.

The Firefighters Symbol.

The Lady With the Lamp

The flame has represented life, love, eternity, hope, mutability, purification, sacrifice, destruction, and renewal in virtually every culture since the dawn of humankind. Ultimately, the flame is both a universal and a personal symbol. In nursing graduation or capping ceremonies, the flame is a symbol of transmission, as the duties and sacred trust of the profession are passed from one generation to the next (see Fig 1.37).

Although guardians making their rounds used candles and lamps to illuminate the darkness of physical places, the lamp is more frequently a metaphorical banishing of the darkness of ignorance. It is a symbol of learning and guidance, the light that brings knowledge and wisdom. The lamp as a contemporary symbol of nursing can be traced to Florence Nightingale. During the Crimean War (1854–56) at Scutari, it was Miss Nightingale's habit to make night rounds to inspect the condition of the patients, the hospital, and the grounds. At such times, she carried a paper accordion lamp containing a candle. (The oil lamp usually depicted with Miss Nightingale is an artistic invention, the more ancient symbol of knowledge substituted for the candle lamp she actually carried.) The soldiers, comforted by her presence, began referring to her as "The Lady with the Lamp." When she returned to England, that title was bestowed upon her by the British public and ultimately the entire Western world (see Fig. 5.11). At the beginning of the 20th century, the association of the nurse with the lamp was so strong that any nurse, particularly in World War I, could be referred to as "The Lady with the Lamp."

The Mother

The word "nurse" has etymological origins related to breast-feeding and nurturing. The mother as a source of life and nourishment is often represented by the Earth Mother, usually an image of a heavy woman with large breasts who is often presented as a fertility goddess. Although both the Nurse Mother and the Earth Mother can represent all mothers, their roles and attributes are quite different.

The Nurse Mother has no aspect whatsoever of fertility or fecundity; sex and reproduction are not associated with her. She is never portrayed as pregnant, but she does appear with children, to whom she provides nourishment and safety. In art postcards, the Nurse Mother often appears as a Madonna figure, in variations of the Pieta tableau. The patient, usually a young man, is gravely ill and may even have recently expired. The Nurse Mother, supporting him, looks down on him with exquisite care and tenderness, symbolic of the nurse who cares for her patient as she would her own child.

In other cases, the Nurse Mother is shown with all humanity as her children. Her devices in this aspect are the globe, which represents all the peoples of the world, and the cloak, which protects them. She enfolds humanity into her cloak as a mother hen takes chicks under her wing in times of danger. This symbolism can be seen in postcards issued by the American Red Cross, which refers to itself as "The Greatest Mother in the World" (see Fig. 3.32).

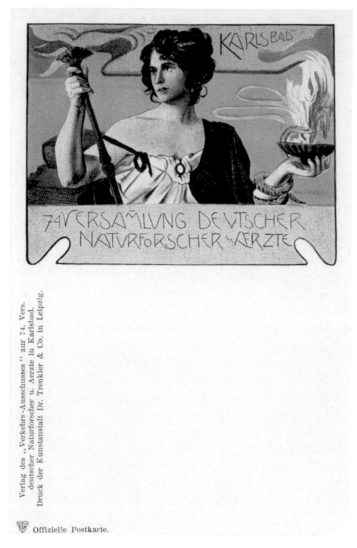

Verlag des „Verkehrs-Ausschusses" zur 74. Vers.
deutscher Naturforscher u. Aerzte in Karlsbad.
Druck der Kunstanstalt Dr. Trenkler & Co. in Leipzig.

Offizielle Postkarte.

Figure 1.2. **Assembly of German Natural Scientists and Physicians.**
Karlsbad, Germany. c. 1902. *(See note.)*

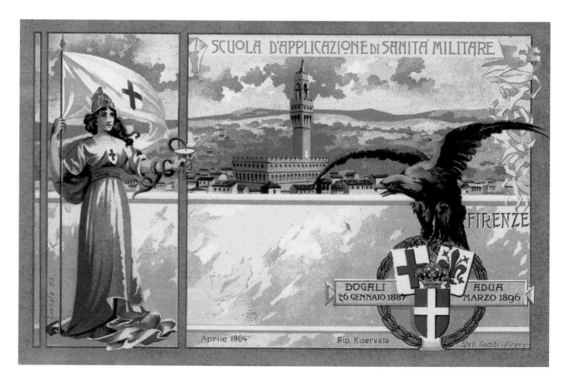

Figure 1.3. **School of Clinical Application of Military Hygiene.**
Florence, Italy. 1904. *(See note.)*

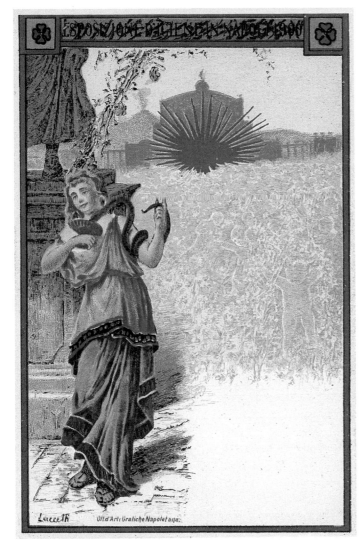

Figure 1.4. **Hygiene Exposition.**
Naples, Italy. 1900. *(See note.)*

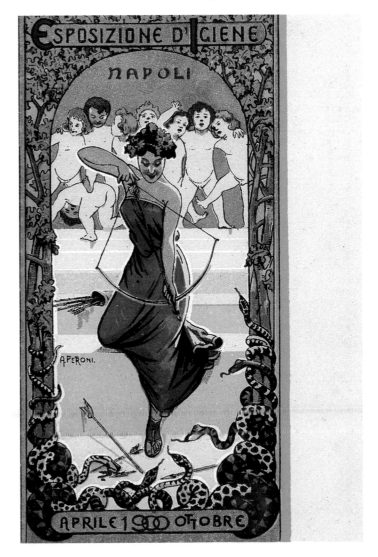

Figure 1.5. **Hygiene Exposition.**
Naples, Italy. 1900. *(See note.)*

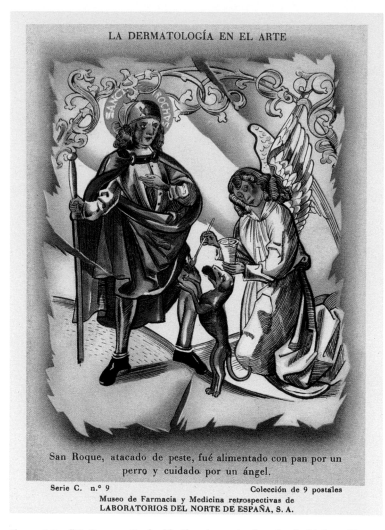

LA DERMATOLOGÍA EN EL ARTE

San Roque, atacado de peste, fué alimentado con pan por un
perro y cuidado por un ángel.

Serie C.   n.º 9   Colección de 9 postales
Museo de Farmacia y Medicina retrospectivas de
LABORATORIOS DEL NORTE DE ESPAÑA, S. A.

Figure 1.6. **"St. Roque, attacked by the plague, is given food with bread by
a dog and care by an angel."**
From the series "Dermatology in Art." Museum of Pharmacology and Medicine, Barcelona,
Spain. c. 1920. (Figures 1.6–1.9 represent an angel–human continuum). *(See note.)*

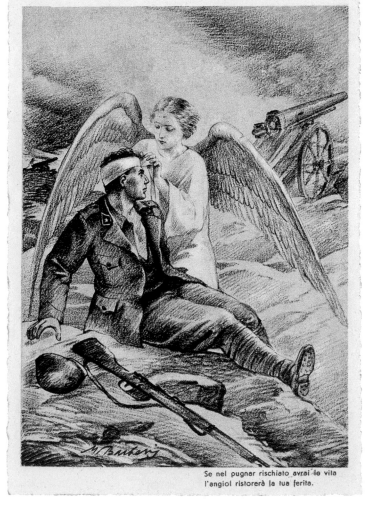

Se nel pugnar rischiato avrai la vita
l'angiol ristorerà la tua ferita.

Figure 1.7. **"If you risk your life in battle, an angel will treat your wounds."**
Italy. 1942. *(See note.)*

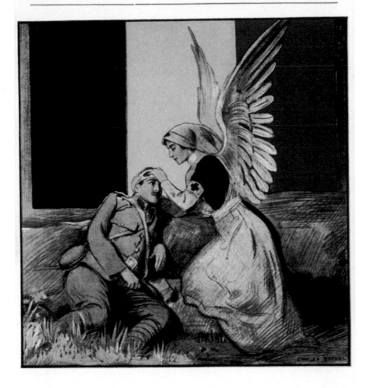

Figure 1.8. **Belgian Red Cross Under the Patronage of Their Majesties the King and Queen of the Belgians.**
Belgium. c. 1916. *(See note.)*

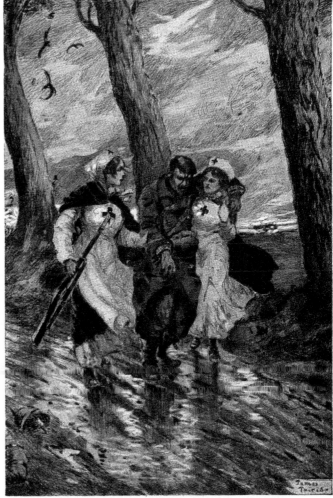

"LES ANGES DES DERNIERS MOMENTS„   *J. Thiriar.*

Figure 1.9. **J. Thiriar. "The Angels of the Final Moments."**
Belgium. c. 1916. *(See note.)*

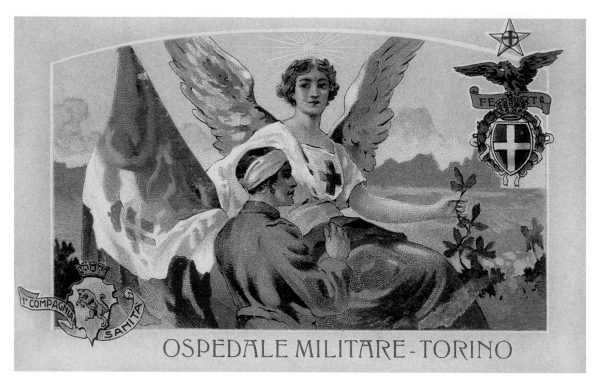

Figure 1.10. **1st Sanitary Company, Military Hospital of Torino.**
Italy. c. 1916.

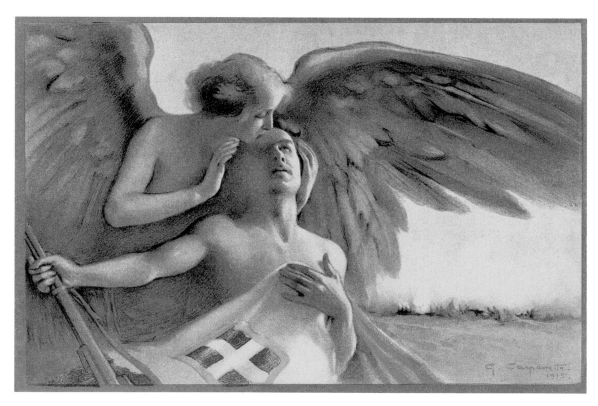

Figure 1.11. **Bologna Committee for the Assistance of War Invalids.**
Italy. 1918.

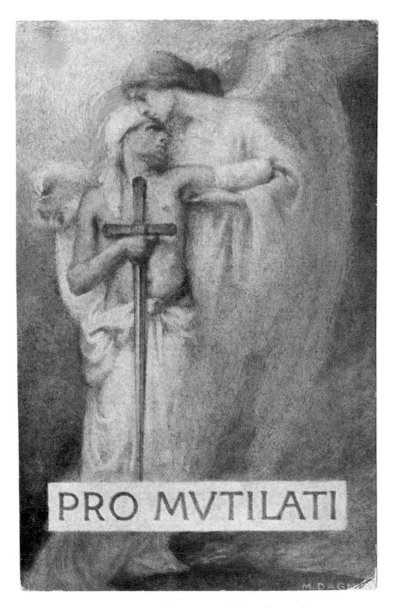

Figure 1.12.   **Torino Regimental Committee of the Italian Red Cross.**
Italy. 1915.

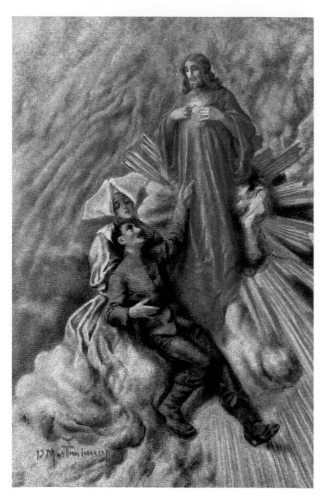

Figure 1.13. **D. Mastroianni (1876–1962). "Charity."**
Italy. c. 1905. *(See note.)*

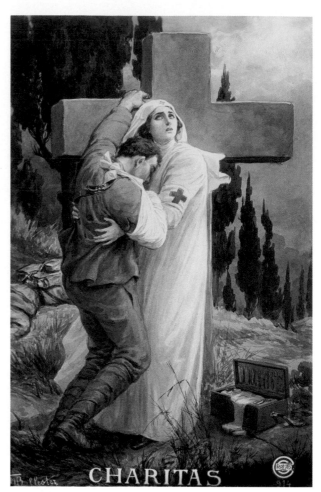

Figure 1.14. **Charity.**
France. c. 1914. *(See note.)*

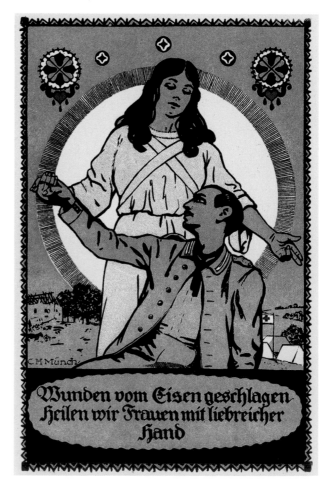

Figure 1.15. **"We women use our loving hands to heal wounds inflicted by iron."**
Germany. c. 1916. *(See note.)*

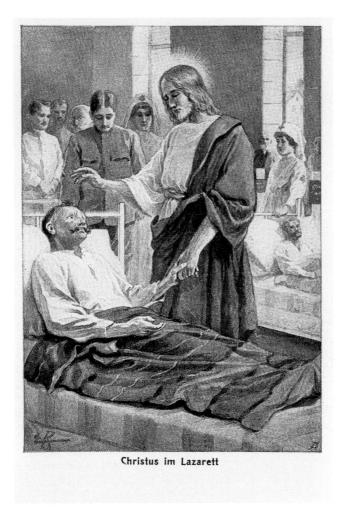

Christus im Lazarett

Figure 1.16. **Christ in the War Hospital.**
Austria. c. 1914.

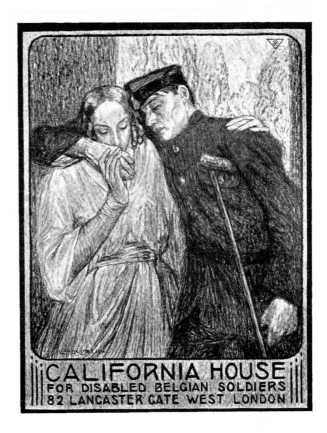

CALIFORNIA HOUSE
FOR DISABLED BELGIAN SOLDIERS
82 LANCASTER GATE WEST LONDON

Figure 1.17. **California House.**
England. 1914. *(See note.)*

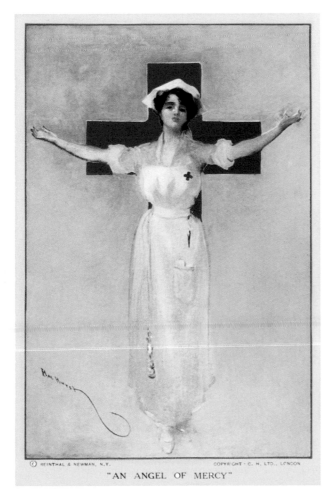

"AN ANGEL OF MERCY"

Figure 1.18. **Hal Hurst (1865–1938). "An Angel of Mercy."**
England. 1917. *(See note.)*

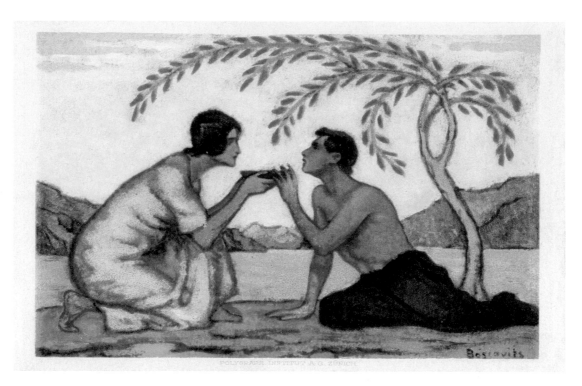

Figure 1.19. **For the Benefit of the Red Cross.**
Switzerland. 1917. (Figures 1.19–1.23 depict the progression of nurse as servant.)
(See note.)

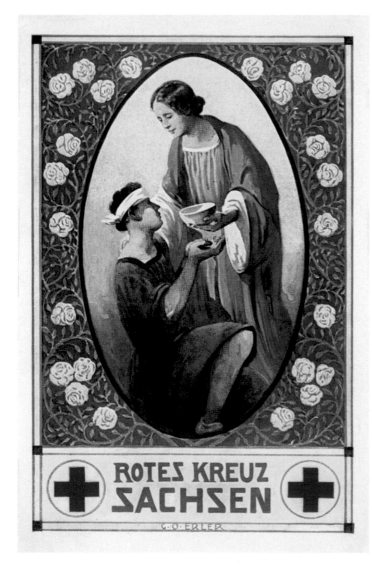

Figure 1.20. **Saxony Red Cross.**
Germany. c. 1912. *(See note.)*

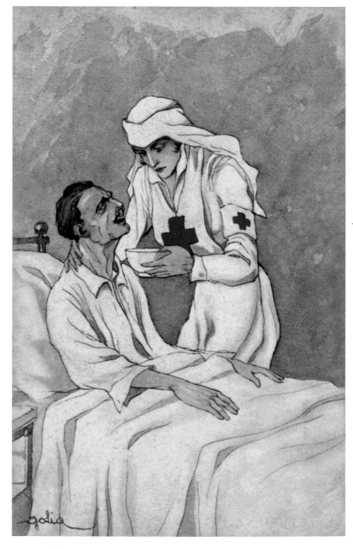

Figure 1.21. **Golia, pseudonym for E. Colmo (1885–1967).**
Italy. 1915. *(See note.)*

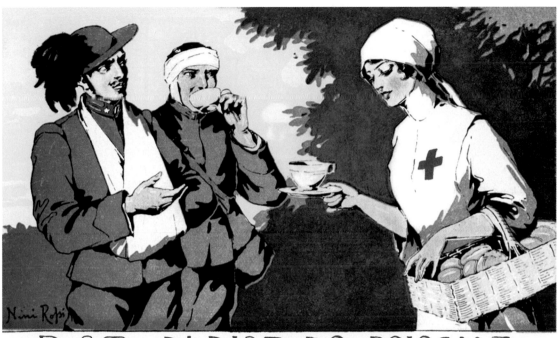

Figure 1.22. **Restoration Post.**
Bologna, Italy. 1916. *(See note.)*

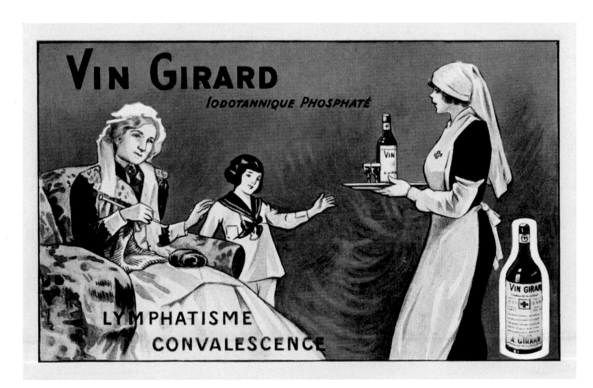

Figure 1.23. **Vin Gerard (Gerard Wine).**
France. 1929. *(See note.)*

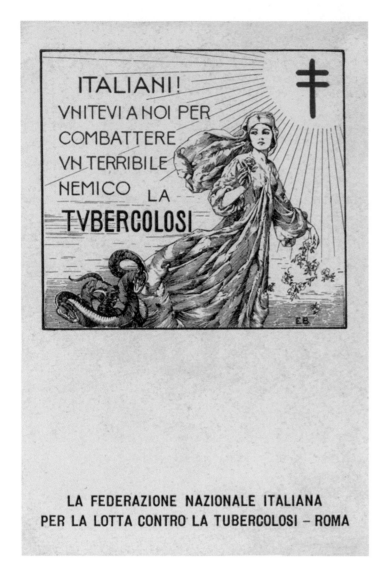

Figure 1.24. **"Italians! Unite with us to fight the terrible nemesis of tuberculosis!"**
Italy. 1912.

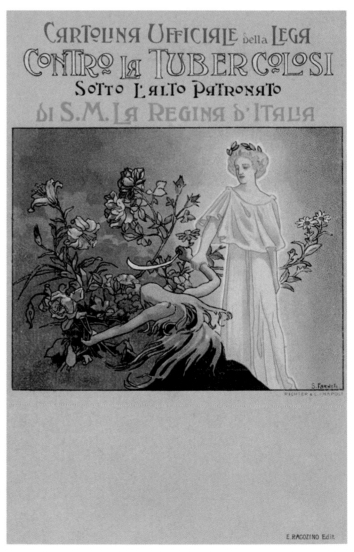

Figure 1.25. **"Official postcard of the League Against Tuberculosis under the Royal Patronage of Her Majesty the Queen of Italy."**
Italy. c. 1900.

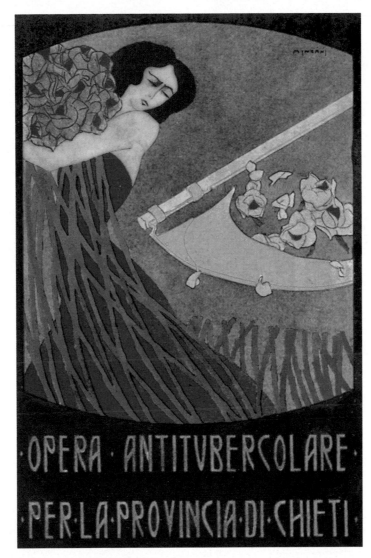

Figure 1.26. **Anti-Tuberculosis Organization of the Province of Chieti.**
Italy. c. 1910.

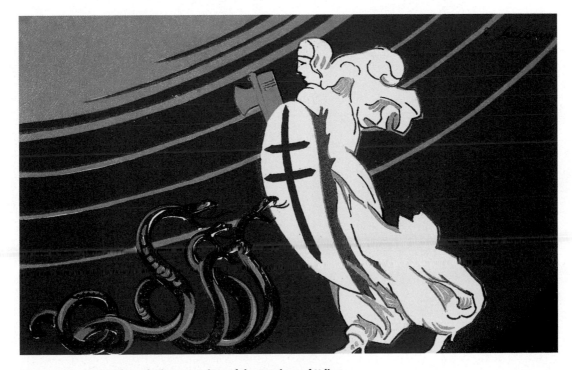

Figure 1.27. **Anti-Tuberculosis Consortium of the Province of Udine.**
Italy. c. 1935. *(See note.)*

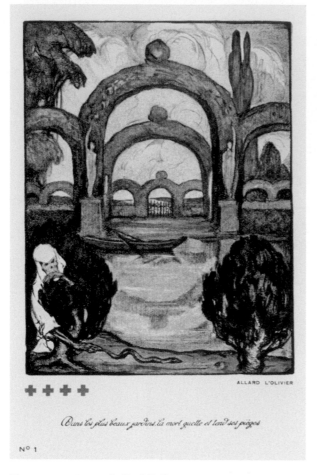

NO 1

Figure 1.28. Fernand Allard l'Oliver.
The Red Cross of Belgium. "In the most beautiful gardens, Death sets its snares." c. 1912. *(See note.)*

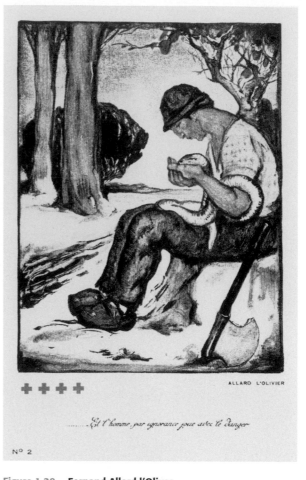

NO 2

Figure 1.29. Fernand Allard l'Oliver.
The Red Cross of Belgium. " . . . and Man, out of ignorance, plays with the danger." c. 1912. *(See note.)*

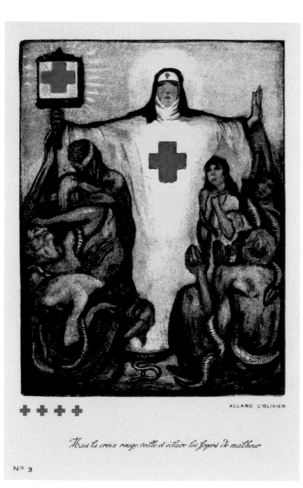

NO 3

Figure 1.30. Fernand Allard l'Oliver.
The Red Cross of Belgium. "But the Red Cross reveals and illuminates the sources of misery." c. 1912. *(See note.)*

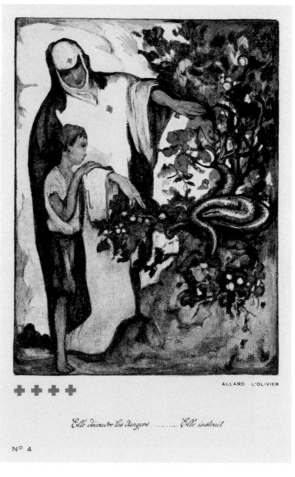

NO 4

Figure 1.31. Fernand Allard l'Oliver.
The Red Cross of Belgium. "It uncovers the danger . . . it teaches." c. 1912. *(See note.)*

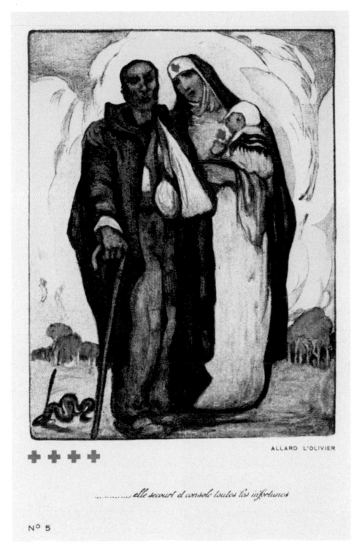

Figure 1.32. Fernand Allard l'Oliver.
The Red Cross of Belgium. " . . . It helps and consoles all the unfortunates."
c. 1912. *(See note.)*

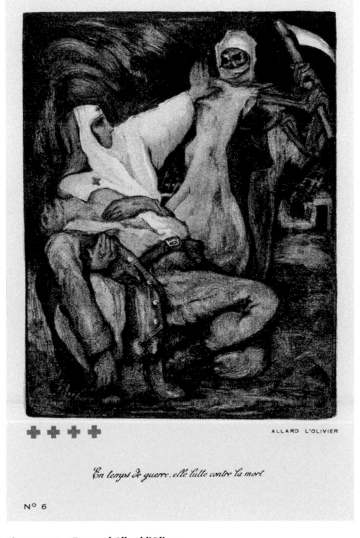

Figure 1.33. Fernand Allard l'Oliver.
The Red Cross of Belgium. "In times of war it fights against Death." c. 1912.
(See note.)

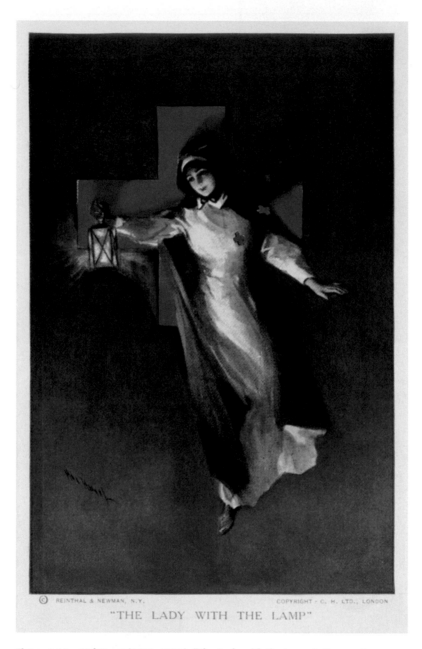

"THE LADY WITH THE LAMP"

Figure 1.34.   **Hal Hurst (1865–1938). "The Lady with the Lamp."** *(See note.)*

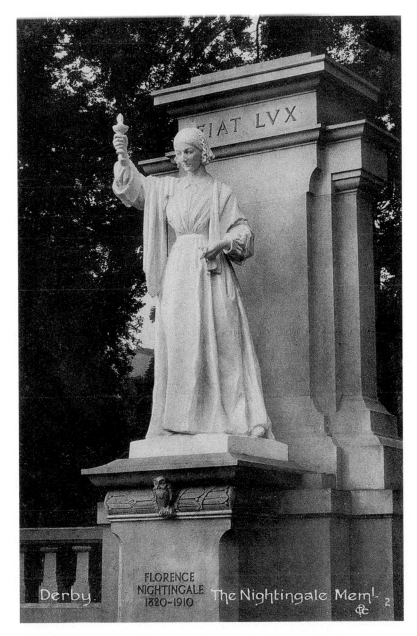

Figure 1.35.
Real photo. England. 1918. *(See note.)*

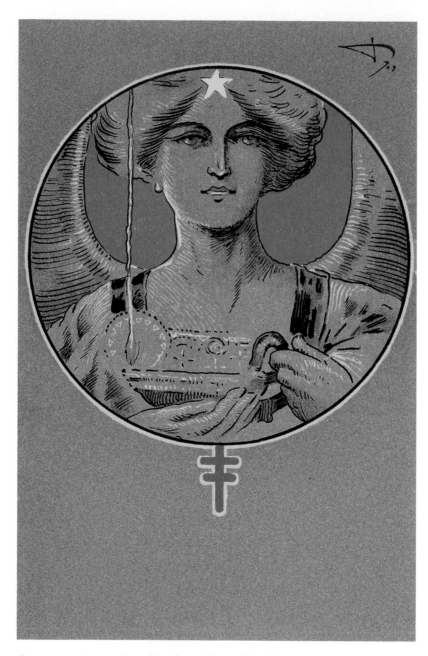

Figure 1.36. **Genova Committee for Soldiers with Tuberculosis.**
Italy. c. 1910. *(See note.)*

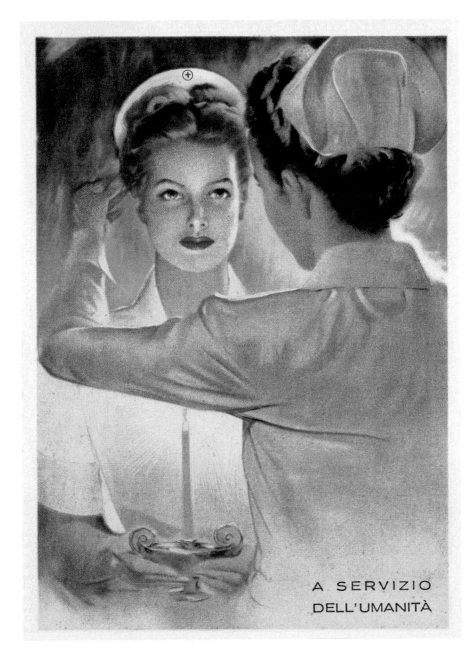

Figure 1.37. **"In Service to Humanity."**
Italy. c. 1950. *(See note.)*

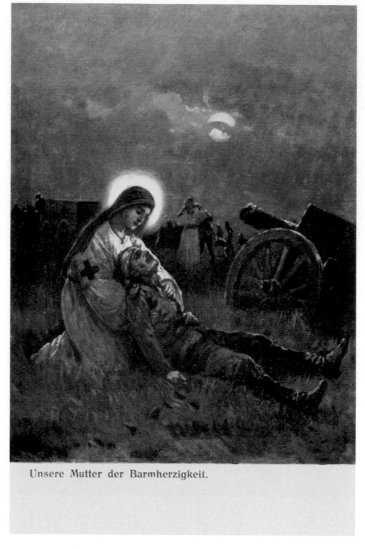

Unsere Mutter der Barmherzigkeit.

Figure 1.38. **"Our Mother of Mercy."**
Germany. c. 1916.

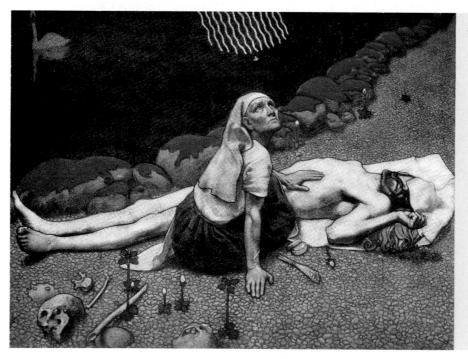

Axel Gallén:
Lemminkäinens
Moder
Lemminkäisen
äiti

Figure 1.39. **Axel Gallén (1865–1931). "Lemminkäinen's Mother."**
Sweden. c. 1920. *(See note.)*

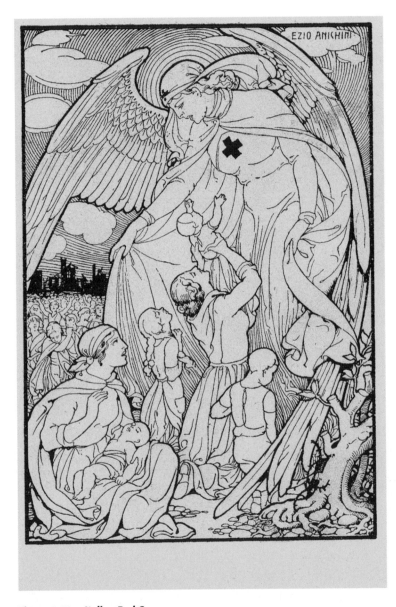

Figure 1.40. **Italian Red Cross.**
Italy. 1916.

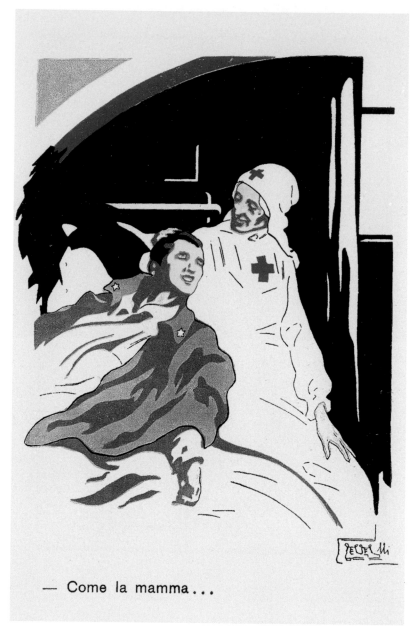

— Come la mamma...

Figure 1.41. "Like Mama."
Italy. c. 1915.

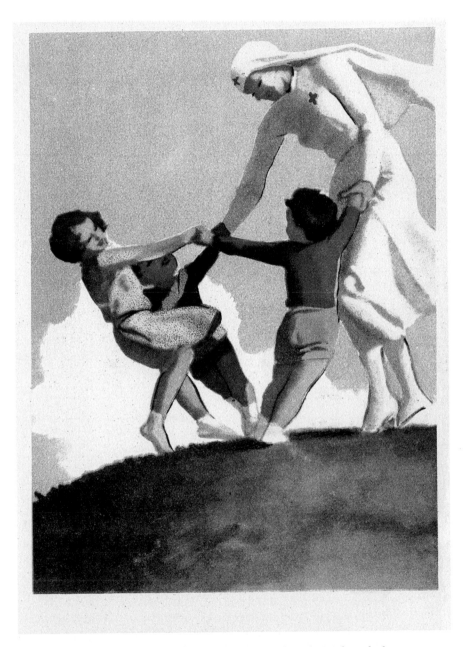

Figure 1.42. **Italian National Fascist Federation for Work Against Tuberculosis.**
Italy. 1936.

1.1. A demure **Hygeia.** She and the serpent are relaxed and accustomed to each other, friends of a sort.

1.2. A torch and a book are added, both symbols of knowledge and authority. **Karlsbad,** literally, *Karl's* (Count Karl William of Baden) *bath,* is the location of a group of European luxury spas, very fashionable at the turn of the 20th century. Although the postcard is German, Karlsbad is actually located just across the German border in what was then Czechoslovakia. The entire area, built around its mineral springs, was dedicated to the promotion and restoration of health. The baths were mentioned in literature as early as the 12th century. The spas were established in the 1850s and are still in operation.

1.3. **Hygeia** dons a battle helmet and bears a standard. She represents the School of Clinical Military Hygiene in Florence. The device featuring the military eagle is the school's emblem. The three shields display the emblems of the Red Cross, the Crown of Italy, and the City of Florence.

Dogali and **Adua** are both towns in Eritrea, bordering Abyssinia (Ethiopia), where the Italians were fighting to gain colonies. In the Battle of Dogali in January 1887, the Abyssinians surrounded and attacked a detachment of 500 Italians, killing 400 of them. In Adua, in March 1896, the Italians lost over 6500 troops. It seems odd to put dates of disastrous defeats on a military school crest, but it is possible that the graduates of the School of Military Hygiene had some heroic hand in rescuing and treating the fallen. Either that, or the school was created to fulfill a need recognized after those battles.

Figures 1.4 and 1.5 are souvenirs of the Hygiene Exposition of Naples, Italy, in 1900.

1.4. This is a classic Hygeia.

1.5. This Hygeia is a blend of symbolism from several eras. The bow and arrow are attributes of **Diana,** the Roman goddess of the hunt. Rather than an agent of healing, Hygeia's serpent has become a Christian symbol of malice, a life-threatening plague that menaces the children in the background. The children are copied directly from Italian Renaissance renditions of the **Holy Innocents,** the children of Bethlehem killed on order of Herod, and representing all innocent victims. Hygeia's dress, the garlands in her hair, and the border elements in the painting are done in Art Nouveau style.

1.6 to 1.9. These postcards represent an angel–nurse continuum. As the images progress, the subjects change in degree of humanity.

1.6. This painting, reproduced as one in a series of nine postcards, represents an event in the life of **St. Roche,** a 14th-century healer. While nursing the sick during the plague outbreak in northern Italy, St. Roche contracted the disease himself. He was miraculously cured through the intervention of an angel and a dog. The angel is a classic angel: it has wings, wears heavenly attire, and is sexless. In this case, it is a miraculous agent associated with a mythical figure, a heavenly saint.

1.7. This angel is more feminine. She wears heavenly garb, but she tends an ordinary man in an ordinary human war. Here she binds wounds, but she could as easily be watching over children.

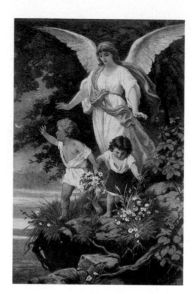

Guardian Angel.

1.8. Now the angel is unmistakably female. She still has wings, but has traded her heavenly attire for the uniform of a Belgian Red Cross nurse. Or, possibly, a human nurse has miraculously sprouted full-fledged angelic wings. Either is equally probable. In this figure, human and divine are completely indistinguishable.

1.9. On the fourth postcard in the series, the figures appear human. Perhaps they are human; we have no way of knowing just by looking at them. Here, the presence of the angel is so subtle that a caption is needed to alert us to it. Without the caption, we might mistake the angels for ordinary humans. The divine and the human are still indistinguishable. These two have appeared to a soldier leaving the battle for the last time. One supports him; the other relieves him of his burden and guides him on his final journey. These are the angels of the final moments. Note the three birds wheeling in the wind, symbols of both the storm (of war) and the soul freed from the body.

1.13. **Domenico Mastroianni** (1876–1962) was an Italian sculptor who worked in Paris. His postcards are based on his bas-relief sculptures, for which the term "photo-sculpture" had to be coined. In this postcard, a nursing sister with a beatific expression supports the soldier as he reaches out to **Jesus of the Sacred Heart,** symbol of the end of suffering.

1.14. This card was issued for the first Christmas following World War I, which had ended only 6 weeks earlier.

1.15. This depiction of a nurse is so Christ-like that she is almost a female Jesus. In case the hairstyle, robe, and circle of light were not enough to inform, the artist added Messianic symbols to the illustration. The hand with two pointing fingers is an iconographic device for a divine blessing, and there is no mistaking the stylized crown of thorns and sacred bleeding heart.

1.17. An example of the nurse as Jesus, this time as a servant. She supports the soldier and appears to be kissing his hand to express tenderness, compassion, and perhaps appreciation of the soldier's sacrifice.

California House was a hospital established in London for the rehabilitation of Belgian wounded soldiers evacuated from the front. Belgian soldiers were evacuated to England, as there was no room for them in the French or Belgian hospitals nearer the front.

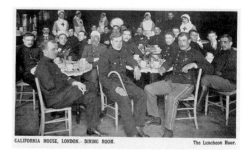

California House.

This postcard of the California House dining room shows the patients in makeshift uniforms assembled from different services, indicating that the scene was from the early part of the war. Complete Belgian uniforms would have been available in England later in the war, as khaki uniforms for the Belgian Army were then being manufactured in England.

1.18. **Hal Hurst's** (1865–1938) paintings and sketches appeared at the turn of the 20th century in British periodicals such as *Judge* and *The Idler,* as well as in children's and adult fiction books. This postcard is from a series of six that show both U.S. and British nurses during World War I. Figure 1-34 is from the same series.

1.19 to 1.23. These postcards show a progression of the Nurse Servant from the spiritual to the commercial.

1.19. This postcard represents one of the most basic acts of human kindness: giving water to a thirsty man. The archetype here is **the Samaritan** and her device is the bowl.

1.20. In this postcard, the woman is now **Hygeia,** giving a restorative to a wounded patient. The bowl has become a form of Hygeia's *patera*.

1.21. Hygeia has become a realistic modern nurse, serving nourishment to a 20th-century hospital patient. **Golia** is the pseudonym for Eugenio Colmo. He was given the nickname because he was very tall: Golia is Italian for Goliath. Colmo started the study of law, but abandoned it to become a caricaturist for humor magazines. In 1914 he began working intensively as an illustrator of children's books.

1.22. This shows the nurse as **waitress,** serving refreshments at a recovery post in Italy. The rooster plume identifies the soldier as a member of a *Bersaglieri* (rifle) regiment.

1.23. The nurse has become a **household servant,** still promoting health, but now endorsing a commercial product.

1.27. The **Nurse Guardian** is armed with the shield and the **Fasces,** a bundle of rods with an ax projecting from it, a symbol of power.

1.28 to 1.33. These six postcards were issued by the Red Cross of Belgium.

1.30. The Lady with the Lamp.

1.31. The Lady of the Lamp without the lamp: the Teacher. (See Fig. 3-69 for another Nurse Teacher.)

1.32. The Nurse Mother.

1.33. The Guardian. Note the progress of the serpent from the just-released young potent snake, to nests of thick vipers, and finally, in Figure 1-32, to a wasted specimen, pinned to the ground through its neck.

1.34. This is one of six postcards from the series by **Hal Hurst.** (See also Fig 1-18.) The lamp carried by this nurse is similar to the one used by Florence Nightingale.

1.35. **Florence Nightingale** has been raised to the level of a demigoddess, her simple accordion candle lamp now having become the Torch Which Illuminates the World. Behind her are the words "Fiat Lux" (Let there be light!). The **owl** is a double reference. Miss Nightingale had a pet owl of that proportionate size named Athena, after the Roman goddess of wisdom. The owl itself is one of the symbols of Athena. (For more on Florence Nightingale, see note 5-11.)

1.36. A beautiful **Art Nouveau Nurse Angel** bearing the Lamp of Knowledge. Note the Cross of Lorraine with the bars modified to create a balanced pendant effect.

1.37. A rare postcard image of a **capping ceremony.** The graduate holds the candle signify

---

ing the transmission of the lineage from nurse to nurse, down through the ages. The candle base is the Lamp of Knowledge.

1.39. Although the postcard is from Sweden, **Axel Gallén** (Akseli Gallén-Kallela, 1865–1931) was a Finnish painter who studied in Paris and Berlin. His art was primarily of mythological subjects, including the now-famous paintings inspired by the Kalevala, the **Finnish national epic,** compiled from old Finnish ballads, lyrical songs, and incantations.

Lemminkäinen was the most adventurous and reckless of the heroes in the Kalevala legends. Heedless of his mother's warning, Lemminkäinen embarked on a daredevil attempt to win the hand of the proud Maid of the North by killing the **Swan of Death,** the immortal bird of ancient legend. The painting shows the mother, after having pulled Lemminkäinen from the River of Death, awaiting the arrival of a bee.

The painting, finished in 1897, is laden with symbols of death: the corpse of Lemminkäinen, the shroud covering his face, the black river, the Swan of Death, the bloodstained stones, the skulls and bones. But the painting also contains symbols of life: the golden sun-rays and the golden bee (just in front of the vertical sun rays). The real hero of the story is the bee: it flew tirelessly across the earth and the heavens to bring a life-restoring balm to Lemminkäinen's mother (Finnish National Gallery, 2002).

The model was **Gallén-Kallela's** own **mother.** Gallén-Kallela stated that doing the painting made him suffer, because in order to get his mother to keep the expression of anguish on her face, Gallén-Kallela had to tell her sad and tragic stories to make her miserable (Gallén-Kallela Museum, 2002).

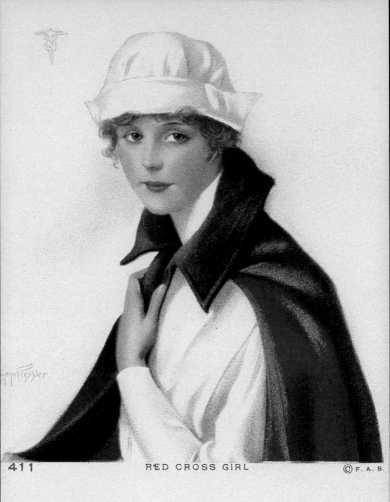

411   RED CROSS GIRL   © F. A. S.

Figure 2.1.   **Gene Pressler (1894–1933). "Red Cross Girl."**

Twentieth-Century *Postcard Art*

*T*his chapter includes the entire range of nurse-related postcard art except poster styles, which will be shown in Chapters 3 and 5. The art on the majority of postcards was produced by unrecognized artists. That is, they were not known during their productive years, apart from small circles of friends and associates, and almost no one has heard of them today. Some of them signed their work with initials or pseudonyms and are completely unidentifiable, even by name. Interestingly, though, what remains of the work of these unknowns often is as good as the works of the recognized artists. Then, as now, the merit of the work alone was not enough to make an artist popular; accessibility to the right people and promotional effort played a large part in success in art, even commercial art. If an artist was both very good and very popular, the demand for new designs increased and thousands of copies were produced with each print run. The artist might stay in the public eye for years, even for decades. On the other hand, a very good unknown artist might publish a few hundred, or even a few thousand, postcard copies of his one or two best works, and never publish on a postcard again.

Postcard art ranges from old-master style to slapstick comic illustration. In general, there is a progression from realism to fantasy. Realism, as used here, does not mean an attempt to mimic a photograph, but that the nurse is depicted with no glamorization and in an approximation of a real setting. Glamour art, the next step in the progression, emphasizes feminine appeal. A caring expression on a nurse's face becomes a bit more sensual, a uniform becomes slightly more fashionable, dark circles of fatigue around the eyes transform to an eye-shadow makeup effect.

Because glamour postcards far outnumber realistic postcards, the glamour postcard had a greater impact on nursing as a profession. For example, when the call for nurses went out in World War I, women who had a distorted conception of nursing rushed to enlist. Their actions were motivated, at least in part, by the visions of glamour and romance the postcard helped promulgate. Whether this ultimately harmed or helped the profession is open to debate, but in the short run it caused a major headache for the nurses responsible for screening the candidates. (See note 5.11, Clara Noyes.)

Little girls, from the turn of the 20th century until now, have enjoyed playing nurse. Some played with dolls and stuffed animals as patients, or ministered to playmates or pets; others actually took care of real babies or elderly grandparents and pretended they were grown-up nurses. A little girl at play might imagine herself nursing a handsome prince or brave soldier back to health. She might pretend that her patient falls in love with her, they get married in a fancy wedding, and, of course, live happily ever after. This vision of the beautiful grown-up nurse, drawn in adult perspective, is what we see in the glamour postcards. Add a handsome male patient to a glamour postcard, and you have a romance postcard. Sometimes the artist depicts the child herself, playing the role of nurse. Some of the most popular of children-as-nurse postcards were done by artists who were best known for illustrating children's books.

Glamour, romance, and children's games are forms of fantasy. In postcard terminology, however, fantasy refers to wider realms of the imagination, where fairy folk and folklore creatures live, where animals dress and act as people, where people cavort on the moon. Fantasy postcards, most of which appeal both to children and adults, shift gradually to themes where the humor is simply not appropriate or even comprehensible to a child. The situation depicted on the postcard may be sexual or political. Furthermore, the appreciation of the image may depend on a caption beyond a child's understanding.

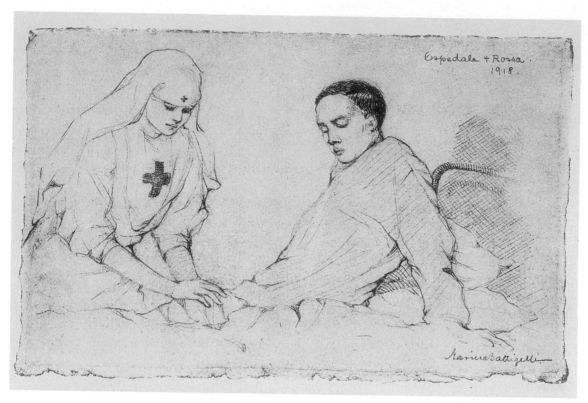

Figure 2.2. **"Red Cross Hospital."**
Italy. 1918.

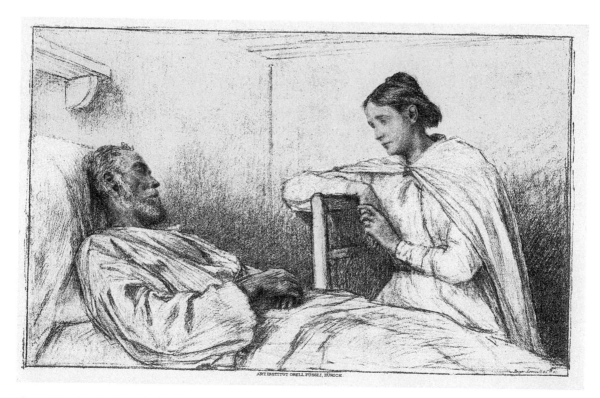

Figure 2.3. **"For the Benefit of Sick Nurses."**
Switzerland. 1927.

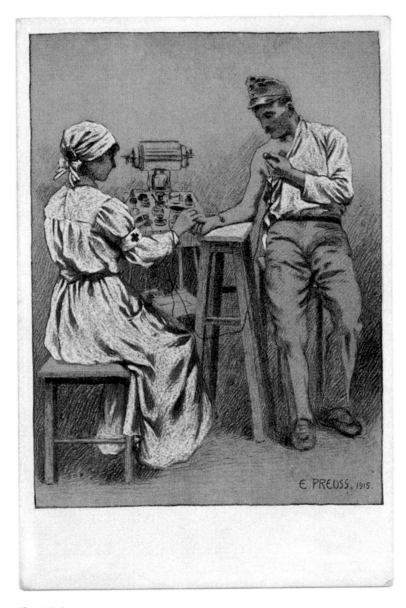

Figure 2.4.
Austria. 1915. *(See note.)*

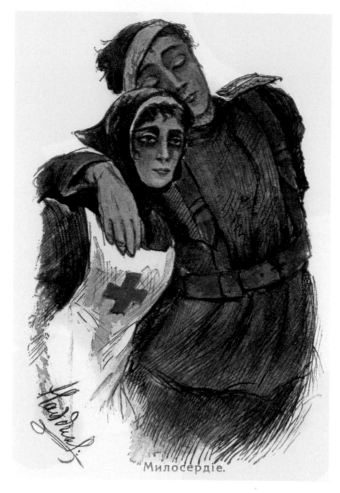

Figure 2.5. **"Compassion."**
Russia. c. 1915 *(See note.)*

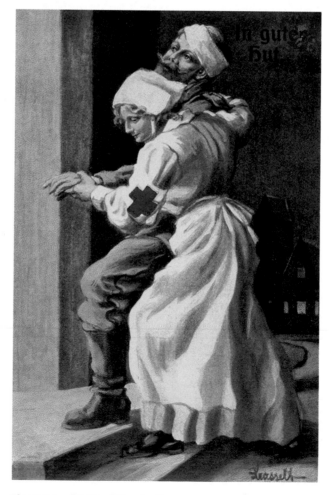

Figure 2.6. **"In Good Keeping."**
Germany. c. 1915.

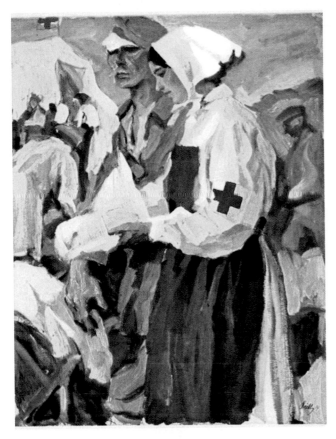

Figure 2.7. **Paul Rieth (1871–1925). "Under the Red Cross."** *(See note.)*

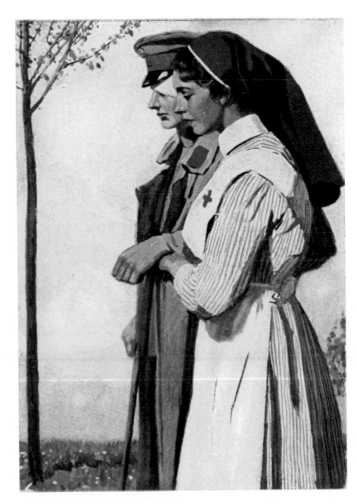

Figure 2.8. **Willy Planck (1870–1956). "In Good Care."** Germany. 1916. *(See note.)*

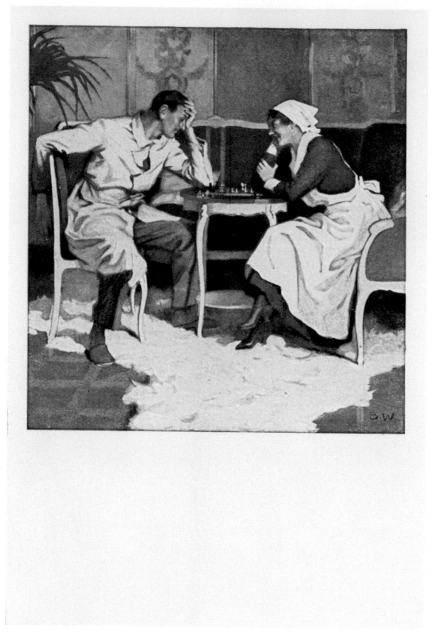

Figure 2.9.   **B. Wennerberg (1866–1950).**
Germany. 1918. *(See note.)*

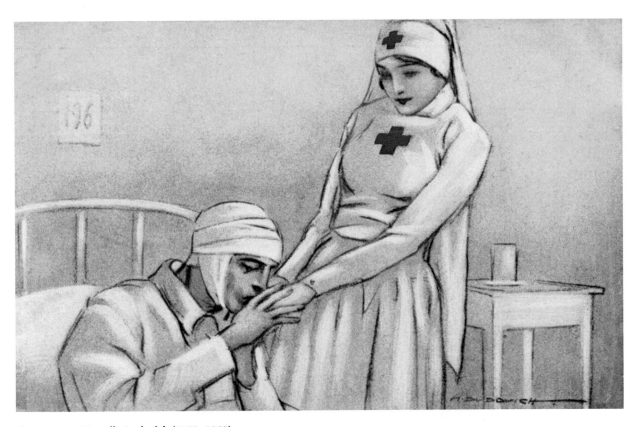

Figure 2.10. **Marcello Dudovich (1878–1962).**
Italy. 1916. *(See note.)*

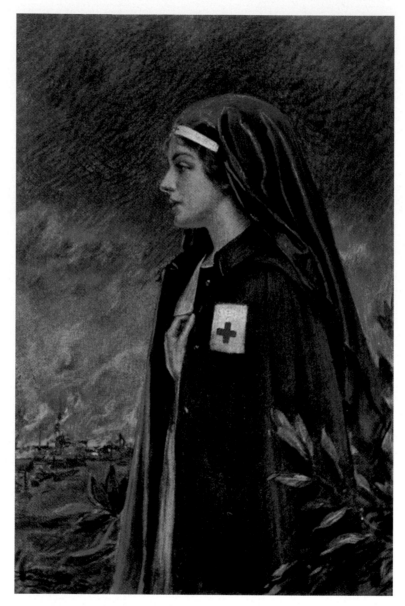

Figure 2.11. **D. Enjorlas. "An Angel."**
Lapina Gallery. France. c. 1916. *(See note.)*

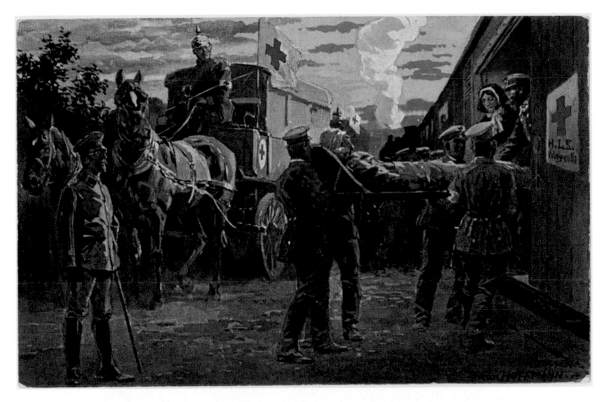

Figure 2.12.
Germany. 1914.

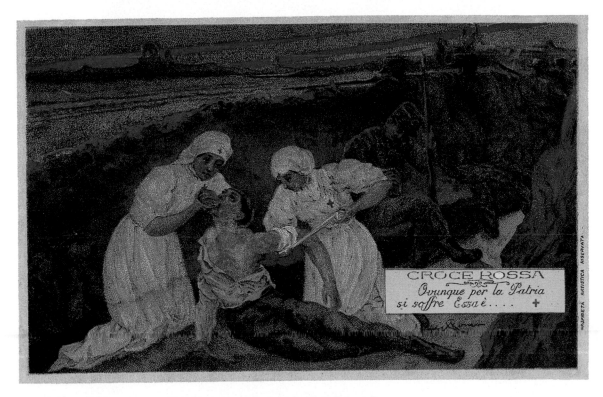

Figure 2.13. **"Wherever one suffers for the country, there is the Red Cross."**
Italy. c. 1914.

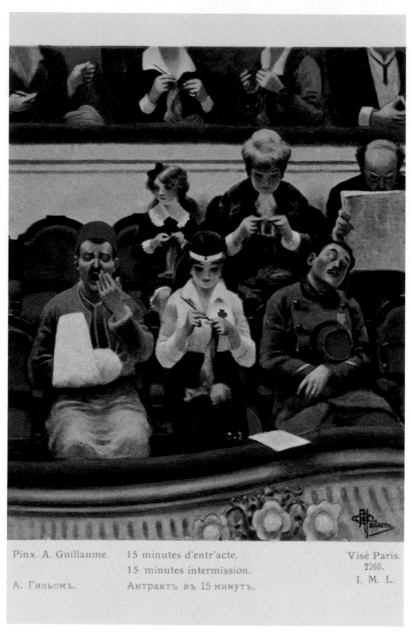

Pinx. A. Guillaume.   15 minutes d'entr'acte.   Visé Paris.
                      15 minutes intermission.   2260.
A. Гильомъ.   Антрактъ въ 15 минутъ.   I. M. L.

Figure 2.14.   A. Guillaume. "15 Minutes Intermission."
Lapina Gallery. France. 1916.

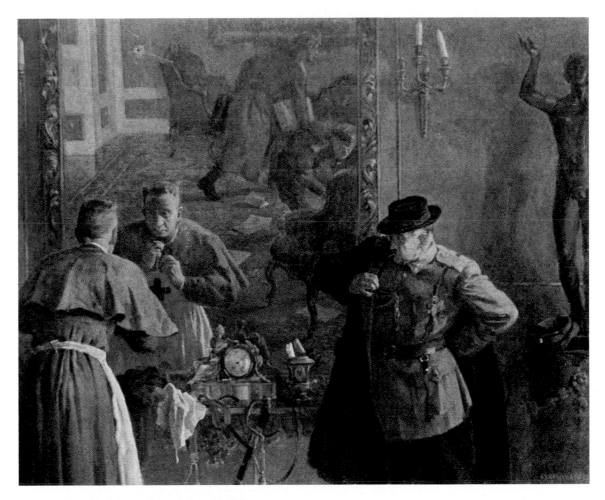

Figure 2.15. Kukryniksy. "Kerensky's Last Exit."
Russia. 1958. *(See note.)*

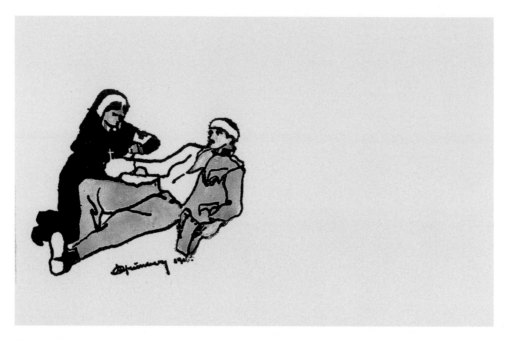

Figure 2.16.
Austria. 1914.

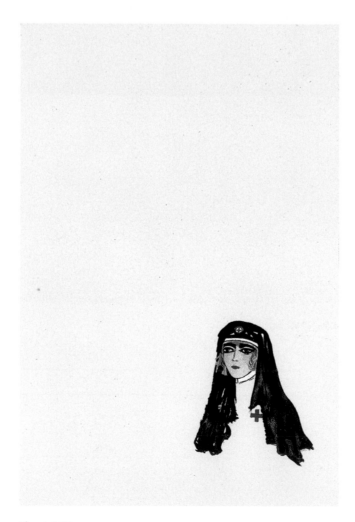

Figure 2.17.
Italy. 1916.

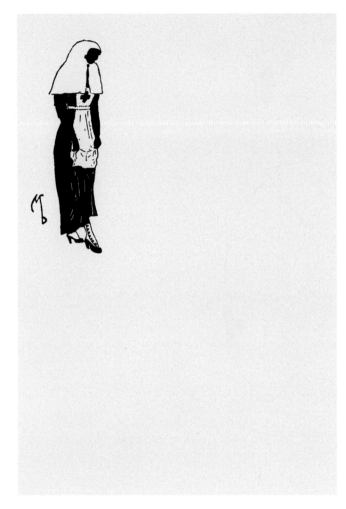

Figure 2.18.
Ukraine. 1921.

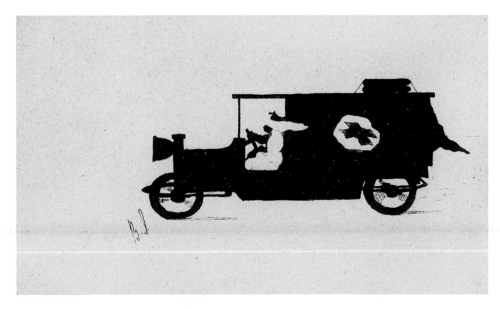

Figure 2.19.
Ukraine. 1922.

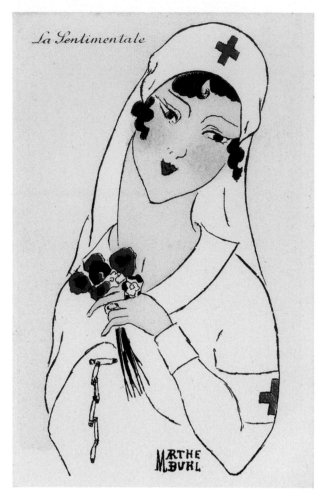

Figure 2.20. Marthe Buhl. "The Sentimental One."
France. c. 1917. *(See note.)*

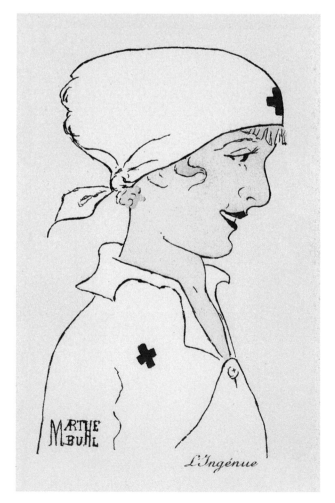

Figure 2.21. Marthe Buhl. "The Ingenue."
France. c. 1917. *(See note.)*

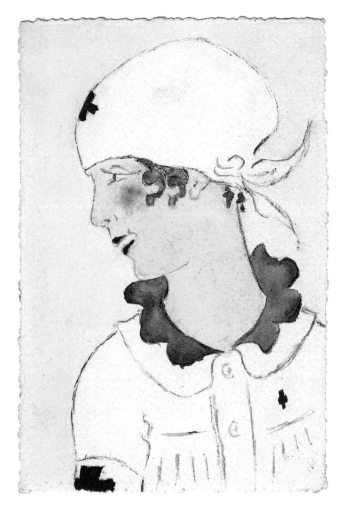

Figure 2.22.   Marthe Buhl.
Handpainted original. France. c. 1917. *(See note.)*

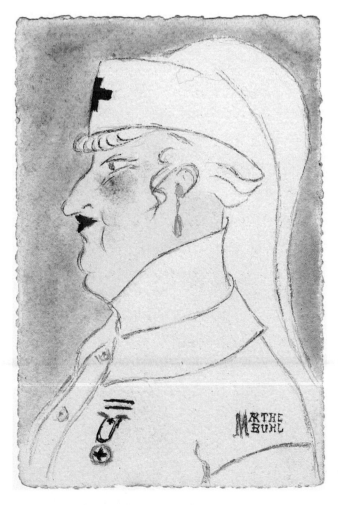

Figure 2.23.   Marthe Buhl.
Handpainted original. France. c. 1917. *(See note.)*

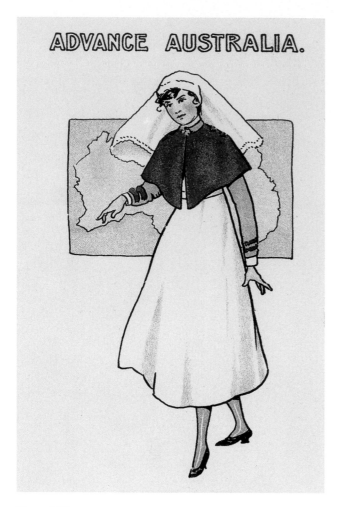

Figure 2.24.
England. 1918. *(See note.)*

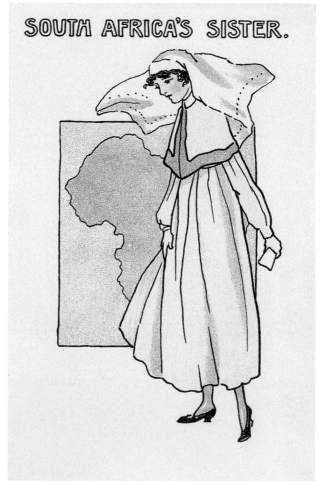

Figure 2.25.
England. 1918. *(See note.)*

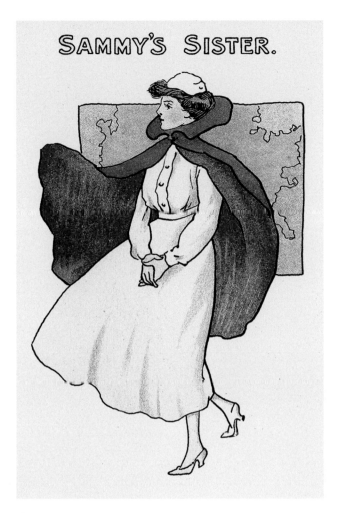

Figure 2.26.
England. 1918. *(See note.)*

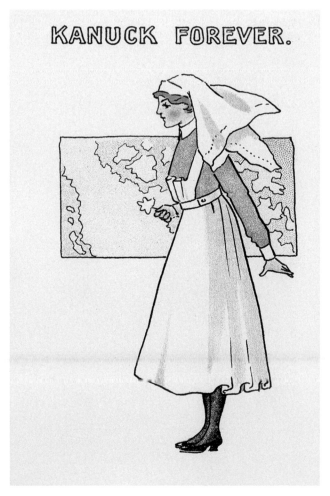

Figure 2.27.
England. 1918. *(See note.)*

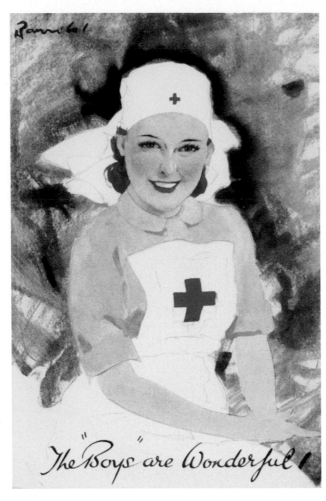

Figure 2.28. **William Barribal (1873–1956). "The Boys are Wonderful."**
England. c. 1940. *(See note.)*

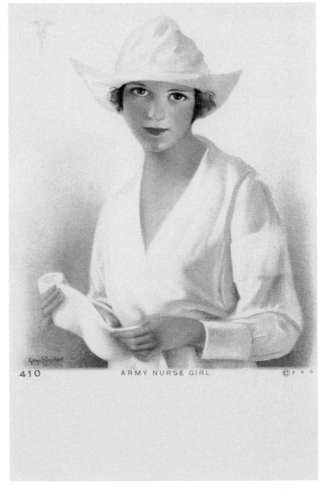

Figure 2.29. **Gene Pressler (1894–1933). "Army Nurse Girl."**
United States. c. 1920 (See Figure 2.1).

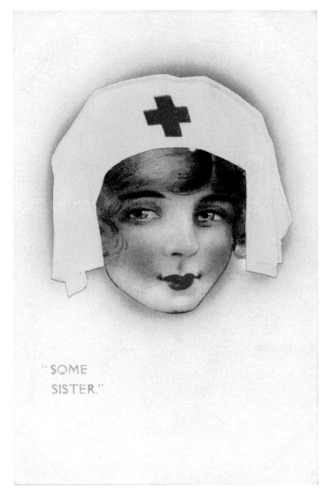

"SOME
SISTER."

Figure 2.30.
England. c. 1916. *(See note.)*

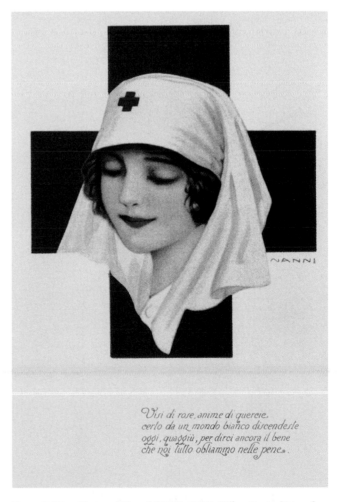

*Visi di rose, anime di quercie,
certo da un mondo bianco discendeste
oggi, quaggiù, per dirci ancora il bene
che noi tutto obliammo nelle pene.*

**Figure 2.31.   Giovanni Nanni (1888–1969). Milan Committee of
Red Cross Publicity.**
Italy. c. 1925. *(See note.)*

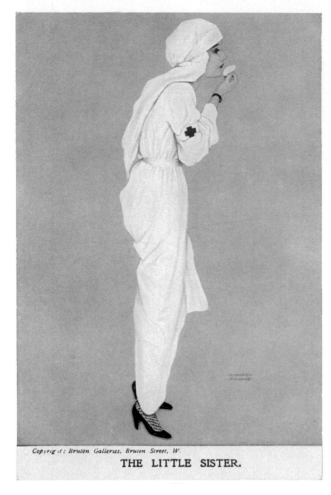

Figure 2.32. **Raphael Kirchner (1876–1917). "The Little Sister."**
England. 1916. *(See note.)*

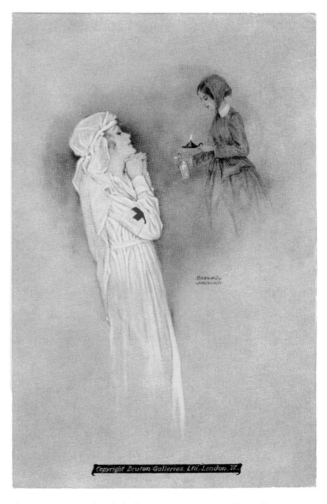

Figure 2.33. **Raphael Kirchner (1876–1917). "The Call."**
England. 1916. *(See note.)*

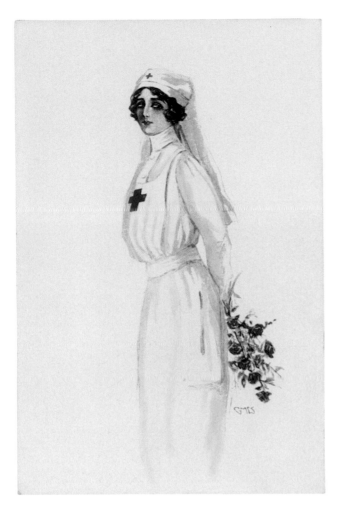

Figure 2.34.
Italy. c. 1920.

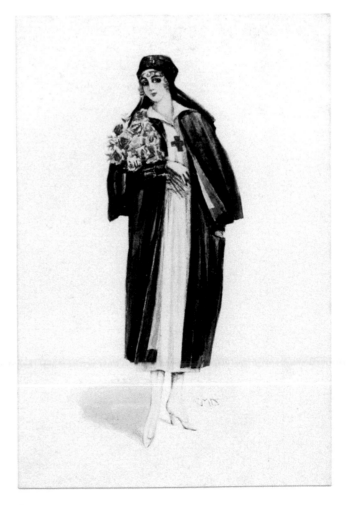

Figure 2.35.
Italy. c. 1920.

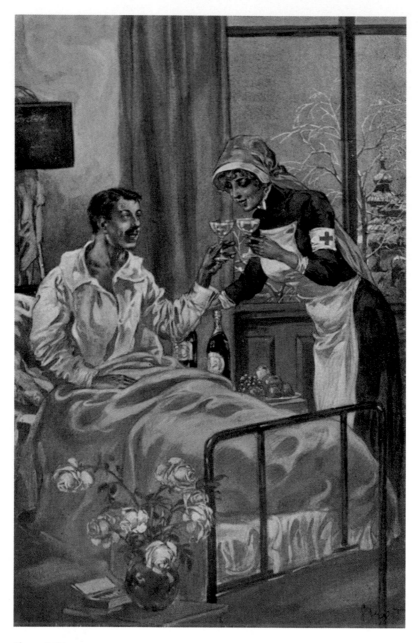

Figure 2.36.
Austria. 1917. *(See note.)*

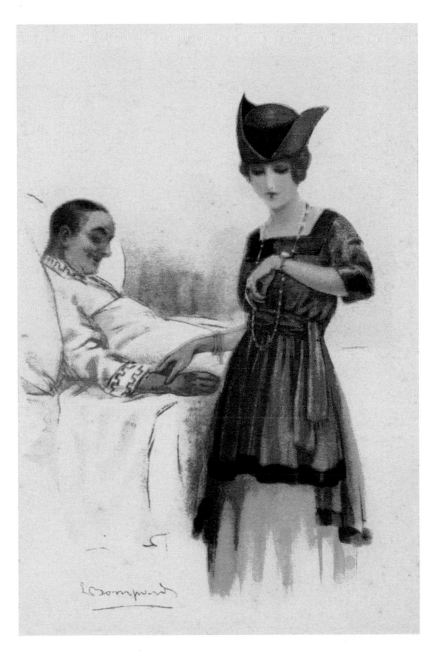

Figure 2.37. **Luigi Bompard (1879–1953).**
Italy. 1907. *(See note.)*

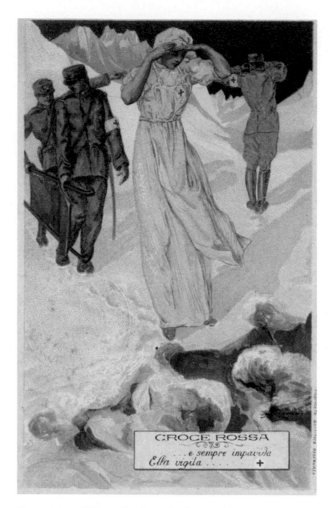

Figure 2.38. **"Always fearless, she keeps vigilant."**
Italy. c. 1917.

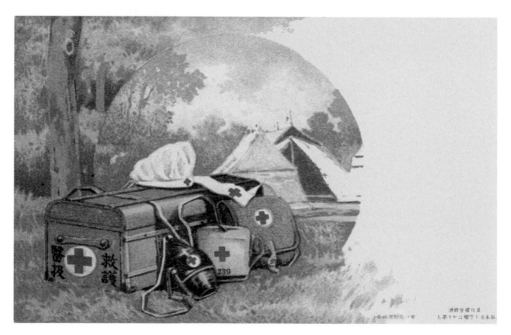

Figure 2.39.
Japan. c. 1915.

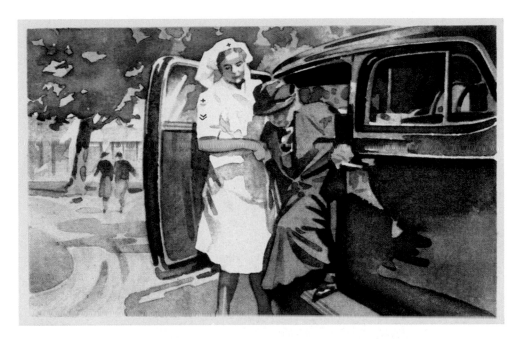

Figure 2.40.
The Netherlands. c. 1940.

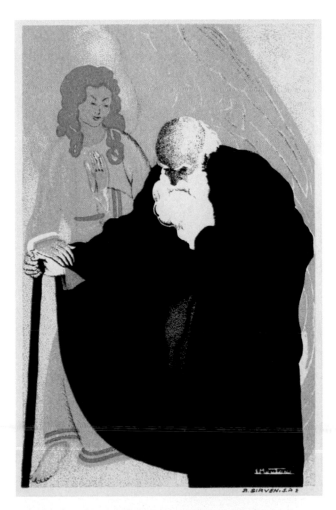

Figure 2.41. **"By assisting those who have worked their entire lives . . ."**
Spain. c. 1930. *(See note.)*

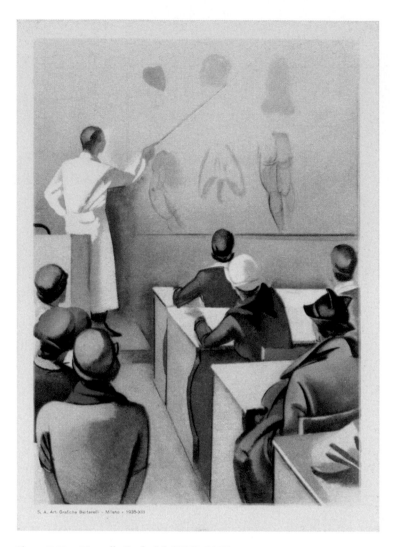

Figure 2.42. **Marcello Dudovich (1878–1962).**
Italy. 1935. *(See note.)*

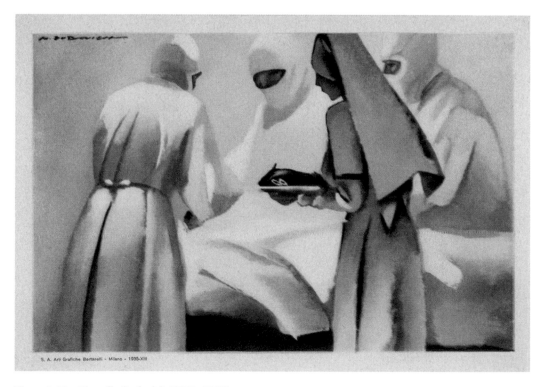

Figure 2.43. **Marcello Dudovich (1878–1962).**
Italy. 1935. *(See note.)*

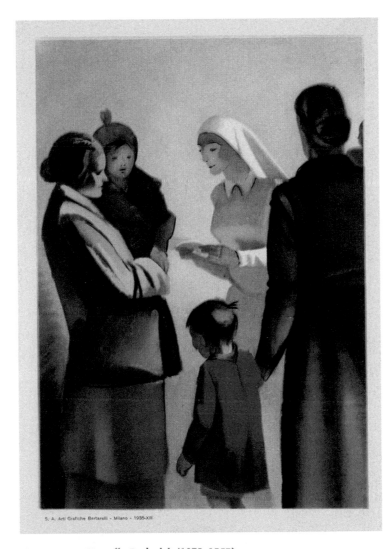

Figure 2.44. **Marcello Dudovich (1878–1962).**
Italy. 1935. *(See note.)*

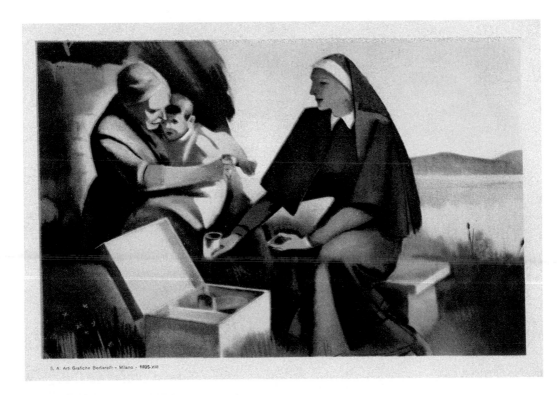

Figure 2.45. **Marcello Dudovich (1878–1962).**
Italy. 1935. *(See note.)*

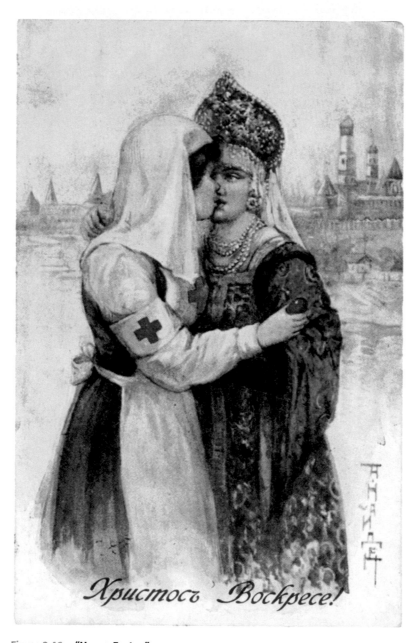

Христосъ Воскресе!

Figure 2.46. **"Happy Easter."**
Russia. c. 1915. *(See note.)*

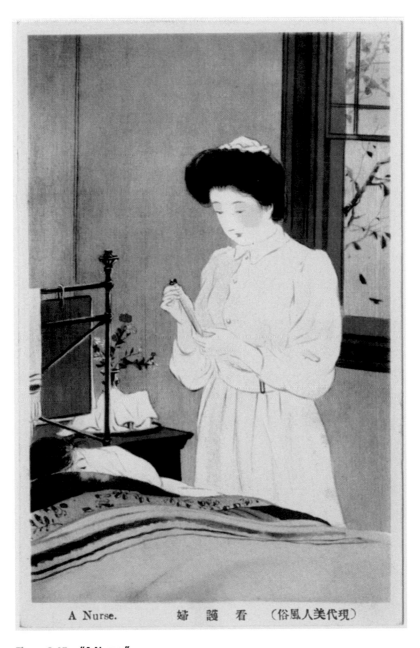

A Nurse.　　　　看　護　婦　　（現代美人風俗）

Figure 2.47. "A Nurse."
Japan. c. 1920.

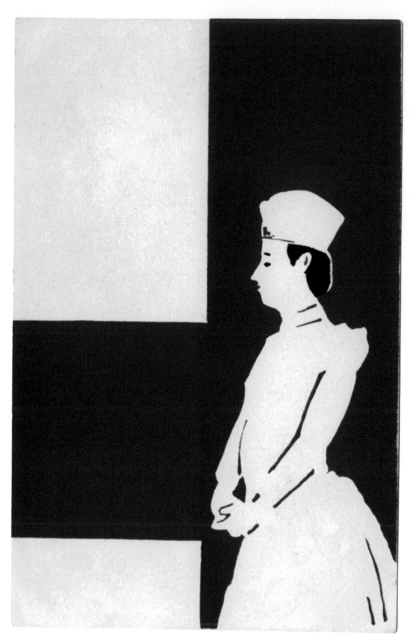

Figure 2.48.
Japan. c. 1912.

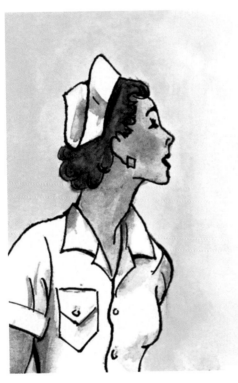

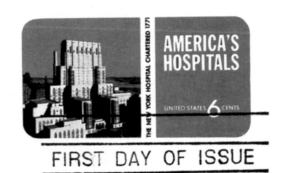

Figure 2.49. **H. Maul (1897–1983).**
United States. 1971. *(See note.)*

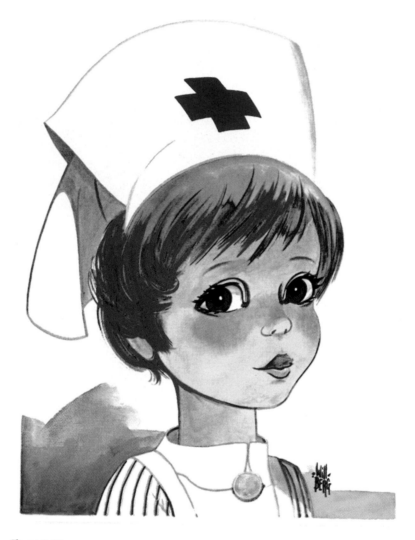

Figure 2.50.
The Netherlands. c. 1960.

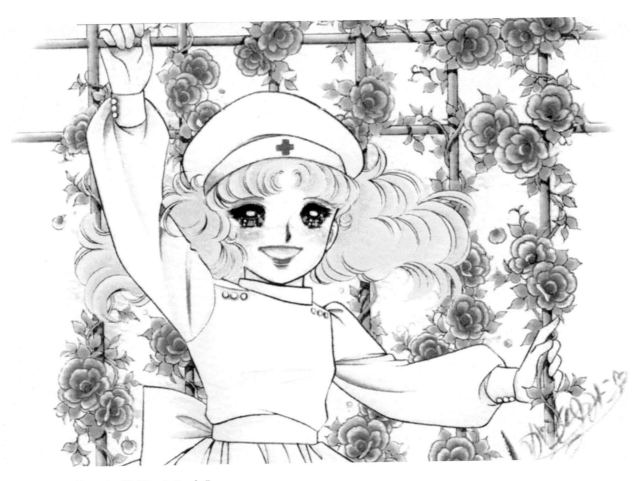

Figure 2.51. Yumiko Igarashi. "Candy Candy."
Japan. 1990. *(See note.)*

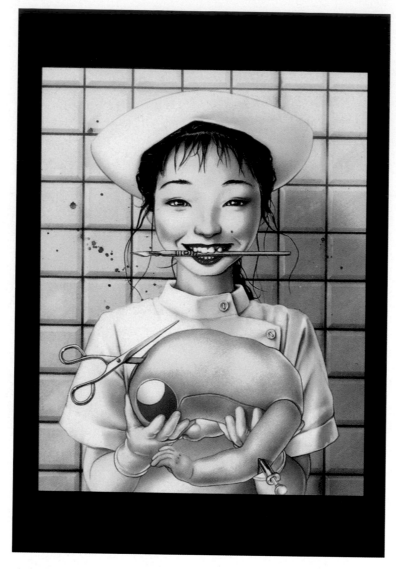

Figure 2.52. **Trevor Brown (1959–). "Nurse."**
Japan. 1996.
©Trevor Brown, used with permission of the artist. *(See note.)*

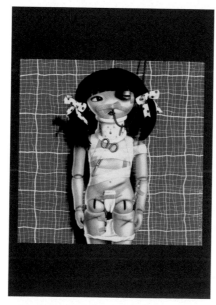

Figure 2.53. **Trevor Brown (1959–).**
"Broken."
Japan. 1996.
©Trevor Brown, used with permission of the
artist. *(See note.)*

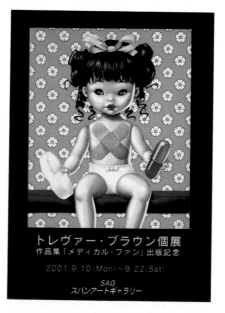

Figure 2.54. **Trevor Brown (1959–).**
Trevor Brown Exhibition commemorating
the publication of his work "Medical Fun"
2001.9.10 Mon.-9.22 Span Art Gallery.
Japan. 1996.
©Trevor Brown, used with permission of the
artist. *(See note.)*

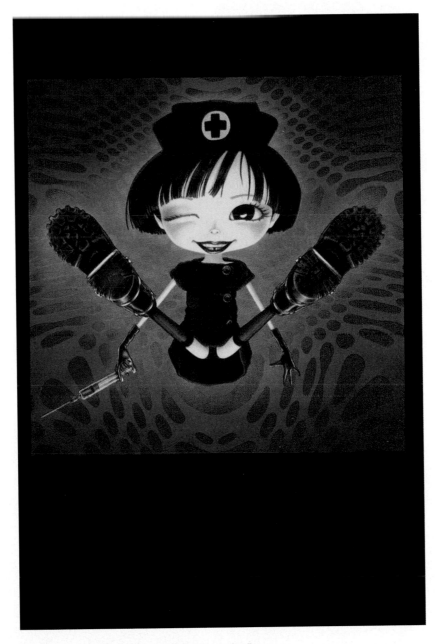

Figure 2.55.   Trevor Brown (1959–). "Mosquito."
Japan. 1998.
©Trevor Brown, used with permission of the artist. *(See note.)*

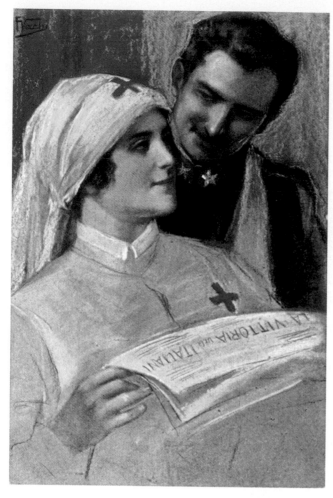

Figure 2.56.
Italy. 1917. *(See note.)*

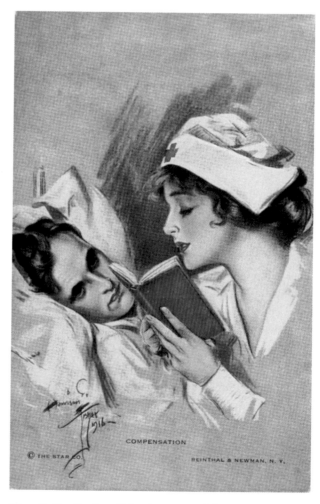

Figure 2.57. **Harrison Fisher (1875–1974). "Compensation."**
United States. 1916. *(See note.)*

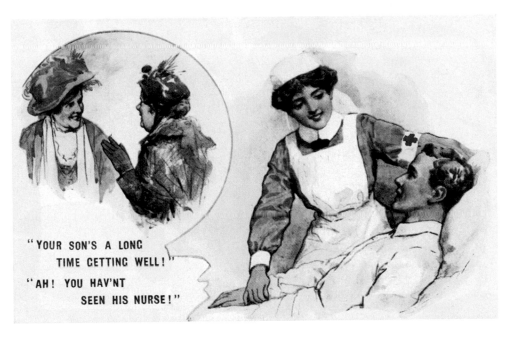

Figure 2.58.
England. c. 1910.

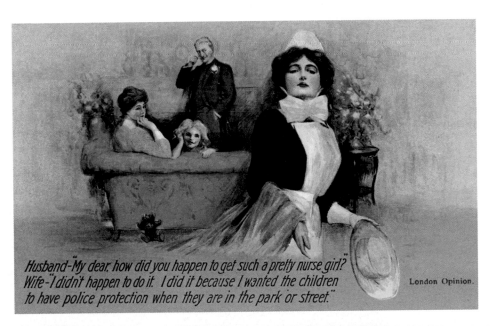

Figure 2.59.
England. c. 1910.

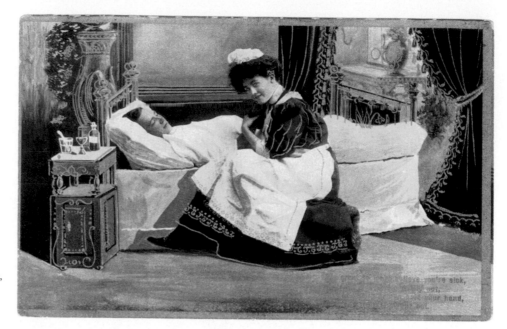

Figure 2.60.
United States. c. 1908.

"It's great to make believe you're sick,
Although you're really not.
And have a nurse to hold you,
And sit beside your cot."

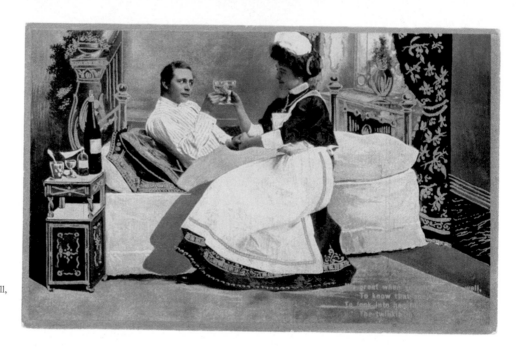

Figure 2.61.
United States. c. 1908.

"It's great when you are getting well,
To know that she's nearby,
To look into her face and see,
The twinkle in her eye."

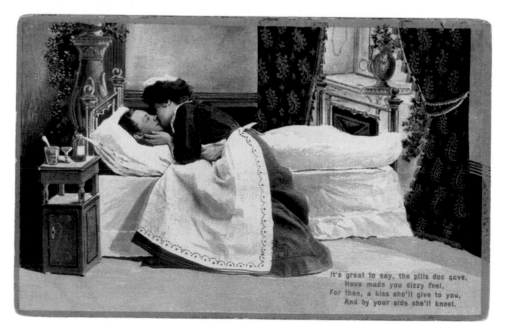

Figure 2.62.
United States. c. 1908.

"It's great to say, the pills doc gave,
Have made you dizzy feel,
For this, a kiss she'll give to you,
And by your side she'll kneel."

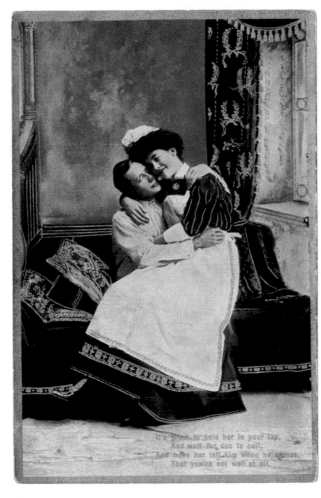

Figure 2.63.
United States. c. 1908.

"It's great to hold her in your lap,
And wait for doc to call,
And have her tell him when he comes,
That you're not well at all."

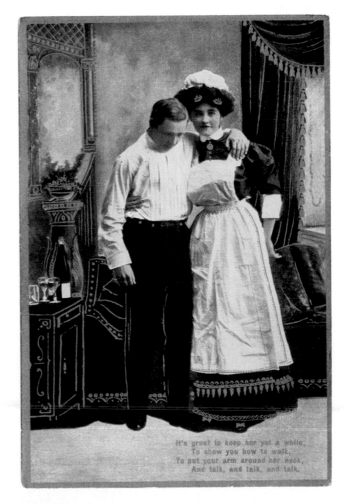

Figure 2.64.
United States. c. 1908.

"It's great to keep her yet a while,
To show you how to walk,
To put your arm around her neck,
And talk, and talk, and talk."

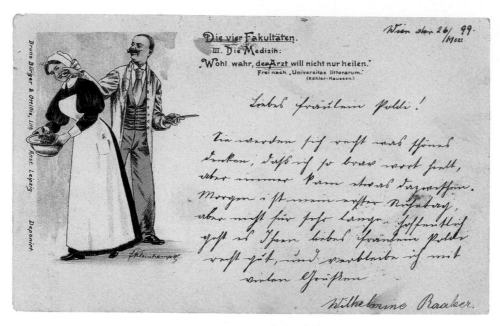

Figure 2.65.   **The four faculties of medicine. Vienna, 26 March 1899. "It's true, the doctor doesn't just want to heal." "Freely adapted from Universitas Literarum (Köhler-Haussen)."**
Austria. 1899. *(See note.)*

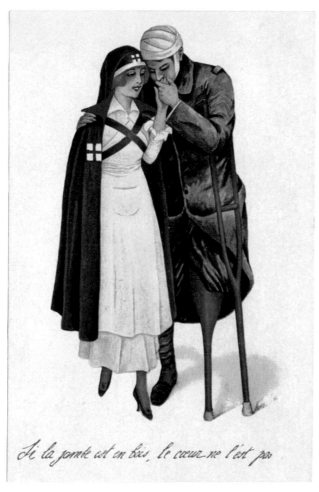

Figure 2.66.   **Xavier Sager (1870–1930). "The leg is injured, but the heart is not."**
France. 1916. *(See note.)*

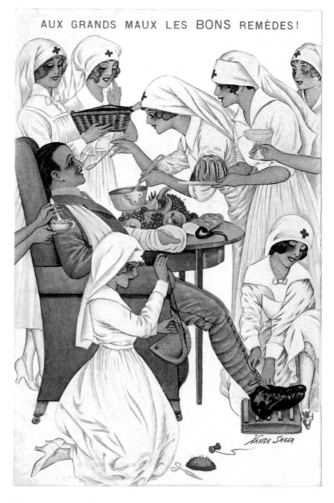

Figure 2.67.   **Xavier Sager (1870–1930). "To great ailments, good remedies."**
France. 1916. *(See note.)*

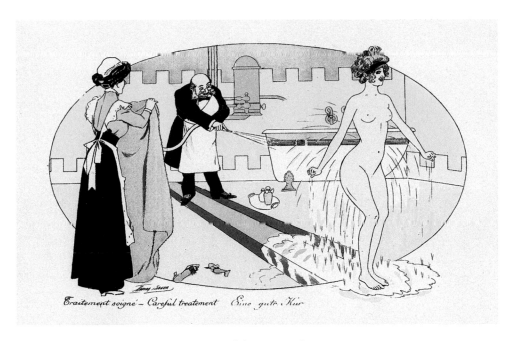

Figure 2.68. **Xavier Sager (1870–1930). "Careful Treatment."**
France. c. 1912. *(See note.)*

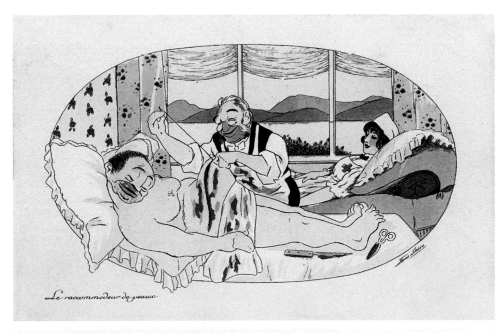

Figure 2.69. **Xavier Sager (1870–1930). "The mending of the skin."**
France. c. 1912. *(See note.)*

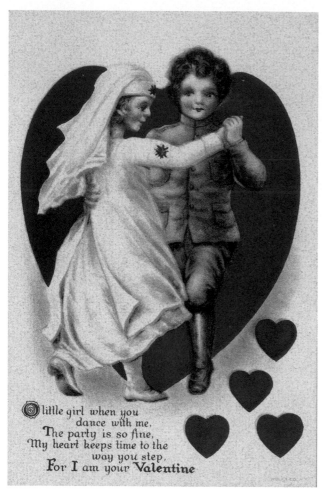

Figure 2.70.
United States. c. 1918.

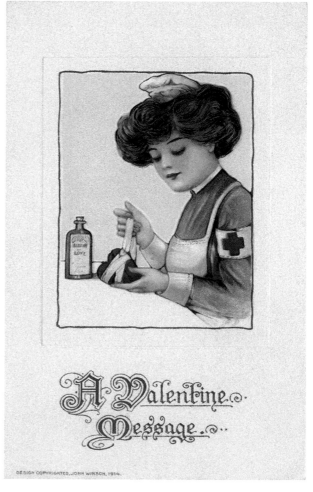

Figure 2.71. **Samuel Schmucker (1879–1921).**
"A Valentine Message."
United States. 1914. *(See note.)*

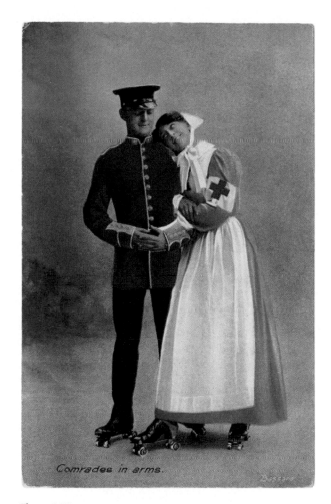

Figure 2.72.
Great Britain. c. 1915.

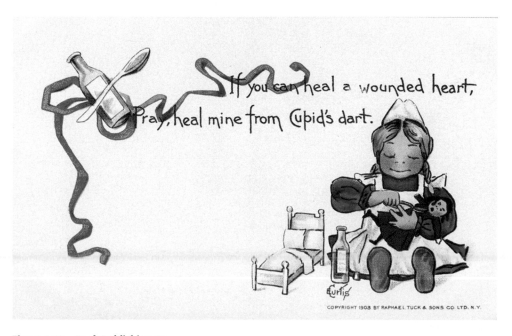

Figure 2.73. Tuck Publishing Co.
United States. 1903. *(See note.)*

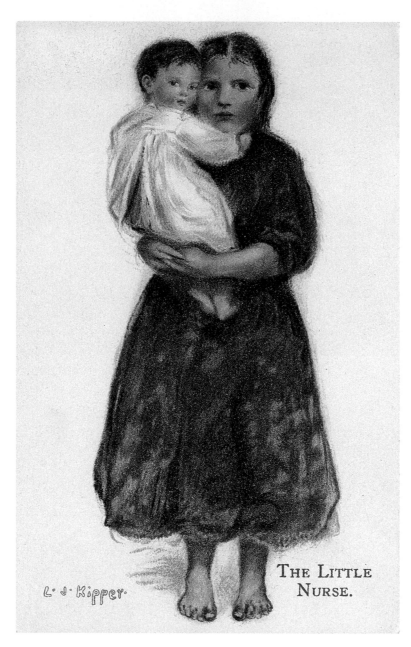

Figure 2.74. L. J. Kipper. "The Little Nurse."
United States. c. 1910.

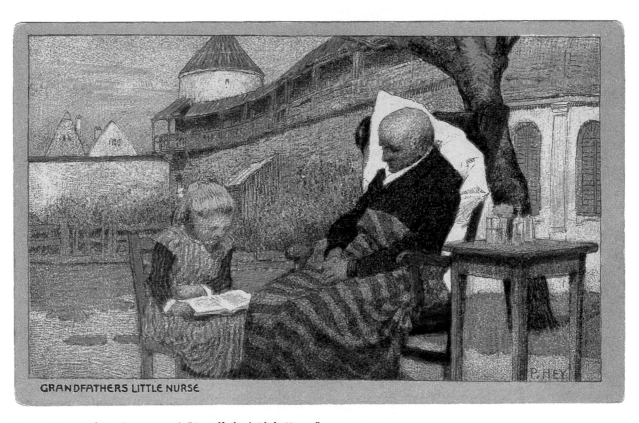

GRANDFATHERS LITTLE NURSE

Figure 2.75. **Paul Hey (1867–1952). "Grandfather's Little Nurse."**
England. c. 1910. *(See note.)*

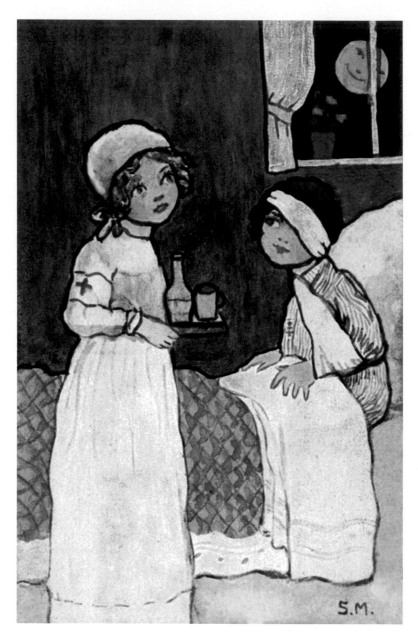

Figure 2.76.
Hungary. c. 1910. *(See note.)*

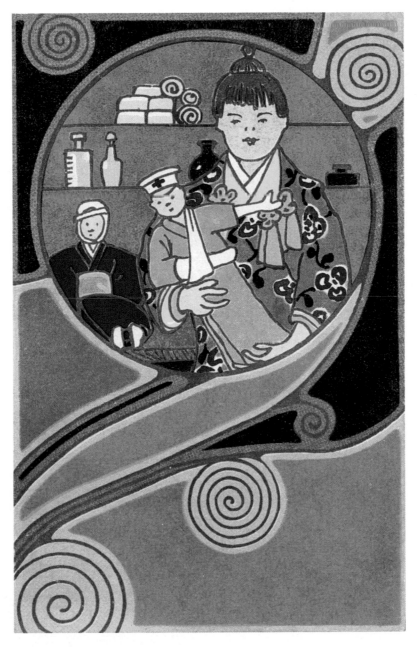

Figure 2.77.
Japan. 1907. *(See note.)*

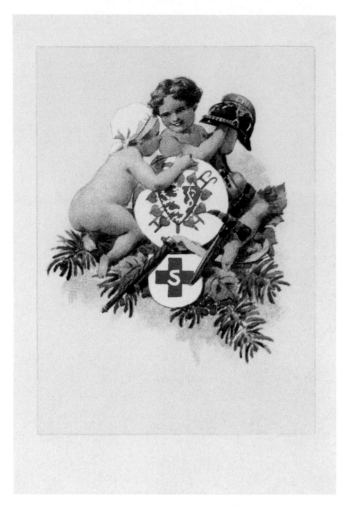

Figure 2.78.
Prague, Czechoslovakia. 1928. *(See note.)*

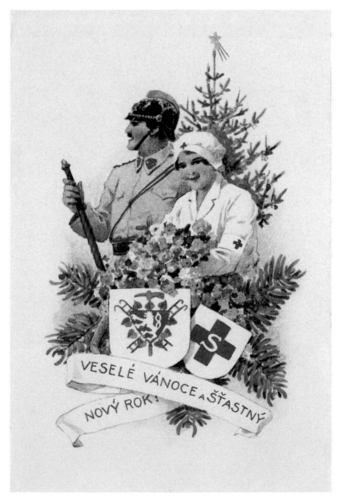

Figure 2.79.
Prague, Czechoslovakia. 1928. *(See note.)*

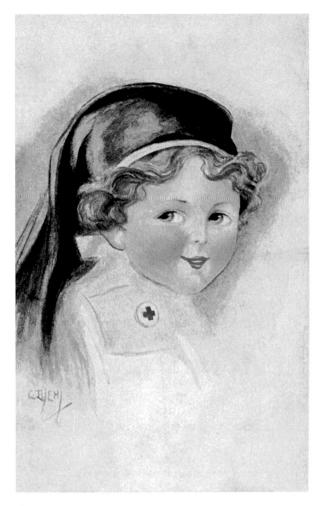

Figure 2.80.
Germany. c. 1916. *(See note.)*

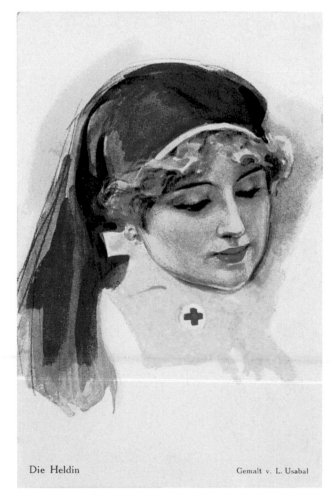

Die Heldin   Gemalt v. L. Usabal

Figure 2.81.   L. Usabel. "The Heroine."
Germany. c. 1916. *(See note.)*

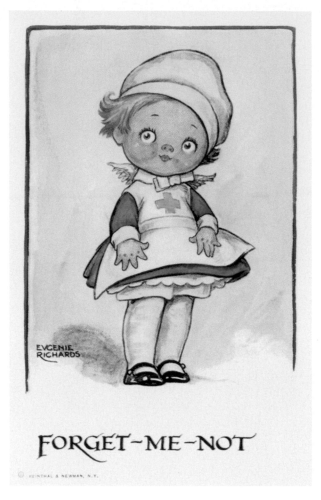

Figure 2.82. **Eugenie Richards (1873–1941). "Forget-Me-Not."**
England. c. 1910. *(See note.)*

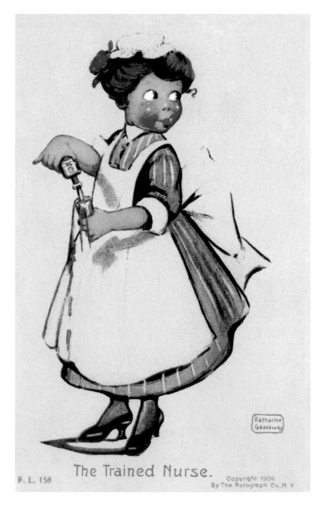

Figure 2.83. **Katherine Gassaway. "The Trained Nurse."**
United States. 1906. *(See note.)*

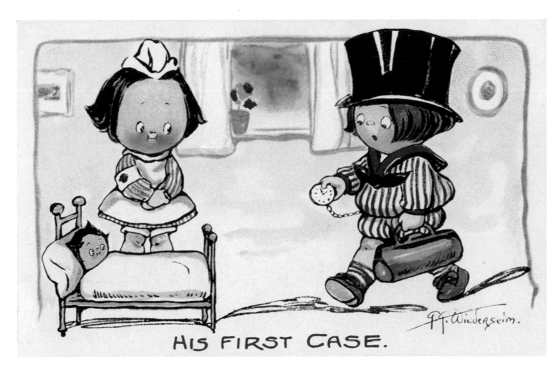

Figure 2.84. Grace G. Wiederseim (1877–1936). "His First Case."
United States. c. 1910. Grace Wiederseim was the creator of the Campbell's Soup Kids.
(See note.)

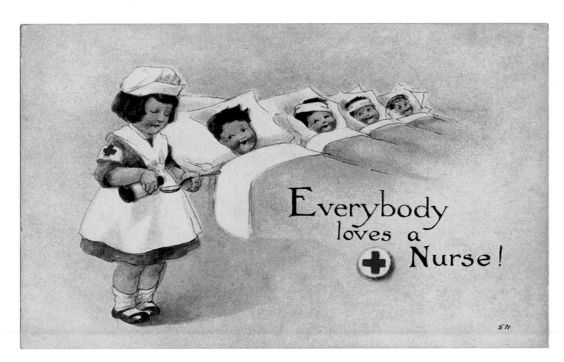

Figure 2.85.
United States. c. 1917. *(See note.)*

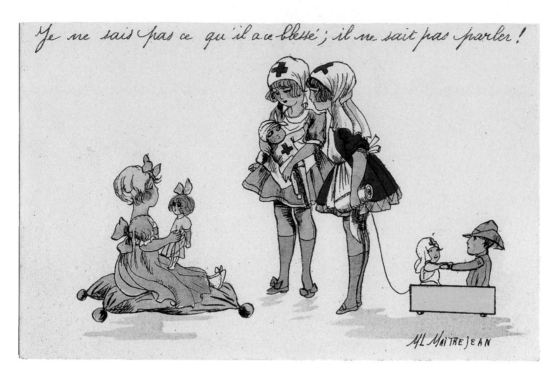

Figure 2.86. **"I don't know if he's wounded; he doesn't know how to talk."**
France. c. 1916.

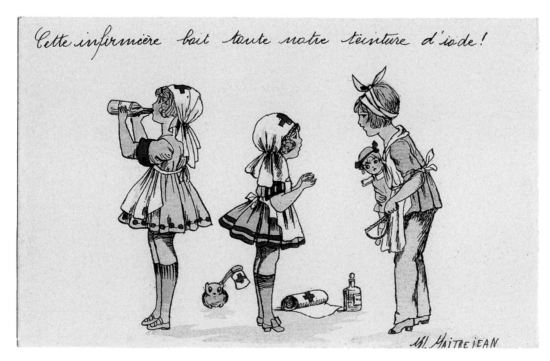

Figure 2.87. **"That nurse is drinking all our tincture of iodine!"**
France. c. 1916.

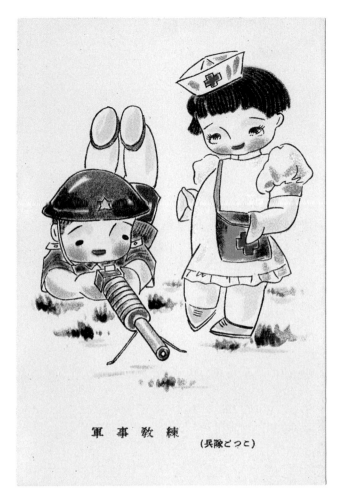

軍 事 教 練
（兵隊ごっこ）

Figure 2.88. **"Playing War."**
Japan. c. 1939.

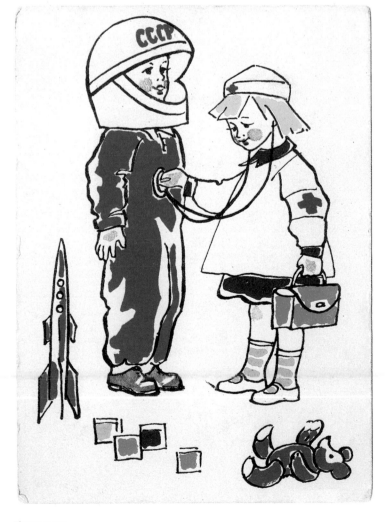

Figure 2.89.
U.S.S.R. 1963. *(See note.)*

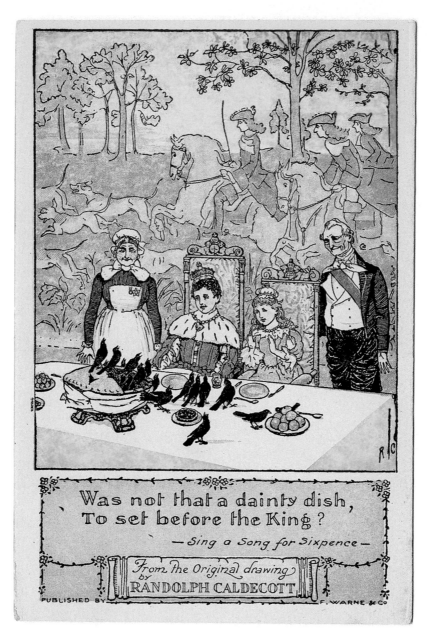

Figure 2.90.   Randolph Caldecott (1846–1885). "Was not that a dainty dish, to set before the King."
England. c. 1910. (See note.)

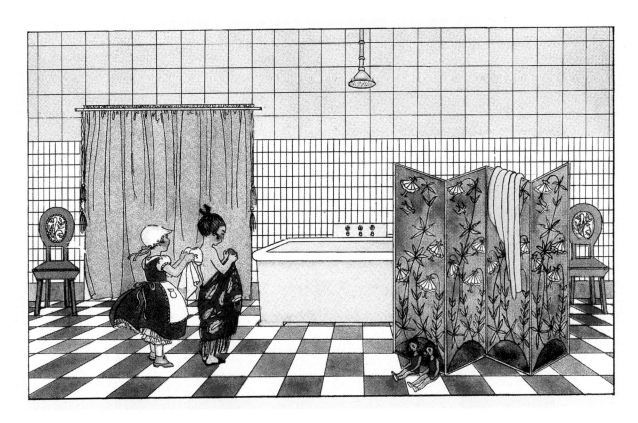

Figure 2.91.
Sweden. c. 1910. *(See note.)*

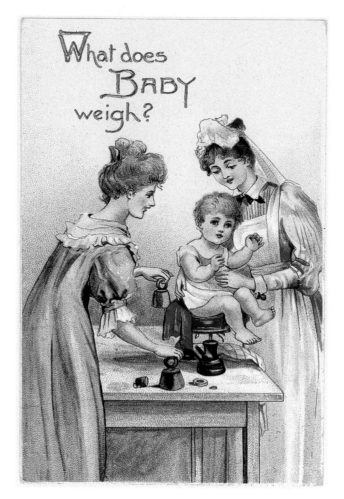

Figure 2.92.
United States. c. 1910.

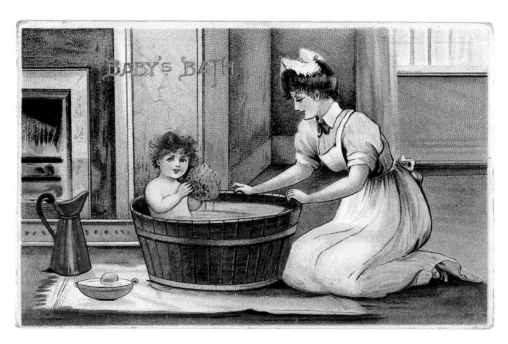

Figure 2.93.
United States. c. 1910.

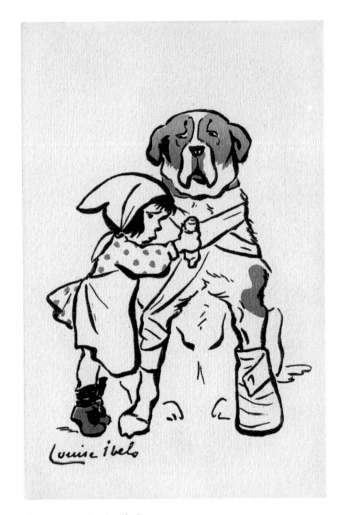

Figure 2.94. **Louise Ibels.**
France. c. 1910. *(See note.)*

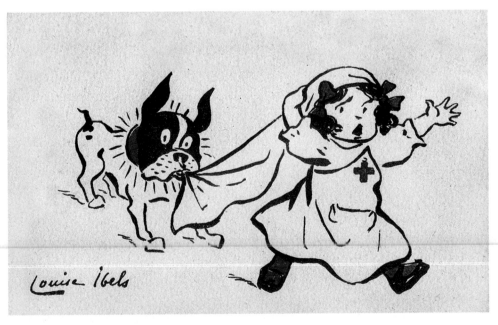

Figure 2.95. **Louise Ibels.**
France. c. 1910. *(See note.)*

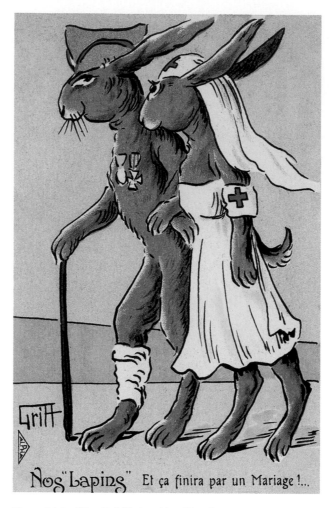

Figure 2.96. **"Our 'Rabbits' and it will end in a marriage!"**
France. 1918.

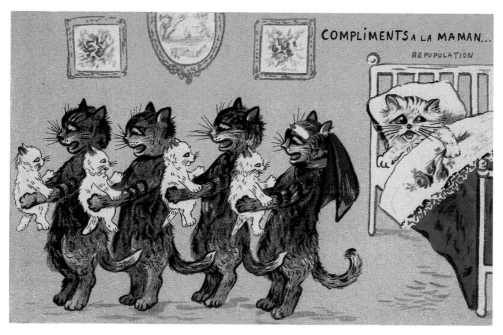

Figure 2.97. **G. Boulanger. "Compliments of Mother."**
France. c. 1910.

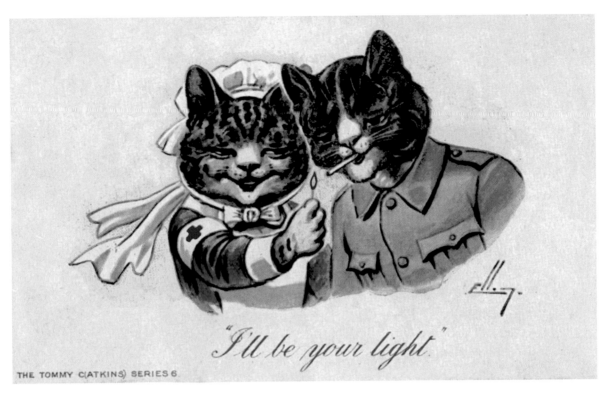

Figure 2.98. William Henry Ellam (1858–1935). "I'll be your light."
England. c. 1916. *(See note.)*

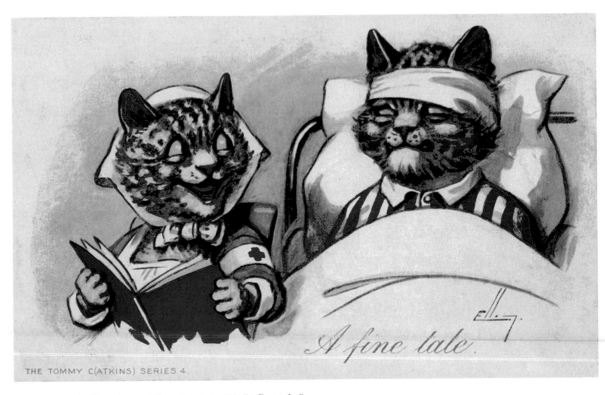

Figure 2.99. William Henry Ellam (1858–1935). "A fine tale."
England. c. 1916. *(See note.)*

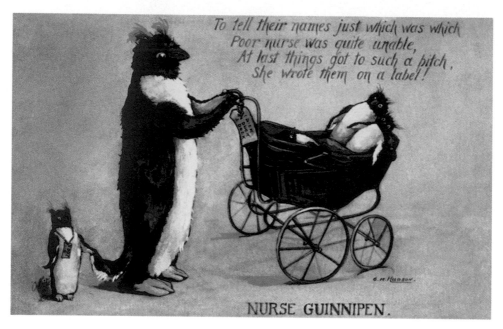

Figure 2.100.
England. c. 1910. *(See note.)*

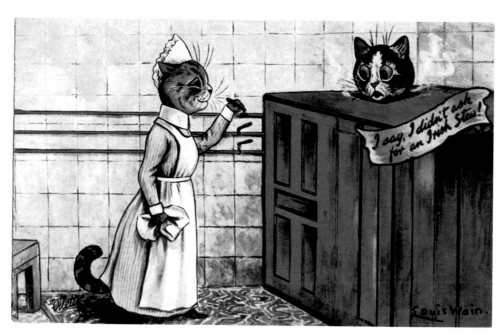

Figure 2.101. **Louis Wain (1860–1939). "I say, I didn't ask for an Irish stew!"**
England. c. 1910. *(See note.)*

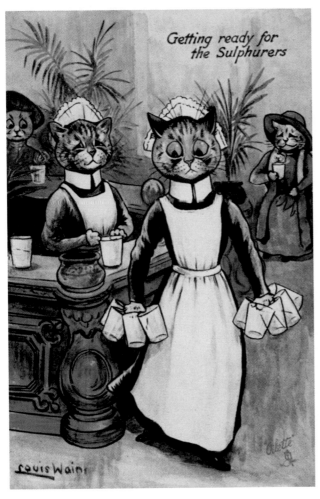

Figure 2.102. **Louis Wain (1860–1939). "Getting ready for the sulphurers."**
England. c. 1910. (Figure 7.23) *(See note.)*

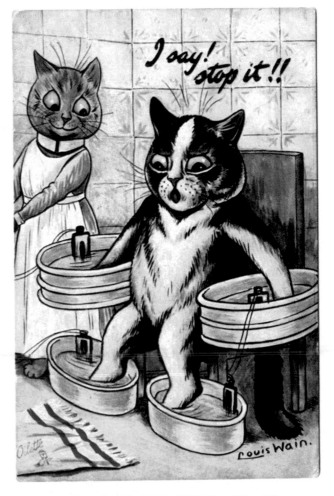

Figure 2.103. **Louis Wain (1860–1939). "I say! Stop it!"**
England. c. 1910. *(See note.)*

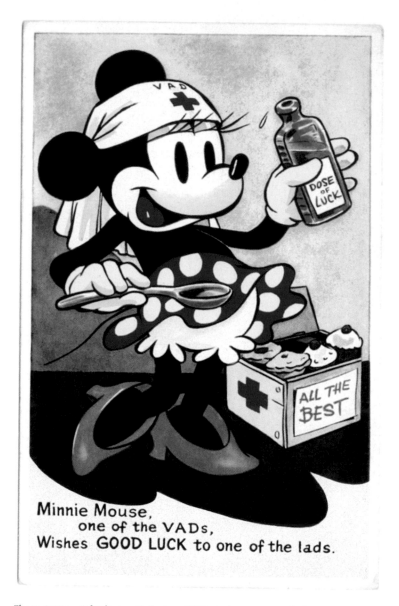

Figure 2.104. **Minnie as a Voluntary Aid Detachment nurse during World War II.**
Minnie Mouse is © Disney Enterprises, Inc., used with permission of Disney Publishing Worldwide.
England. c. 1941.

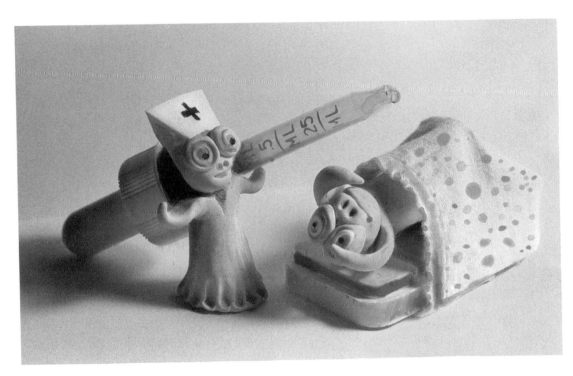

Figure 2.105.   Jane Wiley (1952–). "Nurse Dede's Efficacious Elixir."
© Jane Wiley, used with permission of the artist.
United States. 2002. *(See note.)*

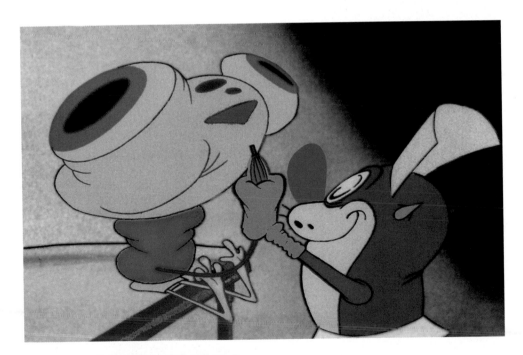

Figure 2.106.   "Nurse Stimpy to the Rescue."
© Nickelodeon, used with permission of Nickelodeon and Penguin, Putnam, Inc.
United States. 1992. *(See note.)*

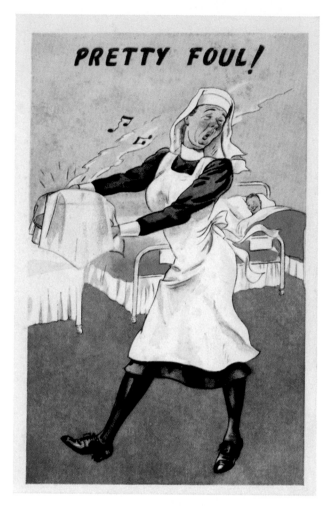

Figure 2.107. **One of two views of mechanical postcard.**
(See Figure 2.108).
England. c. 1914. *(See note.)*

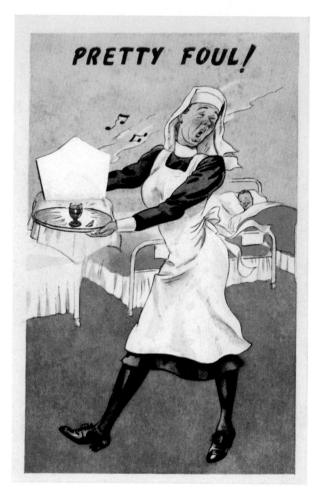

Figure 2.108. **One of two views of mechanical postcard.**
(See Figure 2.107).
England. c. 1914. *(See note.)*

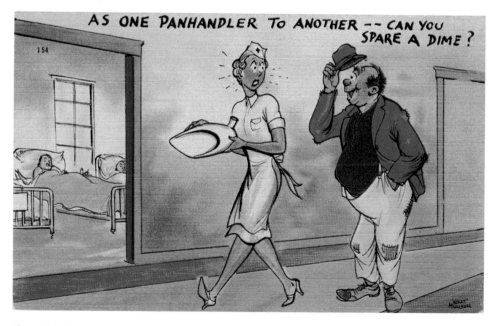

Figure 2.109.
United States. Linen. c. 1940.

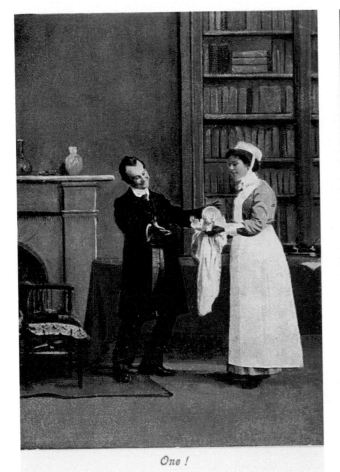

One !

Figure 2.110.
England. 1906.

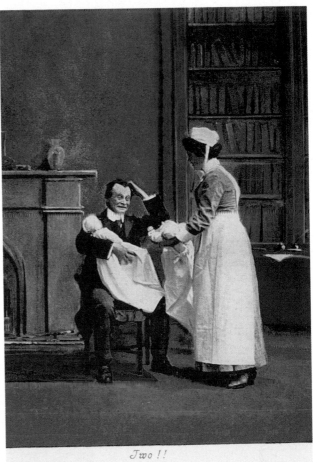

Two !!

Figure 2.111.
England. 1906.

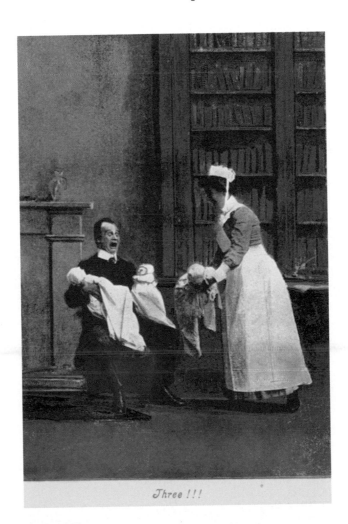

Three !!!

Figure 2.112.
England. 1906.

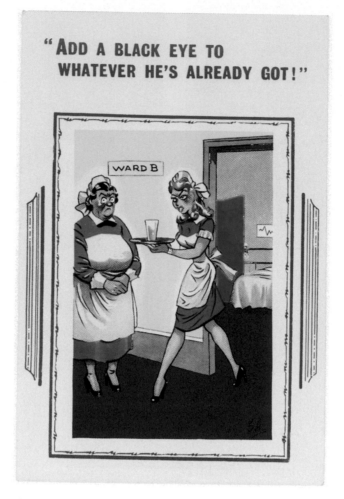

Figure 2.113.
England. c. 1950.

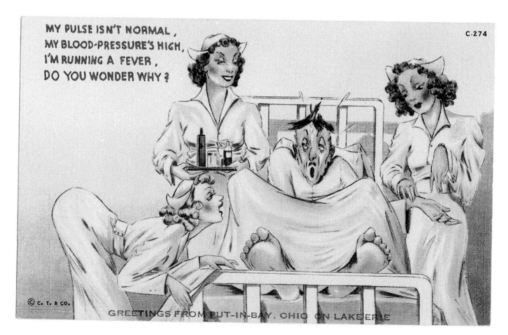

Figure 2.114.
United States. 1937. Linen.

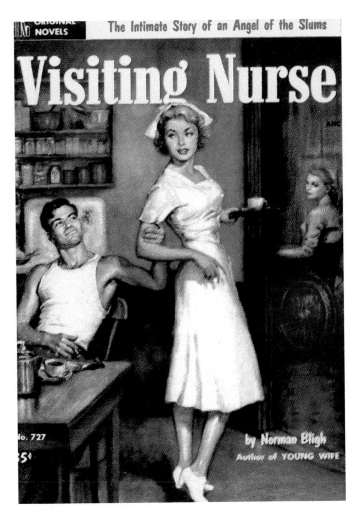

Figure 2.115. **"Visiting Nurse."**
© Philip-Dimitri Galas. United States. 1985. *(See note.)*

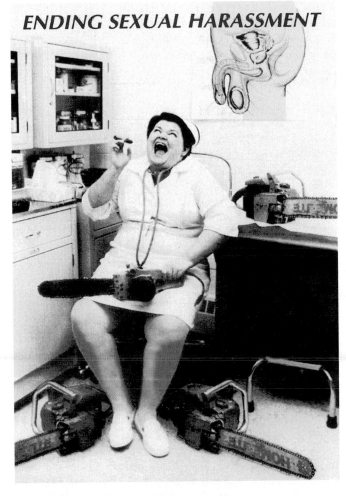

Figure 2.116. **"Ending Sexual Harassment."**
© American Postcard Company, New York. United States. 1990.

2.1. **Gene Pressler** (1894–1933) is best remembered for his artwork on 1920s calendars. He was at the height of his popularity when he was struck down by pneumonia and died at the age of 39, leaving behind a wife and son. His work on postcards is scarce. (See also Fig. 2.29.)

2.4. **Faradic treatment** for muscle rehabilitation. (See note 3.18.)

2.5 to 2.8. These images, all of which show a nurse supporting a patient by his arm, allow for a nice comparison of artistic treatments of the same theme.

2.7. **Paul Rieth** (1871–1925) was best known for his illustrations for *Jugend,* one of the most important early German Art Nouveau periodicals.

2.8. **Willy Planck** (1870–1956) was noted for his illustrations of children's and young adult adventure books, including the Robinson Crusoe series. He was friends with Karl May (1842–1912), one of the most popular and widely read German writers. May's works included stories about the American West, some of which were illustrated by Planck.

2.9. **Brynolf Wennerberg** (1866–1950) studied in Stockholm, Copenhagen, Paris, and Munich. His subjects were most often women, but during the war he also did military propaganda that was published in *Simplicissimus* (1896–1944), a German weekly art and political satire magazine.

2.10. **Marcello Dudovich** (1878–1962) was a renowned Art Deco poster artist and graphic designer. He apprenticed under Leopoldo Metlicovitz (1868–1944), an equally famous Italian artist-lithographer, known for his posters that introduced opera openings. Dudovich worked in Milan, Bologna, Genoa, and Turin. (See also Figs. 2.42 to 2.45.)

2.11. **Lapina Gallery** in Paris was the name used by **Ivan S. Lapin,** a Russian-born Parisian publisher. Lapin specialized in reproductions of salon paintings, like this one. Salon paintings were contemporary oils done in a traditional manner, as opposed to Art Nouveau and impressionism, both of which went against the grain of the Victorian academic art establishment. Since there was not much public enthusiasm for the older, traditional forms, popular artists turned away from them, and salon art was rarely reproduced on postcards. However, Lapin, roaming Paris with its hundreds of galleries, discovered wonderful works by French, Italian, and Russian salon art painters, and put the best of them on quality postcards. His eye and his craft were very good and his postcards became very popular.

Figure 2.14 is another example of a Lapina Gallery postcard.

2.15. Another example of a salon painting. (See also note 2.11.)

Kukryniksy is the collective pseudonym of three collaborating Soviet graphic artists: Mikhail Vasil'evich Kupriyanov (born in 1903), Porfirij Nikitich Krylov (born in 1902), and Nikolaj Aleksandrovich Sokolov (born in 1903). The name was compiled from portions of their first and last names. The Kukryniksy were members of the Academy of Artists of the USSR and People's Artists of the USSR. For over 25 years, the Kukryniksy collaborated in caricatures, posters, illustrations, and paintings, forming "an example of deep-principled collective labor based on original creative friendship" (Soviet Encyclopedia, 1952). Each of the Kukryniksy also worked individually.

Aleksandr Feodorovich Kerensky (1881–1970) was a lawyer and Russian revolutionary. He joined the Socialist Revolutionary party after the February Revolution of 1917 that overthrew the czarist government. He became minister of justice, then war minister in the provisional government of Prince Lvov. He succeeded Lvov as premier in July 1917. One of Kerensky's first acts as prime minister was the suppression of the Bolshevik party led by Lenin, who went into hiding in Finland. Other Bolshevik leaders, including Leon Trotsky, were arrested.

However, the Bolsheviks managed to overthrow Kerensky's government later in 1917, due to his insistence on remaining in World War I and his failure to deal with urgent economic problems. Kerensky fled to Paris, where he continued as an active propagandist against the Soviet regime. In 1940, he entered the United States where he lectured on political and social science. Kerensky died in New York City on June 11, 1970.

2.20 to 2.23. Figures 2.20 and 2.21 are from a series of six postcards printed by **A. Noyer,** a well-known Parisian postcard printing firm. Figures 2.22 and 2.23, however, are **hand-painted originals,** done with watercolor, pencil, and ink. Blank postcards were available for this purpose. The hand-painted postcards may have been among the ones Buhl submitted to Noyer for reproduction, or simply additional renditions that she sold or kept in her private collection. **Marthe Buhl** was one of the many unknown artists of the time.

2.24 to 2.27. From a series of six postcards showing uniforms of nursing services of the Commonwealth and the United States. Here Australia, South Africa, the United States, and Canada are represented, each with a map of the corresponding country in the background.

2.28. **William Henry Barribal** (1873–1956) was born in Worcestershire, England in 1873. He studied at Worcester Art School and later at the Julian Art School in Paris. One of his fellow students, Raphael Kirchner, became another artist familiar to Art Nouveau collectors (see also Figs. 2.32 and 2.33). Barribal's first design appeared in 1905. The model in this figure, as in over 200 of his 300 total designs, is **Barribal's wife,** Gertrude, better known as Babs (who was actually a brunette, not a redhead). Babs is also the model for the nurse in Figure 5.14; Barribal himself is the model for the patient, though his deformed right hand, a result of an injury when he was 6 years old, is not depicted.

Most of Barribal's works were elegant, fashionable female portraits, but he was proficient in other areas as well. He designed advertising posters, patriotic postcards, magazine illustrations, and a wide range of playing cards. Above all, Barribal was a commercial artist: he could not afford to be otherwise because he had a family to raise. Although he professed an ambition to be a significant figure in the art world, he chose to become an illustrator, which offered less fame but a more steady income (Edwards, 1999).

2.30. A play on the word **"sister."** The artist is suggesting that, with such a glamorous nurse, it might be difficult to keep one's thoughts strictly on the platonic level.

2.31. One example from a striking series of six **Art Deco glamour** postcards by **Giovanni Nanni** (1888–1969), another of Italy's well-known painter-illustrators. Verse on nursing postcards was usually doggerel, really not much different from greeting card verse today. This is one of the better examples, and it probably gained something in the translation.

> "Faces of Roses, souls of oaks
> Certainly from a white world you descend
> Today, to remind us again of the good
> That we all forget when we are in pain."

2.32 to 2.33. Born in Vienna, **Raphael Kirchner** (1876–1917) was one of the most popular and influential postcard artists of the 20th century. After attending the Vienna Academy of Art, he earned his living as a book illustrator and painter of portraits of women from Viennese high society. He settled in Paris at the turn of the century and stayed there until the beginning of World War I, when he moved to the United States.

Kirchner's most frequent model was his wife, **Nina;** she was often shown in various states of undress, but always saucy, charming, innocent, and lovable. Florenz Zeigfield, captivated by the charm of Kirchner's work, commissioned him to liven up the foyer of the Century Theater, and to produce playbills and other illustrations for Zeigfield's productions. When Kirchner died suddenly from complications of appendicitis in 1917, Zeigfield was desperate to find someone to replace him. Zeigfield turned to an unknown young artist named **Alberto Vargas** (1896–1982). Vargas deeply admired Kirchner, and his works were the natural continuation of Kirchner's: the poses, the techniques, even his signature was the same style. In 1940, Vargas went to work for *Esquire* magazine, replacing **George Petty** as Esquire's centerfold artist. Esquire shortened his name to Varga and so created the Varga Girl, considered to be the most well-known pinup girl of the 20th century. The Kirchner Girl, therefore, can be seen as the direct forerunner of the **American pinup** (Dell'Aquila, 1996).

Sadly, when Kirchner died, Nina, out of grief, turned to opium and died an addict within a few years. Kirchner's postcards number over 1000 designs; the only two that depict nurses are shown here.

2.36. A glamour rendition of a nurse and a patient sharing a traditional drink at the New Year's hour. Compare the glamour rendition to a more realistic, more sedate depiction of the same theme, also from Austria, issued in the same year.

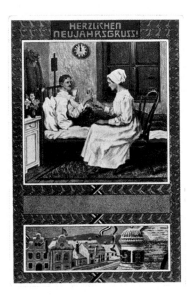

Austria. 1917.

2.37. **Luigi Bompard** (1879–1953), as well as being a painter, book illustrator, and commercial artist, was also a fashion designer. Here he has transformed the nurse's uniform into a trendy modern outfit, using all the nurse uniform elements, including apron, sash, collar and cuffs, rosary (Italian nurses were mostly Catholic sisters), and even the winged cornet.

2.41. From reverse: "By assisting those who have worked their entire lives when they no longer have anything more, we perform our Christian and social duty." (Women's Social Action Program Savings Pension Plan. Same series as Fig. 3.77.)

2.42 to **2.45.** From a series of 12 postcards titled "The Nurse's Mission," produced for the National Federation for the Work Against Tuberculosis. Compare Dudovich's Deco style in the 1930s to his work in Figure 2.10, done two decades earlier.

2.46. The **exchange of eggs** in the springtime is a custom that was centuries old when Easter was first celebrated by Christians. A great many pagan religious customs celebrating the return of spring became associated with **Easter,** probably due to Constantine, who arranged for Easter to be celebrated at the same time as the pagan ceremonies, to appeal to the Roman populace. Easter itself is named after Oester, a pagan goddess of the dawn, fertility, and spring, who also provides the etymological origin of "estrus" and "estrogen."

It is the Russian custom to give a red Easter egg to someone special, held in high esteem. It was not uncommon for a patient to give one to his nurse. Here, in a highly metaphoric gesture, the nurse shows the esteem in which royalty was held by the nursing profession. Whatever else the Russian aristocracy might have been accused of, there is no question of its regard for and contribution to nursing.

2.49. **A First Day Cover** (FDC) is an envelope or card bearing a stamp that is canceled on the day the stamp is issued. Often an artist will design a small picture, called a cachet, to be placed on the envelope to add interest (and value) to the item. Cachets come in three types: printed, hand painted, and hand drawn. The printed cachets are usually produced in large quantities, all identical. Hand-painted cachets are printed only in black and white, so the artist can color them by hand, adding a distinctive touch to each one. Finally, hand-drawn cachets are one-of-a-kind originals, drawn and colored individually on the cover.

Herman Maul (1897–1983) was an exceptional cachet artist who only produced one-of-a-kind originals. He gave most of them away, since making cachets was a source of pleasure for him. An architect, he once remarked that when he worked on a cachet it was a relief to be drawing something other than straight lines. The example shown in 2.49 was issued in New York as a tribute to America's hospitals, in connection with the 200th anniversary of New York Hospital.

2.51. **Candy Candy** appears in two forms, **manga** (comics) and **anime** (animation video). The overwhelming majority of anime are based on manga, and Candy Candy is no exception. Candy Candy was written by Ms. Kyoko Mizuki and drawn by Ms. Yumiko Igarashi between 1975 and 1979. The highly popular manga resulted in 115 anime episodes, which aired on television in Japan, the United States, and Great Britain.

Candy's courage and endurance, her warm and caring spirit, and her ever-cheerful smile endeared her to the hundreds of thousands of children and teenagers who followed her during

the height of her popularity. She was a role model to many of them, especially those who could identify with her tribulations. She may well have influenced some of her readers to aspire to nursing: Candy's dream was always to be a nurse, and nursing is presented as an expression of everything good in Candy's character. Today Candy Candy still has admirers who keep her in their hearts (and on their Web sites).

2.52 to **2.55.** **Trevor Brown** (1959–), a British artist most known for producing CD covers for *Whitehouse Recording*, took up residence in Japan in 1993. His art has been exhibited in galleries in Japan, the United States, and Italy. *Evil (Hear No, See No, Speak No)*, the first major book collection of his work, was released by NG Publications in 1996. His most recent book at the time of this writing is *Medical Fun*, published in 2001 by Editions Treville Co. Ltd. Another of Brown's postcards appears in Figure 3.87.

2.56. **Patient-nurse romance** is a fantasy that has caused the profession difficulty, not because the fantasy was completely false, but because it has been blown ridiculously out of proportion. During wartime, there certainly were romantic encounters between nurses and their male patients. The nurses and patients, often the same age, were in a foreign country during desperate times. It would have been natural for a young soldier, well enough to walk but still not fit to return to duty, to flirt with his nurse. For the most part, the nurses would turn the flirting aside, and the soldiers respected the nurses too much to press the issue. Matrons did their best to curtail anything other than strictly professional behavior, on or off hospital grounds. Sometimes, however, romance blossomed and affairs occurred. Unfortunately, postcards issued during the war gave the impression that romance was a natural, expected outcome of being wounded in war—a reward for service, if nothing more.

2.57. **Harrison Fisher** (1875–1934) was born in Brooklyn, New York. He moved to California in 1881 and attended the San Francisco Art Association and the Mark Hopkins Institute of Art. Fisher was a major influence on the illustration world, and his depiction of the American Girl made his name well known to all magazine readers after 1900. Fisher filled the gap when **Charles Dana Gibson,** creator of the Gibson Girl, retired in 1905. Fisher was one of the most prolific of all American illustrators.

Of the hundreds of postcard designs by Fisher, only two show nurses. The card shown in Figure 2.57, published by Reinthal and Newman of New York, is a comparatively common one. The rarest of the Fisher cards, however, is also a nurse, reproduced by a French publisher in 1920 from one of the better-known Fisher posters (see also Fig. 5.10).

2.65. This is the **earliest example of a nurse stereotype** on a postcard. This particular stereotype, the nurse-doctor romance, is not as common as the nurse-patient romance, but it can still be found today, popping up now and then in comic strips, daytime television soap operas, and prime-time series. Now, it is given far less credence than when it first appeared, but at the turn of the 20th century, doctor-nurse romance was seen as almost inevitable. In fact, right up until the HMO/managed care era, it was considered "a good catch" for a young woman to marry a medical student or doctor, and the pursuit of this "catch" has been the subject of many a film and romance novel.

2.66 to **2.69.**   Xavier Sager (1870–1930) was a French caricaturist. Some of this work is simply romantic (such as Fig. 2.66), but Sager is best known for his rather gross depiction of medical practice. These illustrations often showed surgeons as happy butchers, with blood everywhere, which never seemed to bother the patients because they were always smiling, conscious or not. There was almost always a bawdy element. The physician is often shown examining the female patient's anatomy with more than purely professional interest. The nurses are always willing participants in this scenario. Patients, doctors, and nurses might all be on the bed together, although the images stopped short of pornography.

Other than the dates of his birth and death, virtually nothing else is known about the biographical details of Sager's life, in spite of the fact that over 3000 designs and 3 million postcards are attributed to him (Neudin, 1991).

2.71.   **Samuel Schmucker** (1879–1921) was born in February 1879 in Reading, Pennsylvania and died unexpectedly of heart failure at the age of 42 on Long Island, New York. His one great passion was art, even though his right (dominant) arm had been crippled from polio in childhood. In 1896, he enrolled in drawing and still-life painting at the Pennsylvania Academy of the Fine Arts (PAFA) in Philadelphia. He studied at the Howard Pyle Institute at Drexel from 1899 to 1900. (Pyle's students included Maxfield Parrish, Jessie Willcox Smith, and N. C. Wyeth.) Schmucker fell deeply in love with **Katharine Rice,** another student at the PAFA. Katharine's image, with upswept hair, high cheekbones, and wide-set eyes, was the inspiration for most of his work. He worked for the **Detroit Publishing Company** in 1907 and the **John Winsch Company,** 1909–1915. Winsch published many of his postcards as greetings for all the major holidays: Valentine's Day, Thanksgiving, Christmas, Halloween, and so forth. Schmucker's works are unsigned, or signed only with the monogram "S.L.S." His stunning women and Art Nouveau designs make his work among the highest-priced of the American postcard artists, even though he never realized widespread recognition in his own lifetime (Davis & Davis, 2001).

2.73.   The publisher is **Raphael Tuck & Sons,** the best-known English postcard publisher. Tuck was the only postcard company to be issued a royal warrant (a testimony of service and distinction) from the Royal House of England. Tuck also had a New York branch, which issued this design. No information could be found on E. Curtis, the artist.

2.75.   **Paul Hey** (1867–1952), etcher, painter, and illustrator, was born in Munich and studied at the Academy there. He made study trips throughout much of Europe and created paintings of the places he visited, especially Italy. He also created large lithographic plates depicting fables and folklore. Hey is most known for working in **pointillism,** a form of impressionism in which tiny colored dots are placed close together to form secondary colors. The term pointillism was first used with respect to the work of Georges Seurat, the artist most closely associated with the movement. Although the postcard was issued circa 1910, the work is probably from the 1890s.

2.76.   This work, one of my personal favorites, is by an unknown artist from Hungary working in children's fairy-tale illustrator style.

2.77.   From a series of four postcards issued on June 5, 1907 by the **Japanese Red Cross** in honor of the 15th Grand Meeting of the Japanese Red Cross. The art is a blend of Art Nouveau and Japanese wood block design.

2.78 and **2.79.**   These are New Year cards issued by the **Slovakian Association of Firefighters and the Red Cross.** The two organizations were combined in Czechoslovakia, and firemen are often seen with nurses, and vice versa, on Czech postcards. Figure 2.78 shows two children; Figure 2.79 shows them as adults.

2.80 and **2.81.**   Another child and adult comparison. In this case, the child version was almost certainly based on a copy of Usabel's adult version, since **Usabel** was a noted artist and his work was widely distributed.

2.82.   **Eugenie Richards** (1873–1941) was raised in a family involved in the design and manufacture of lace, Nottingham's major industry at that time. She enrolled at the Nottingham school of Art and Design, where she became a remarkably talented and multifaceted artist, producing children's book illustrations, stained glass, alphabet design, life drawings, plates, wallpaper, illuminated pages, and more. She continued her studies there for 10 years, and then accepted a teaching position under the leadership of the principal, Joseph Harrison, one of the most powerful influences in design education in his day.

Richards is remembered as an awesome and domineering woman who spoke in resounding patrician tones, enunciating every word and radiating an intimidating air of grandeur (Cope, 2000). Nevertheless, there must have been a soft spot, for she is best known for her delightful illustrations of nursery rhymes (eg, "Simple Simon," "Dicky Bird, Dicky Bird," "Mary, Mary, Quite Contrary") reproduced in the Sissons and Parker *Humpty-Dumpty Nursery Rhymes Readers* series and on postcards.

2.83.   Not much is known about **Katherine Gassaway** except that she did children's illustrations for a number of prominent postcard firms from 1906 to 1909. Compare Figure 2.83 to the following, postmarked 1909, and decide which came first, the comic photo or the Gassaway drawing.

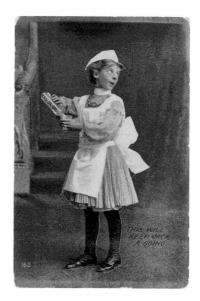

United States. 1909.

2.84.   **Grace Wiederseim's** life was not a happy one. The following is reprinted, with kind permission of Susan Brown Nicholson, from her *Encyclopedia of Antique Postcards* (Nicholson, 1994).

Viola Grace Gebbie was born in Darby, PA in 1877. Her father was a successful art book publisher. She had two sisters, Janet, who died at the age of 20, and Margaret who became an artist as well.

Grace drew from an early age. The darling children she created were actually perfected from early childhood self-portraits. Grace reported, "I kept on making round roly-polys, consulting the mirror from time to time. Eventually I had created a type that was as much a part of me as myself . . . When I thought of a career I found I had one in keeping alive these youngsters I had created in and from my own childhood."

When Grace was a teenager her father died, causing the family financial distress as well as the loss of a loved one. At seventeen,

Grace accepted professional art assignments to keep the family going. By eighteen, she had a cover assignment from *Truth* magazine, but for a long time after that no magazine purchased her work.

Grace married her first husband, Theodore Wiederseim, in 1900 when she was twenty-two. Her artistic break came when Seymour Eaton started *The Booklover's Magazine*. Although she received no pay, her work was in the public eye. After her first illustration appeared in 1903, the New York American Magazine offered her a two-year contract. In 1904 she began her twenty-year relationship with Campbell's Soup Company.

She divorced her first husband in 1911 and later that year married W. Heyward Drayton, III. Drayton was very wealthy and socially prominent. They had a winter home in Florida and traveled a great deal. The marriage ended in divorce in 1923 and Grace never remarried.

Grace's work was signed Grace Gebbie, G. G. Wiederseim and Grace Drayton. Her work was prolific not only on postcards, but in books written and illustrated with her sister Margaret. She designed embroidery pieces and dolls. One of her most successful endeavors was her series of Dolly Dingle paper dolls, published in magazines.

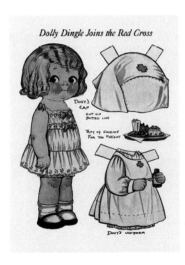

"Dolly Dingle Joins the Red Cross."

By December 1933, Grace was poverty stricken after losing her job with King Features. She wrote to Bernard Wagner, her background artist, "I have no work and am almost down and out. I have tried everything . . . I feel so bad whenever I look at our empty studio. To add to my agony, I lost my only dearly beloved sister a few weeks ago. So I am now all alone and poverty stricken in heart as well as pocket. . . . Nevertheless I try to keep my pug nose in the air . . ." She died two years later in 1936, at age 58, of a heart attack. She was buried in Philadelphia in an unknown location.

2.85. From a series of 12 postcards titled "War Nurses," published in the United States, all featuring the little girl nurse shown here.

2.89. The postcard was issued in 1963. At the time of its appearance, only eleven men and one woman had been in space, but the world's imagination had been captured. Boys wanted to grow up to be cosmonauts and astronauts and, as the postcard reflects, little girls wanted to be their nurses.

2.90. **Randolph Caldecott** (1846–1885) transformed the world of children's books in the Victorian era. He was born in Chester, England, and taught himself drawing as a child. In 1878 Caldecott began an association with Edmund Evans, a publisher. The agreement was that the artist would produce two books annually, to sell for one shilling. By 1884, sales of Caldecott's Nursery Rhymes had reached 867,000 copies and he was internationally famous. He became known as "Lord of the Nursery" (Randolph Caldecott Society, 2000).

Caldecott illustrated novels and accounts of foreign travel, made humorous drawings depicting hunting and fashionable life, and drew cartoons and sketches of the famous inside Parliament and out of it. He also exhibited sculptures and paintings in oil and watercolor in the Royal Academy and in numerous galleries. However, Caldecott's health was generally very poor, and he suffered from gastritis and a heart condition going back to childhood. His health, among other things, prompted his many winter trips to warm climates. It was on such a tour in the United States that he died. He and his wife Marian had sailed to New York and traveled down the East Coast. They reached Florida during an unusually cold February, and Caldecott was taken ill. He died at St. Augustine on February 12, 1885, only 39 years old.

In 1937, René Paul Chambellan designed the **Caldecott Medal.** It is awarded annually by the Association for Library Service to Children, a division of the American Library Association, to the artist of the most distinguished American picture book for children.

The postcard was printed circa 1910, reproduced from a Caldecott drawing from one of his Christmas shilling books, *Sing a Song for Sixpence,* which was published in 1880. When Caldecott produced this book, the nursery rhyme on which it was based seemed to be just a children's song. But only 60 years previously, when the rhyme first appeared, it was full of political significance, based on the **"Cato Street Conspiracy"** of 1820 in which 24 men, at dinner one night, plotted to murder the entire Cabinet. When they were discovered, many of them began to tell about the others in the hope of saving their own lives—hence "the birds began to sing" (Randolph Caldecott Society, 2000).

2.91. This postcard is drawn in a style known as and associated with a decorative trend called **Japonism.** Two little girls are playing a game, in which one is a nursemaid. The hairstyle and the decor reflect the influence that the Japanese had on European fashion. Art Nouveau, already in vogue, had borrowed heavily from the Japanese wood block print, but the Art Nouveau forms themselves were distinctly western. However, on March 14, 1885, in the presence of the Duke and Duchess of Edinburgh, "The Mikado" was presented for the first time. One of Gilbert and Sullivan's most popular operas, in its initial run, it played for a record 672 performances over the course of 2 years. From that point, Japanese fashion started to insert itself into European society.

Japonism reached its peak with the **Japan-British Exhibition** held in London in 1910. (See also Fig. 4.125.) The Exhibition in London in 1910 was a great celebration of more than 50 years of close collaboration between Japan and Britain. The exhibition attracted a staggering 8 million visitors and ran for approximately 5 months. This was the first time Japan had taken part in such a major international event. It soon became quite fashionable for the wealthier European families to decorate entire sections of the residence in Japanese style, an affectation that lasted until World War I.

2.94 to 2.95. Prior to World War I, **Louise Ibels** painted children, animals and fantasy subjects. During the war she painted lighthearted caricatures, and was active in book illustration as late as the 1930s.

2.98 to 2.99. William Henry Ellam (1858–1935) was known as a man of astute wit and elegant style. He earned a great deal of money from his prolific output of artwork. He appeared to spend it as soon as he earned it; he readily indulged his taste for fine clothes and high living, dressing with studied elegance in fashionable suits, hats, and spats and carrying a hallmark silver-topped cane (Cope, 2000). He loved to be in the presence of children and many of his postcards are designed to please them.

2.100. From the **"Guinnipen the Penguin"** series, showing her in different roles.

2.101 to 2.103. At the turn of the 20th century, **Louis Wain** (1860–1939) was perhaps the most visible artist in England. His irrepressible cats and their kittens could be seen on a thousand bedroom walls, in a thousand schools. His cats reflected every aspect of Edwardian style, from the classroom to the health spa, sports, walking about town, commerce on a busy street, courtrooms, symphonies, and so on. Most of his work was wonderfully humorous. The Louis Wain Annual was a perennial bestseller; his designs adorned countless postcards and filled the pages of newspapers, books, and periodicals. The Wain cat was everywhere, prompting H. G. Wells to remark "English cats that do not look like Louis Wain cats are ashamed of themselves" (Cox, 2001).

Louis Wain was born on August 5, 1860, the only boy in a family of six children. He was a sickly child and kept from mixing with others on medical advice. An attack of scarlet fever at the age of 9 left Wain oddly healthier. Now an unruly, strong-headed child, Wain rarely attended school, preferring to wander the streets of London where he sought out factories and stood transfixed by the workings of their vast, intricate machineries. In his own words, he was "strong and pugnacious and difficult to control." He roamed the countryside, climbing trees and collecting trophies (Wainsworld, 2002).

Wain's father died in 1880, and the family managed to survive on savings until Wain, then attending classes at the West London School of Art, was able to graduate and begin teaching there. He was not a successful teacher: he was shy and disliked his job, preferring "to search for knowledge rather than impart it" (Nicholson, 1994).

Following his marriage to Emily Marie Richardson, the governess employed to look after Wain's youngest sister, Wain became estranged from his family, which had not approved the match. Nevertheless, in January 1884, Wain, age 23, married Emily, who was 10 years his senior. They obtained a black and white kitten named Peter, and shortly thereafter Louis started to visit the then-popular Cat Shows. It was Emily who urged Wain, who at this point was drawing all sorts of animals *but* cats, to use Peter as a model.

The first Cat Show was held at the Crystal Palace London on July 16, 1871. Mr. Harrison Weir had conceived the idea while pondering the large numbers of cats living in London. The day was a resounding success, with over 300 cats entered, and the Show has been held ever since. In 1887, Weir founded the **National Cat Club,** with Louis Wain one of the founding members. Weir remained its president until 1890, when Wain replaced him, and continued as president until 1907. Wain designed the logo for the club, still in use today.

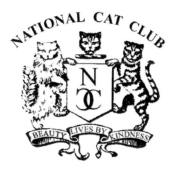

"National Cat Club."

In 1881, the *Illustrated Sporting and Dramatic News* published Wain's first signed illustration of bullfinches, mistitled "Robin's Breakfast." In 1886, the editor of the *Illustrated London News,* persuaded by Wain's wife, featured Wain's now famous **"Kittens Christmas Party,"** in the *News'* Christmas Edition, and that marked the start of his immense popularity. In the 1887 Christmas Edition, Wain produced over 20 pictures of various cats up to mischief. Sadly, in the same year, his wife Emily, already bedridden with breast cancer, died. After only 3 years of marriage, Wain was a widower at age 26. He had lost the source of his inspiration and the one person who, above everyone else, nourished his abilities.

Wain carried on. Gradually, his uncanny knack of giving cats human expression and characteristics made him extremely popular. He also became a crusader for cats. His own words describe how cats were regarded before his pictures caught the public's imagination: "When I was young, no man would have dared acknowledge himself a cat enthusiast. . . . the man who would take an interest in the cat movement was looked upon as effeminate—now even MPs [Members of Parliament] can do so without fear of being laughed at" (Cope, 2000).

By 1890, Wain was famous and much loved, but not at all wealthy. He was still living financially close to the edge, given the number of people depending on him. His shyness and aversion to business resulted in a failure to copyright his drawings; as a result, anyone could reprint them from pre-existing sketches without ever paying him. Wain was also a soft touch for any request concerning donations to cat organizations, giving thousands of pounds to their causes. His mother and sisters were managing his affairs, and they apparently did not consult any financial or legal experts.

In 1900, Wain's youngest sister Marie, suffering from horrifying delusions, including the "knowledge" that she had leprosy and her teeth were falling out, was committed to a lunatic asylum. In 1907, Wain traveled to the United States where he remained for 2 years, traveling to cat shows and doing drawings for Hearst's *New York American.*

In 1910, while he was still abroad, Wain's mother died, and Wain returned to England. In 1913, Marie died, still confined to the asylum, and this had another profound effect on Wain. In 1914, he suffered a concussion after being thrown from a horse-drawn bus, which once again disturbed his mental equilibrium, necessitating several months' rest.

The subsequent war years (1914–1917) saw a reduced popularity for Wain's works as the public preference shifted from cat drawings to illustrations of the war. In 1917, Carolyn, another sister, died, and it seems that from this point on he began acting out in a manner that attracted attention to his mental instability. Having always been an eccentric and private character, the gravity of his illness seems to have gone unnoticed for a time. Now he began to assert that his family had been plotting against him, stealing from him, and attempting to undermine his well-being. (His sisters had, in fact, been selling pieces from his private collection without his permission, to help ease their financial burden.) Wain grew to believe that spirits were directing malign energies at him. He ruminated on the idea that he was filled with electricity, and that the ether was a source of evil and was present in his food. He became alternately withdrawn and manic. Finally, he became so agitated he had to be confined. He was certified insane with dementia praecox (schizophrenia) on June 16, 1924, at age 64, and committed to the pauper ward of a South London asylum.

Following a month of withdrawal, he again began to draw and paint cats by the hundreds, giving them to fellow inmates and warders as presents. He had been interned just over a year when, by chance, the bookseller and ward visitor Dan Rider noticed a number of sketches and remarked to him, "Good Lord, man, you draw like Louis Wain." "I am Louis Wain." "You're not, you know." "But I am," said the artist. And he was (Serial-design.com, 2001).

After notification by Rider, an appeal was launched by Mrs. Cecil Chesterton in the September, 1925, issue of the magazine *Animals,* which produced an immediate response from the public. When **H. G. Wells and King George V** (both avid Wain collectors) heard of his bankrupt circumstances, they organized a national collection to pay for Wain's hospital treatment and the supply of drawing materials during the remainder of his life.

The last 15 years of his life were spent in asylums where Wain was given private quarters. While there, Wain executed, along with hundreds of his more "normal" style drawings, a series of dazzlingly colored and patterned "psychotic" cat drawings. Wain died on July 7, 1939; he was buried alongside his family in St. Mary's Roman Catholic Cemetery, Kensal Green, London (Serial-design.com, 2001).

Louis Wain remains the most renowned cat artist of the Western world. His works are still highly collectible. Figures 2.101 to 2.103 depict experiences at a traditional European luxury health spa. Figure 2.102 shows the head nurse directing the placement of glasses in each guest room before the guests arrive. Water therapies of all sorts were central to the spa experience, including steam bath therapy (Fig. 2.101) and **Schneebath** therapy (Fig. 2.103; see also Fig. 7.24). Both therapies could be unexpectedly painful, and one can easily imagine a well-bred English gentleman reacting exactly the same way as the cat on the postcard.

2.105. **Jane Wiley,** born in 1952, studied art at Carnegie-Mellon University and the Massachusetts College of Arts in Boston. Her studio is in Boston. She has shown her work at the Cornwall Gallery, Noonan Gallery, Footlight Club, and the Federal Reserve Bank of Boston Gallery. She works in a variety of media including painting, printmaking, black and white photography, and sculpture; her sculptures may be constructed of anything and everything. This postcard, for example, is a hand-tinted photograph of sculpture made from plastic clay, paper, fabric, a medicine dropper, and a spice box lid.

2.106. This postcard appeared in *The Ren and Stimpy Show: Postcards Over the Edge,* a Putnam-Penguin book consisting of 32 perforated postcards featuring scenes from actual episodes of the popular Nickelodeon animation series, chronicling the zany adventures of Ren, the maladjusted Chihuahua, and Stimpy, the gullible feline. Caution: do not attempt the technique shown unless you have completed the in-service on **full-body sphygmomanometry** and have it approved on your competencies list.

2.107 to **2.108.** By 1910, postcards were so popular and the field so competitive that in order to increase sales, some companies used gimmicks to make the cards more novel. Real human hair was added to portraits of women; actual buttons were sewn on for eyes. Postcards were printed on leather, wood, and metal. Some had die-cut openings through which light would shine when the cards were held up to a light bulb, and some had moving parts. The cards with moving parts were called **mechanicals,** and included pop-up postcards, sliding-part postcards, postcards with rotatable paper wheels, and simple hinged postcards like this one. In this card, with the hinge down, one sees the nurse carrying something that smells awful. When the hinge is lifted, we see it is an old egg! Were you expecting something else?

2.115. This card is the reproduction of an actual pulp novel cover of the 1930s.

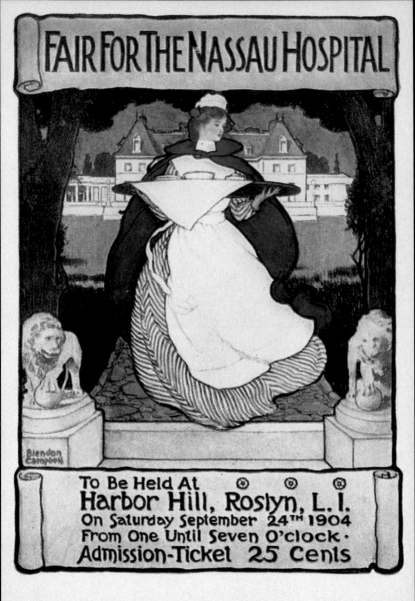

Figure 3.1. **Blendon Campbell (1872–1969). "Fair for the Nassau Hospital."**
Nassau, New York. 1904. Private mailing card. *(See note.)*

As Advertised

CHAPTER 3

The Nurse on the Advertising Postcard

*O*ur culture is a melange of spiritual values, ethics, commerce, and style. The ethics and spiritual values, though mutable, remain relatively stable; however, all of commerce ebbs and flows with innovation and changing preferences. Since advertising postcards remained popular even when other types of postcards were in decline, they provide an excellent and thorough documentation of commerce and style for the entire span of the 20th century. By regarding the nurse on advertising postcards, we can see how she was used to promote, how she was presented to and thus perceived by the public at any given time, and how advertising itself developed over the course of the century.

Americans are exposed so frequently to advertising that we cannot process most of it. We tune much of it out, but it affects us nonetheless. To some extent, it determines not only what we think, but also the rhythm of the way we think it, since advertising ubiquitously manipulates the frequency and duration of the information we receive. Advertising ranges from unsophisticated flyers hand-lettered by school children to multibillion dollar, multimedia corporate and political campaigns. Nevertheless, all advertising, regardless of the level of sophistication, is an attempt at behavior modification.

Professional advertising is based on principles that have been in development for over a hundred years. Advertising agencies, account executives, market research firms, professional copywriters, and so forth were well established by the turn of the 20th century. A world-class advertising agency today can employ psychologists, sociologists, statistics and trends analysts, campaign specialists, linguists, ex-military propagandists and intelligence officers, market researchers, and other behavioral scientists, whose common goal is to cause a defined population (the target) to respond in a manner benefiting the advertiser (the client). Advertising makes an interesting study, if only to confer a little immunity from the ads themselves. Also, there is beauty in ads, both in the images themselves, and in the elegance of the applied psychology.

The mirror that advertising holds up is distorted; the situation and people appear real, but they are not. For one thing, there is a noticeable lack of flaws, unless a "before" picture is being offered to show the necessity for the product. People are impeccably dressed; blemishes are absent; and there is never litter on the street. There is nothing unpleasant that might turn a person away. The resemblance to humans is close enough so that viewers can identify with the characters, but they will never be able to achieve the promised perfection. This unattainability is one of the reasons advertising can be considered harmful. To cite just one widespread deleterious effect, women are caused needless pain and anguish trying to fit the advertised criteria for attractiveness. They do so because satisfaction (love, romance, security, fulfillment) is tied to an ideal that is made to appear attainable but is spurious to begin with.

It must be said that the majority of picture postcard advertisers did not spend a lot of money on market research. Some used a graphics designer who had some experience with ads. Some simply paired a product with a popular image. Some used images that had proved to sell in the past. Others just went with their instinct. Still, even the most unsophisticated advertising has to fulfill a few basic conditions to be effective.

Two obvious requirements for any graphics ad are that it be seen, and that the viewers recognize what is being promoted. However, just because the image is in full view and the viewer's eyes are pointing at it does not mean it will be observed; as noted, there are too many advertisements for an individual to process them all. Something in the image, not necessarily the product itself, must capture the viewer's attention, or the image will be relegated to visual background noise. Thus, the product will be unnoticed.

Today, we know that an advertisement works best if it provokes an emotional response, and that it does not matter whether the response is positive or negative. The stronger the emotional response, the more the content of the ad is likely to be retained. At the turn of the 20th century, the same principle applied, but, with the exception of certain types of propaganda, only a positive response was intended.

The nurse appears in advertising throughout the 20th century and into the 21st century. Why is this so? When the advertising is being aimed at nurses themselves, of course, or to sell a medicine, the answer is obvious. However, why use a nurse to advertise a fan, or a beer, or a stove? The answer is found in the principle of associative conditioning: if the image actually registers, in the moment of pause, the viewer forms an association between whatever caught his eye and whatever else is in the image. If a nurse captures the viewer's attention, the product in the ad will become associated with nurses. There were (and are) good reasons to associate a product with nurses. A 1915 textbook, *Advertising: Its Principles and Practice* (Tipper, 1915) states, "In our own day, experiments have shown in quite definite ways the relative strengths of various appeals which can be used as selling points in advertising copy. Of special interest is the following [list] of persuasiveness, which shows the relative strength of various sorts of selling points for the educated classes of our present day, when the results for men and women are combined."

Appeal (The top 10, listed from the most persuasive to the least.)
Healthfulness
Cleanliness
Scientific Construction
Time Saved
Appetizing
Efficiency
Safety
Durability
Quality
Modernity

The nurse is associated with more than half of the top 10 persuaders, including the two most likely to sell: healthfulness and cleanliness.

The nurse fulfills all the criteria for a good ad image. Her costume and her insignia are striking, making her instantly recognizable. In fact, the red cross was deliberately selected for the purpose of immediate recognition. A nurse evokes a double emotional response, one negative and the other positive. The entire recalled experience (eg, sickness, hospitalization) is negative, but the nurse's presence in that experience is associated with comfort, relief, and healing.

If the nurse in an ad is associated with the product, the reverse is also true: whatever appears with the nurse influences the public awareness of the nurse. For example, if a nurse is shown serving a beer, then serving beer is perceived as what a nurse does. If a nurse is shown selling war bonds, nurses are perceived as patriotic, possibly even militaristic.

Images on advertising postcards (and postcards in general) are either artist-drawn or photographed. Whereas photographic advertising postcards were dominant in the United States, the artist-drawn varieties were dominant in Europe. The Europeans did not have the same easy access to photo processing enjoyed by American advertisers. Also, since the most popular art styles of the time originated in Europe, Europeans were not only familiar with artist-drawn advertising, there was already a demand for it. European advertising postcards are in effect miniature posters, designed as much for the poster aficionado and art connoisseur as for the consumer.

Postcard advertising went into decline after World War I. It reappeared in the late 1930s with the introduction of high-speed presses and cheap paper. The rag-content threads in the paper formed a grid pattern on the surface of the cards, giving them a linen-like appearance, and the postcards became popularly known as *linens*. Linens were inexpensive and became extremely popular with owners of motels, diners, restaurants, and roadside attractions. They could be found in virtually any place a tourist or traveler might stop on a trip across the country. They were also popular with manufacturers of consumer items, especially automobiles, household items, and clothing. The nurse was not well represented on the linen postcard, being confined mostly to the endorsement of shoes and uniforms and the occasional hospital that sold postcards in its gift shop.

Linen advertising postcards remained popular until World War II. By 1940, however, good quality color graphics could be incorporated into magazines, newspapers, and other print media, and postcard advertising dollars were more effectively spent elsewhere. The onset of World War II, with its conservation of materials and its other priorities, brought postcard production in general almost to a stop, the exception being comic and advertising linens, which persevered.

The next postcard resurgence came in the 1950s, with the availability of inexpensive color photography. Although the process of color film photography had been introduced to the mass market in the mid-1930s, it was not until the 1946, with the introduction of Kodak's Ektachrome film, that color photography became commercially feasible. *Color chromes,* as they were called, rapidly replaced postwar linens and black-and-white printed postcards. Companies producing other types of postcards either changed to chromes or went out of business.

From the 1950s through the 1990s, most color postcards were produced from slides or color prints using offset presses. The 1990s saw the introduction of another printing process, the digital press, which printed images directly from computer files. At the same time, a specialized form of advertising postcard appeared: the rack card or freecard. So named because they are set out in racks and available for free, they are placed in restaurants, drugstores, bookstores, theaters, and a wide variety of retail chain stores. Rack cards advertise anything that might interest their target market: consumers with high discretionary income, 18 to 35 years old. They are, in part, responsible for the current resurgence of interest in postcard collecting.

Nurses on contemporary postcards are scarce. Although still recognizable, the nurse has lost some of her visual uniqueness and impact along with her starched white uniform, cap, cape, and red cross. She is rarely used in advertisements apart from those promoting aspects of healthcare. On the other hand, the nurse has remained strong as an associative endorser. In an early 2002 Gallup News Service poll ranking the honesty and ethics of professionals, nurses were listed second. (Firefighters were listed first, in part because of their role in the September 11 attacks.) It was concluded that Americans trust nurses more than doctors, pharmacists, engineers, dentists, and clergy (McCafferty, 2002).

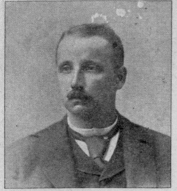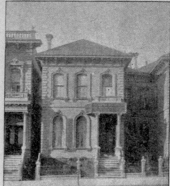

PLEASE KEEP THIS CARD: You or your friends are at any time liable to be taken sick and need an experienced nurse.

The object of this Agency has been to obtain reputable and competent nurses of the intelligent standard requisite for family practice. segregating the good from the indifferent in a just and impartial manner, grading the former, and pushing the most apt, according to their ability and training and satisfaction given to patrons. For the results, the proprietor, who himself has had nearly 9 yrs. private experience, respectfully refers you to any leading physician or surgeon of your acquaintance in this city; suffice to say that he now furnishes employment to over two hundred picked people, whereas in the beginning, less than four years ago, he had not sufficient for twelve. Any further information concerning it will be cheerfully given at the Main Office, where all letters or complaints should also be addressed.

F. E. GOODBAN. Proprietor.

The Main Office, Van Ness near Post, S. F.

"Alpha" Male & Female Nurses', Dressers' and Masseurs' Agency,

(Established July, 1889. Registered at Sacramento, February, 1892.)

Main Office. 1117 Van Ness Ave., near Post, S. F., Cal.   Long Distance Telephone 2579.

Branches: 33 Grant Ave. (open all night) 434 Sutter, 340 Geary, 1113 & 2000 Market Sts. **San Francisco;** cor. Seventh & Market and 1201 Broadway Sts., **Oakland;** B & Second Ave., **San Mateo;** Fourth & K Sts., **Sacramento;** 248 Main St., **Stockton;** E. Santa Clara & Second Sts., **San Jose;** 40 Pacific Ave., **Santa Cruz;** Fourth & C Sts., **San Rafael;** Park St. & Santa Clara Ave., **Alameda;** and Center & Shattuck Sts., **Berkeley.**

Experienced and reliable MALE or FEMALE Professional Nurses (with or without diplomas), Dressers or Masseurs furnished for every kind of disease, at ANY HOUR of the DAY or NIGHT, to all parts of the city or country.   NO FEE CHARGED FOR FURNISHING THEM. OVER TWO HUNDRED PICKED NURSES of all ages, religions, nationalities and training (from the best hospitals in America and Europe) on its list.

N. B.—No attention should be paid to nurses who state that they are members of this Agency, unless endorsed at the Main Office, as many represent themselves as such, whose applications have not been received, or whose names through some fault on their part have been removed from its list.   INVALID GOODS FOR SALE.

Figure 3.2.   "Alpha" Male and Female Nurses.
San Francisco, California. 1893. *(See note.)*

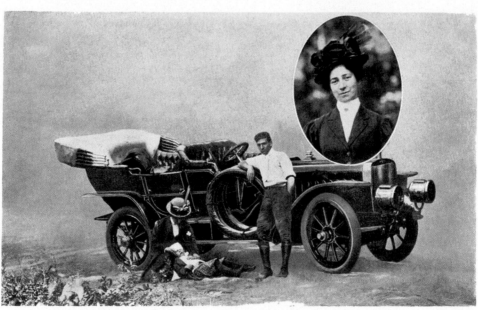

SOUVENIR, BRISTOL VISITING NURSE ASSOCIATION.

Figure 3.3.   Bristol Visiting Nurse Association.
Bristol, Connecticut. 1909. *(See note.)*

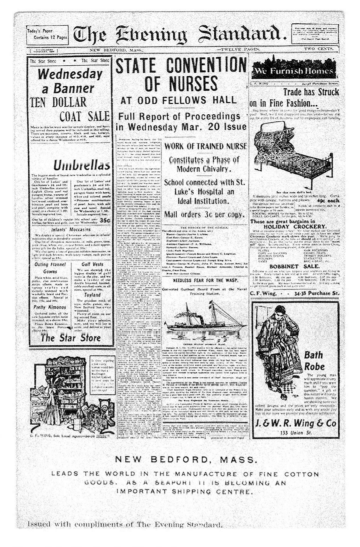

Figure 3.4. **The Evening Standard.**
New Bedford, Massachusetts. c. 1904. *(See note.)*

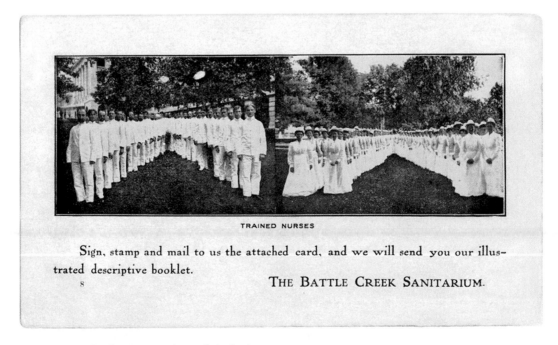

Figure 3.5. **Trained Nurses, Battle Creek Sanitarium.**
Battle Creek, Michigan. *(See note.)*

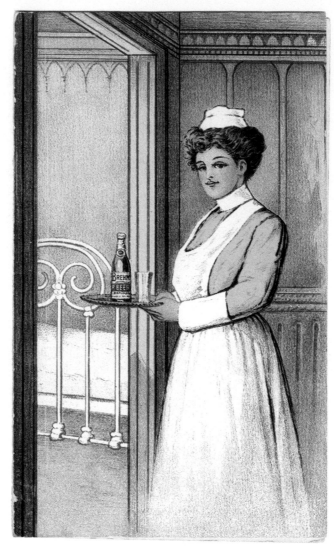

Figure 3.6. **Brehm Beer. George Brehm and Son.**
Baltimore, Maryland. c. 1905.

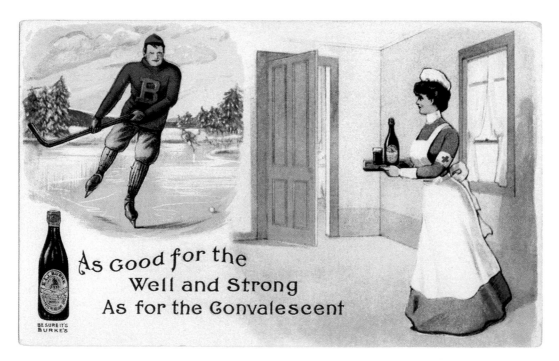

Figure 3.7. **E & J Burke Guinness Foreign Stout.**
1908. *(See note.)*

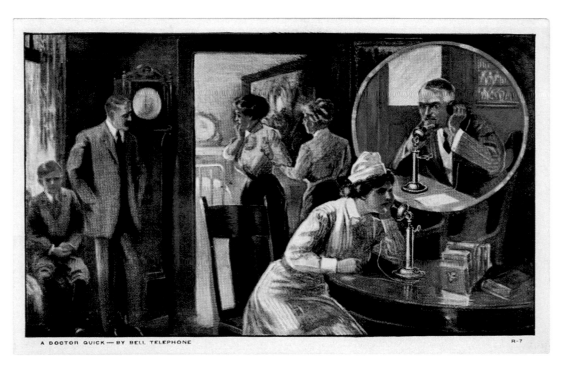

Figure 3.8. **"A Doctor Quick!"**
Bell Telephone. c. 1905. *(See note.)*

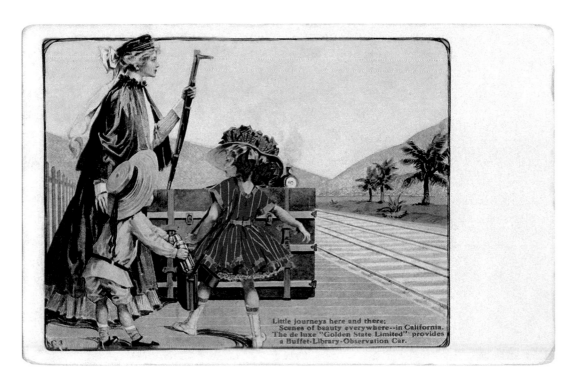

Figure 3.9. **Rose O'Neill (1874–1944).**
Advertising for the Rock Island Railroad. 1909. *(See note.)*

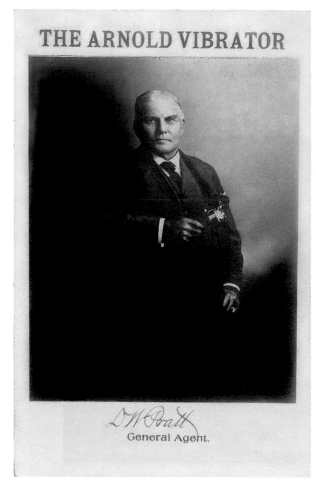

Figure 3.14. **The Arnold Vibrator. D. H. Pratt, General Agent.**
c. 1910. Real photo. *(See note.)*

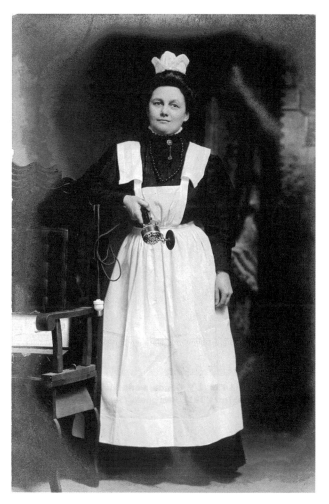

Figure 3.15. **The Arnold Vibrator.**
Galesburg, Illinois. c. 1910. Real photo. *(See note.)*

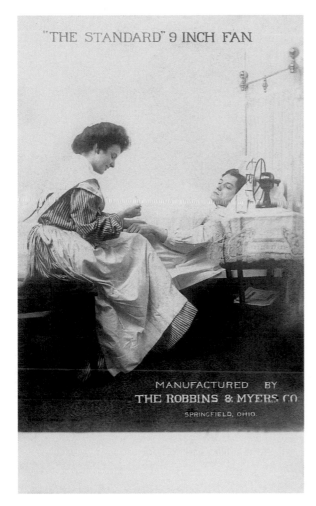

Figure 3.16. **"The Standard" 9-inch fan.**
Robins & Myers Co., Springfield, Ohio. 1908. Real photo.

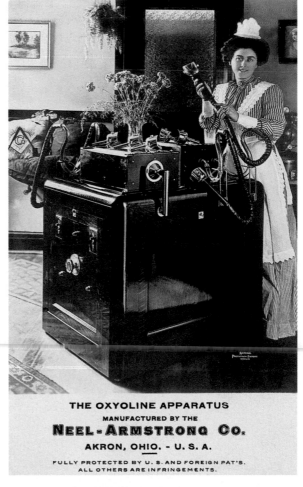

Figure 3.17. **"Oxyoline Apparatus."**
Neel-Armstrong Co. Akron, Ohio. Real photo. c. 1908. *(See note.)*

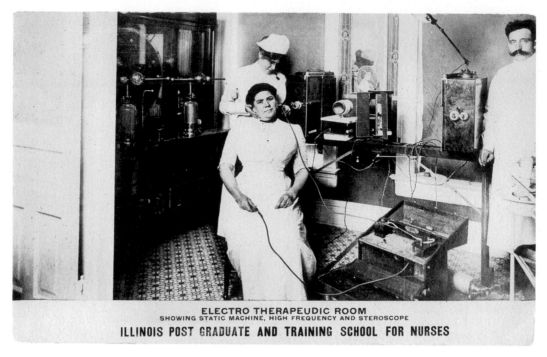

ELECTRO THERAPEUDIC ROOM
SHOWING STATIC MACHINE, HIGH FREQUENCY AND STEROSCOPE
ILLINOIS POST GRADUATE AND TRAINING SCHOOL FOR NURSES

Figure 3.18. **Electro Therapeutic Room. Illinois Post Graduate and Training School for Nurses.**
Chicago. 1914. Real photo. Courtesy of Jane Pepper. *(See note.)*

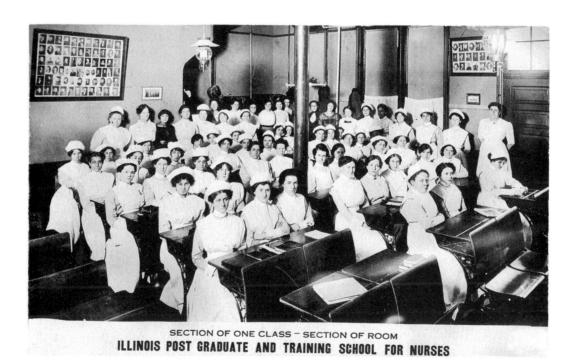

SECTION OF ONE CLASS – SECTION OF ROOM
ILLINOIS POST GRADUATE AND TRAINING SCHOOL FOR NURSES

Figure 3.19. **Classroom. Illinois Post Graduate and Training School for Nurses.**
Chicago. Real photo. 1914. *(See note.)*

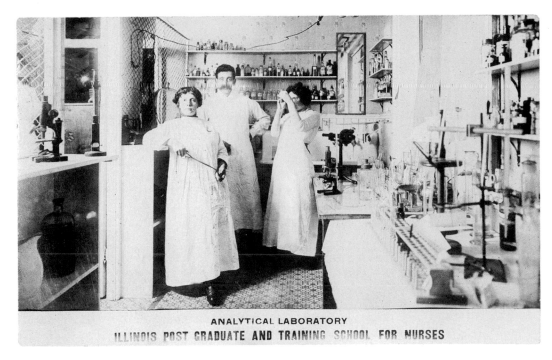

ANALYTICAL LABORATORY
ILLINOIS POST GRADUATE AND TRAINING SCHOOL FOR NURSES

Figure 3.20. Analytical Laboratory. Illinois Post Graduate and Training School for Nurses.
Chicago. 1914. Real photo. Courtesy of Jane Pepper. *(See note.)*

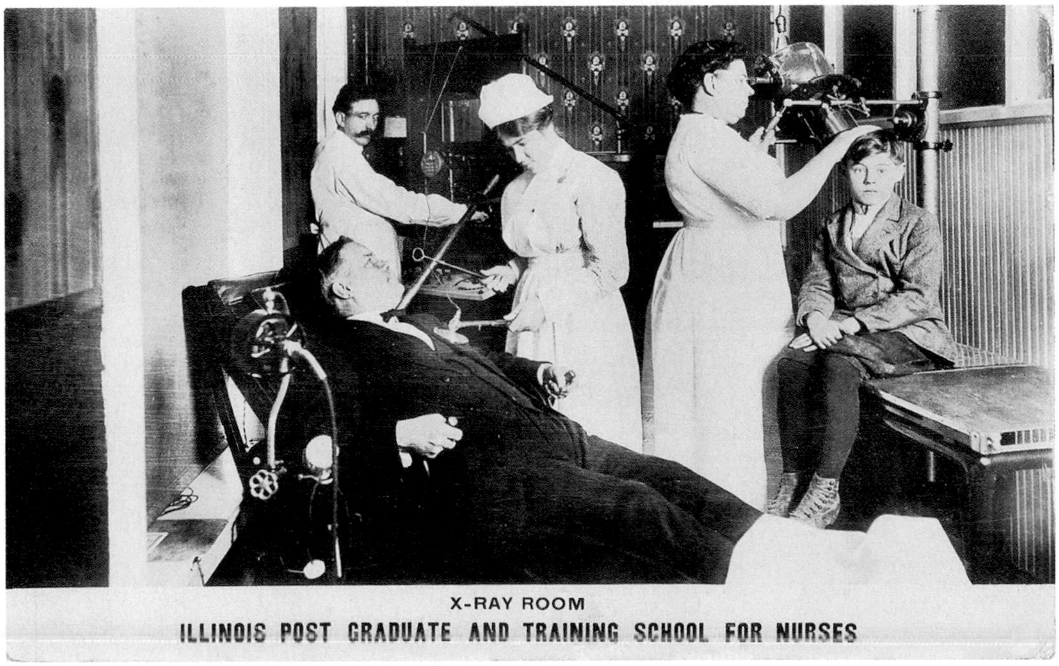

X-RAY ROOM
ILLINOIS POST GRADUATE AND TRAINING SCHOOL FOR NURSES

Figure 3.21. X-Ray Room. Illinois Post Graduate and Training School for Nurses.
Chicago. 1914. Real photo. Note the lack of shielding. *(See note.)*

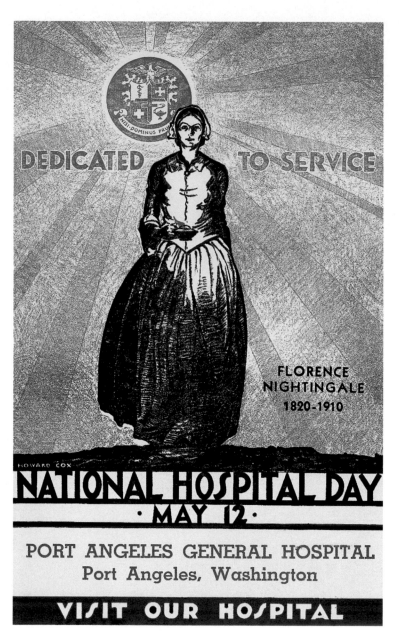

Figure 3.22.   **Howard Cox. "Dedicated to Service."**
Port Angeles General Hospital, Washington. 1937. *(See note.)*

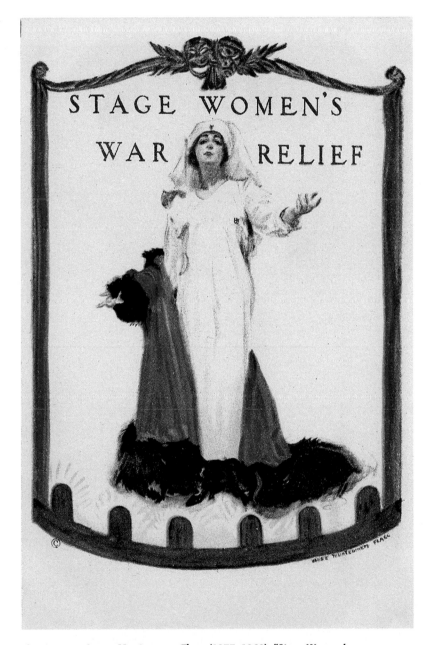

Figure 3.23. **James Montgomery Flagg (1877–1960). "Stage Women's War Relief."**
1918. *(See note.)*

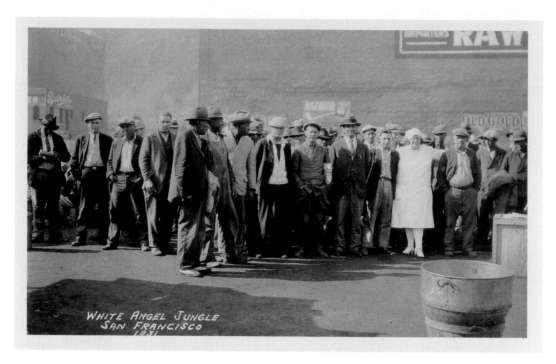

Figure 3.24. **White Angel Jungle.**
San Francisco. 1931. Real photo. *(See note.)*

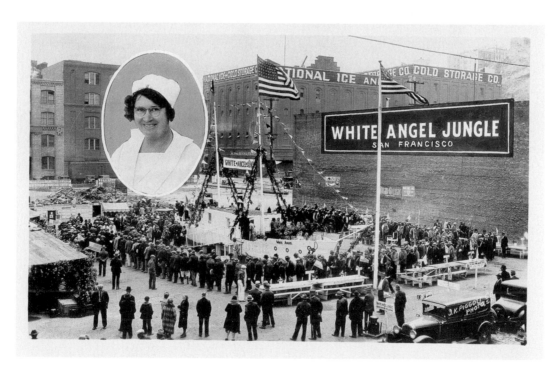

Figure 3.25. **White Angel Jungle.**
San Francisco. 1931. Real photo montage. *(See note.)*

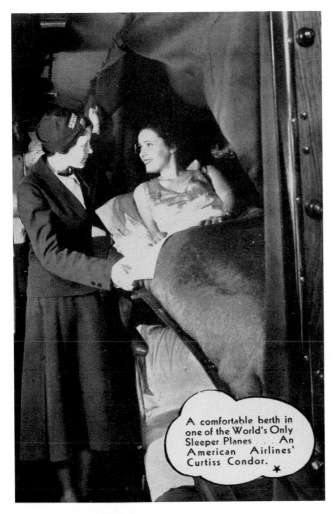

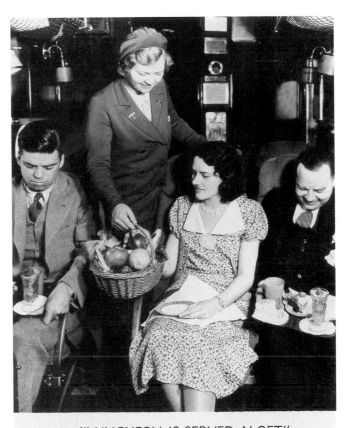

Figure 3.26. **American Airlines.**
c. 1935. From the collection of Don and Newly Preziosi, used with permission. *(See note.)*

Figure 3.27. **United Airlines.**
c. 1935. From the collection of Don and Newly Preziosi, used with permission. *(See note.)*

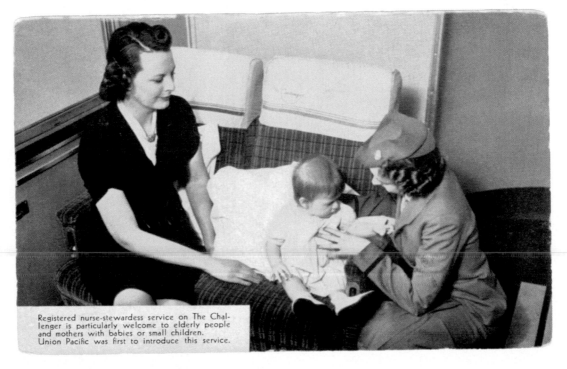

Figure 3.28. **Union Pacific Railroad.**
Omaha, Nebraska. 1938. *(See note.)*

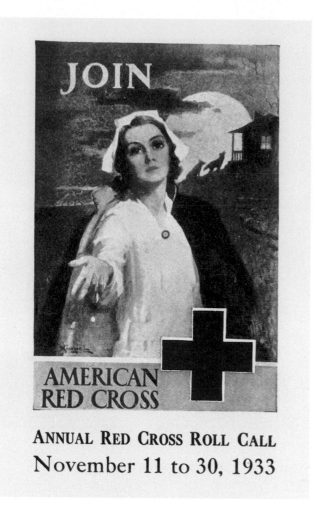

Figure 3.29. **Lu Kimmel. "Join."**
1933 Red Cross Roll Call. American Red Cross. 1933. *(See note.)*

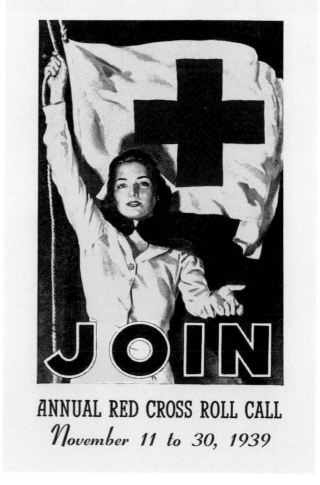

Figure 3.30. **1939 Red Cross Roll Call.**
American Red Cross. 1939. *(See note.)*

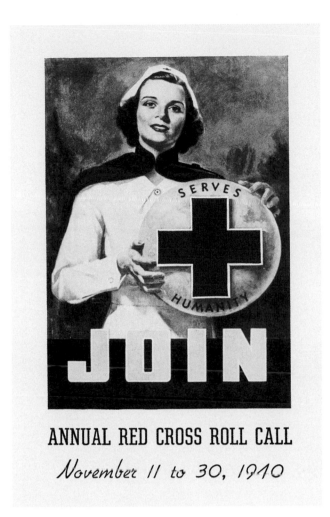

Figure 3.31. **1940 Red Cross Roll Call.**
American Red Cross. 1940. *(See note.)*

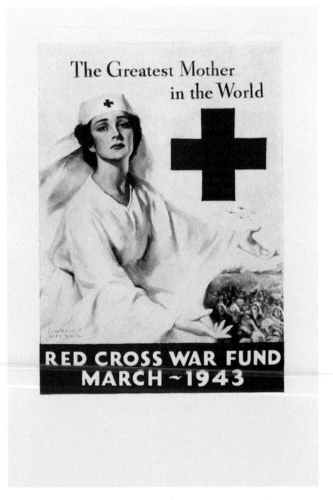

Figure 3.32. **Lawrence Wilbur (1897–1988). "The Greatest Mother in the World."**
1943 Red Cross War Fund. American Red Cross. 1943. *(See note.)*

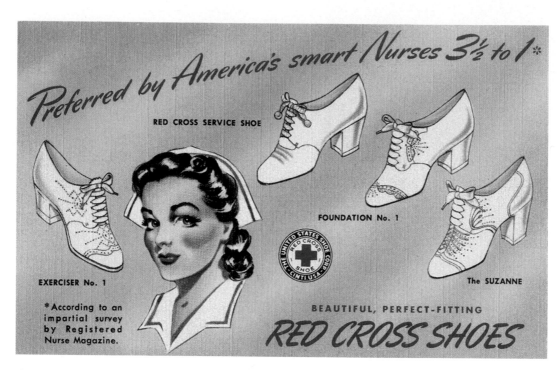

Figure 3.33. Red Cross Shoes.
Linen. 1941.

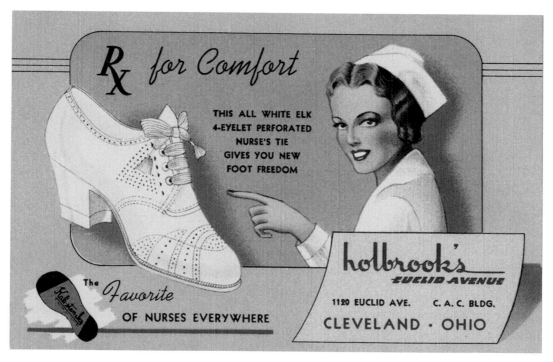

Figure 3.34. Holbrook's Shoes.
Linen. 1939.

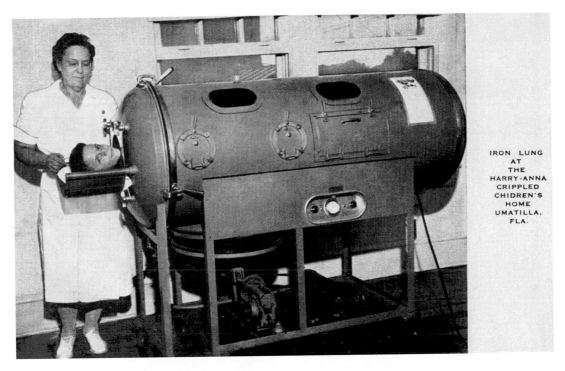

IRON LUNG
AT
THE
HARRY-ANNA
CRIPPLED
CHIDREN'S
HOME
UMATILLA,
FLA.

Figure 3.35. **Harry-Anna Crippled Children's Home.**
c. 1942. Linen. *(See note.)*

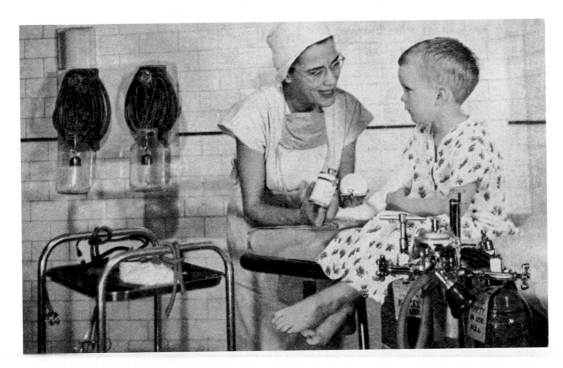

Figure 3.36. **U.S. Army Nurse Corps.**
"Nurse anesthetists find a wide variety of practice in U.S. Army hospitals. The Army Nurse
Corps offers a 12 month course in anesthesiology leading to the certificate for the American Association of Nurse Anesthetists."
1951. *(See note.)*

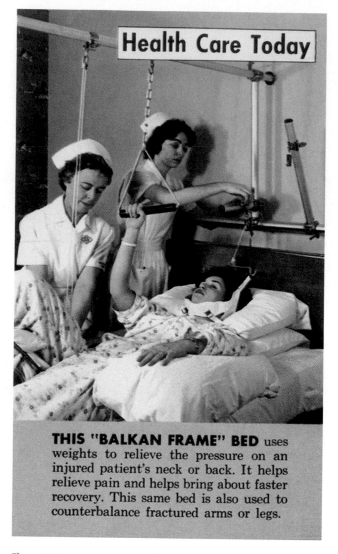

Figure 3.37.   **American Republic Insurance Company.**
Des Moines, Iowa. c. 1950.

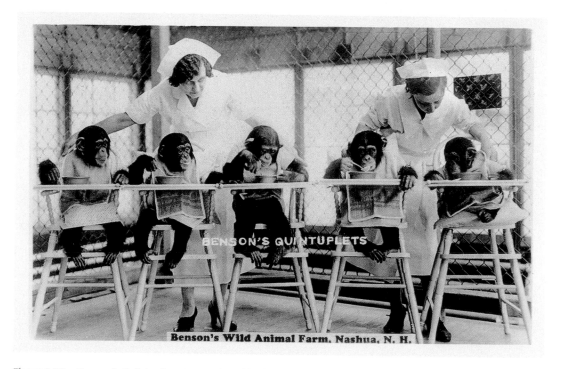

Figure 3.38.   **Benson's Quintuplets. Benson's Wild Animal Farm.**
Nashua, New Hampshire. c. 1950. Real photo. *(See note.)*

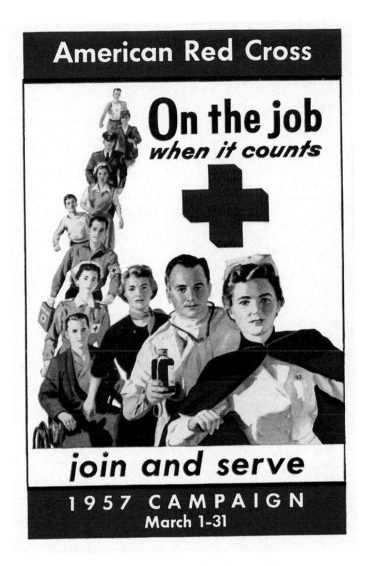

Figure 3.39.   **John Gould. "On the Job When it Counts."**
American Red Cross. 1957. *(See note.)*

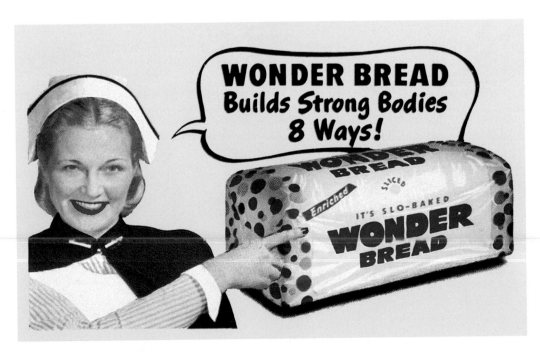

Figure 3.40.   **Wonder Bread.**
Interstate Brands West Corporation. Kansas City, Missouri. 1951.

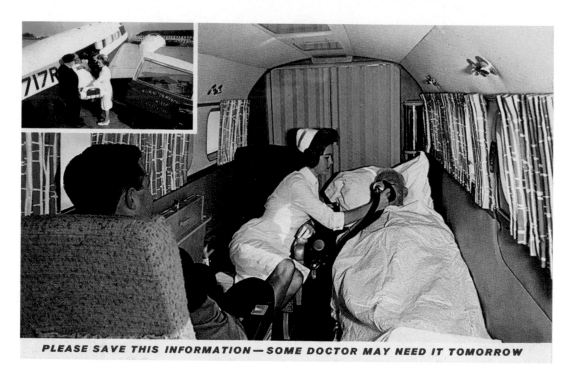

PLEASE SAVE THIS INFORMATION — SOME DOCTOR MAY NEED IT TOMORROW

Figure 3.41. **Special Air Services.**
Washington, D.C. 1958. *(See note.)*

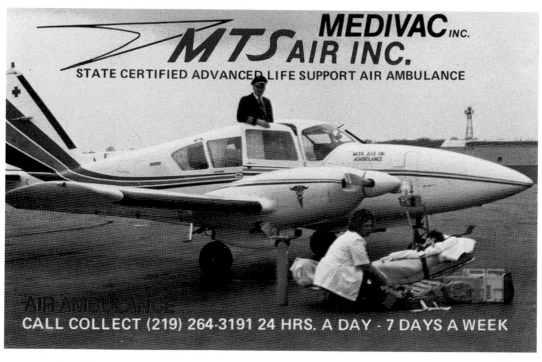

Figure 3.42. **MTS Air Incorporated.**
Elkhart, Indiana. 1979. *(See note.)*

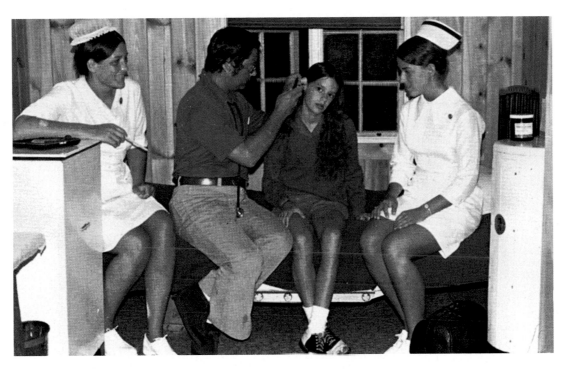

Figure 3.43. **Camp Tapawingo.**
Sweden, Maine. c. 1975. *(See note.)*

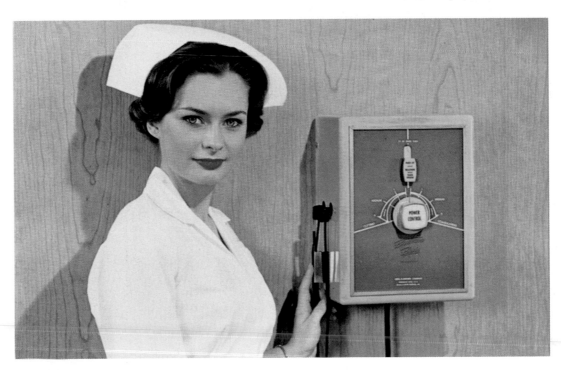

Figure 3.44. **Bovie Corporation.**
c. 1980. *(See note.)*

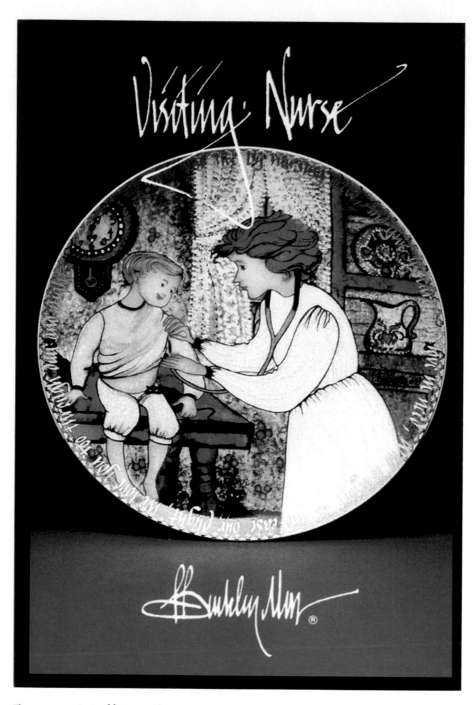

Figure 3.45. **P. Buckley Moss (1933–). "Visiting Nurse."**
Matthews, Virginia. 1993. *(See note.)*

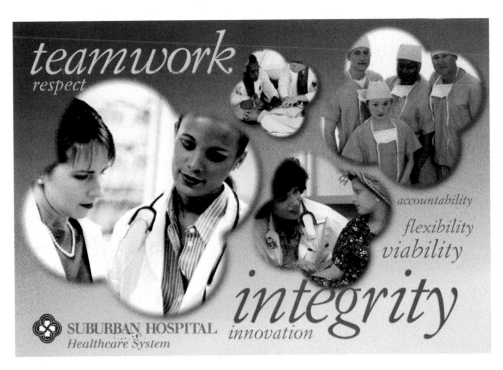

Figure 3.46. **Suburban Hospital.**
Bethesda, Maryland. 1999. *(See note.)*

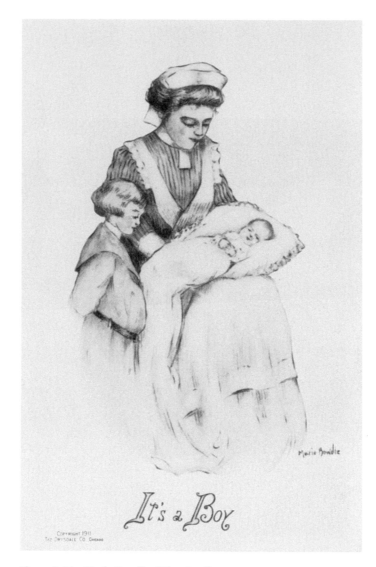

Figure 3.47. **Marie Bowdle. "It's a Boy."**
Chicago. 1911.

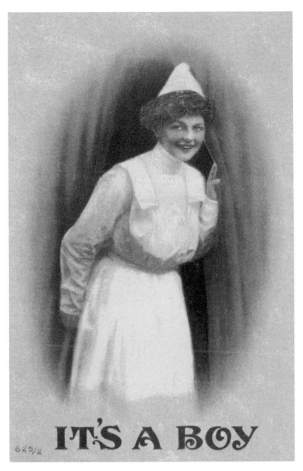

Figure 3.48.
United States. c. 1910.

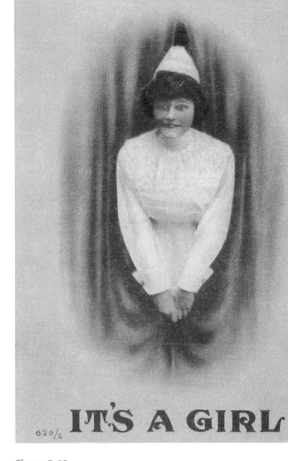

Figure 3.49.
United States. c. 1910.

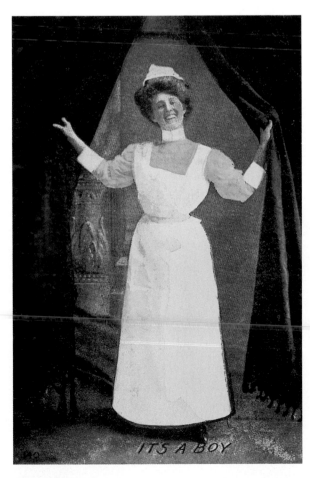

Figure 3.50.
United States. c. 1910.

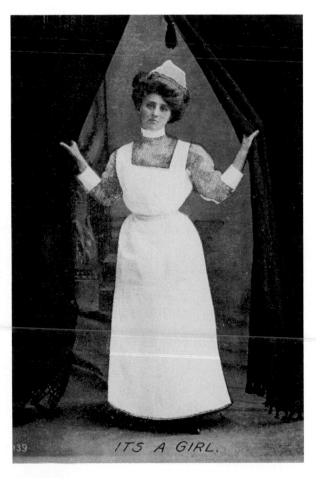

Figure 3.51.
United States. c. 1910.

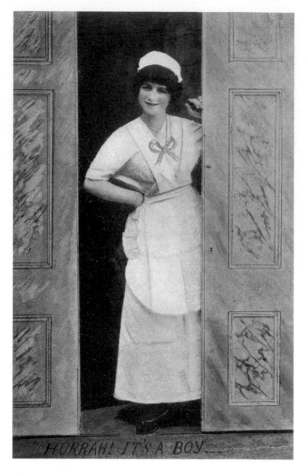

Figure 3.52.
United States. c. 1910.

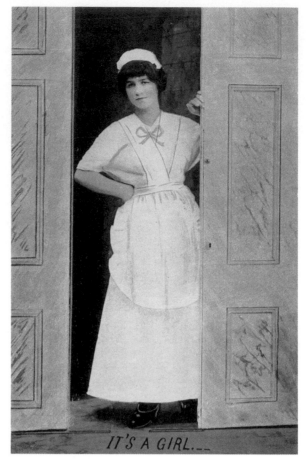

Figure 3.53.
United States. c. 1910.

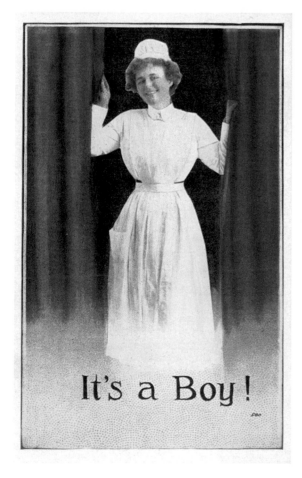

Figure 3.54.
United States. c. 1910.

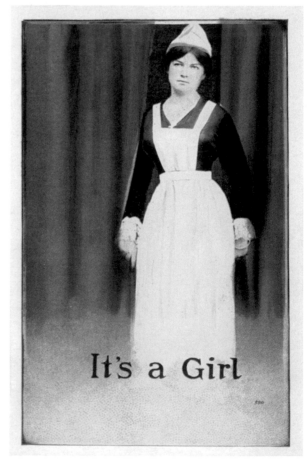

Figure 3.55.
United States. c. 1910.

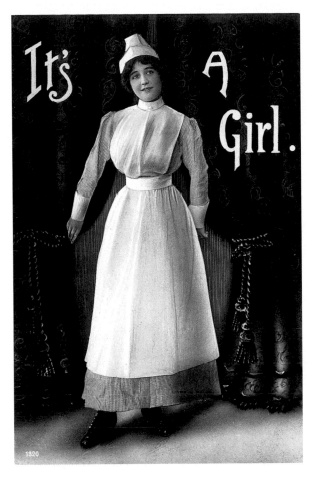

Figure 3.56.
Real photo. United States. c. 1910.

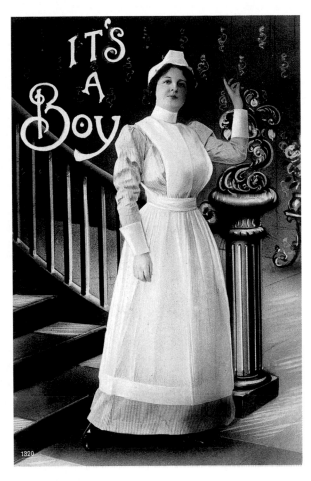

Figure 3.57.
Real photo. United States. c. 1910.

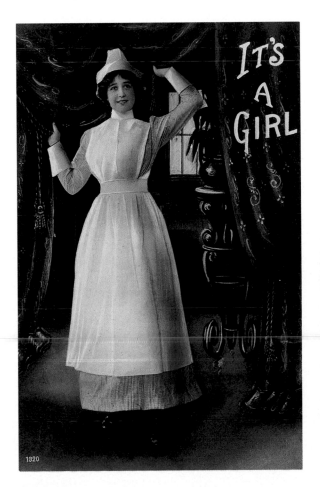

Figure 3.58.
Real photo. United States. c. 1910.

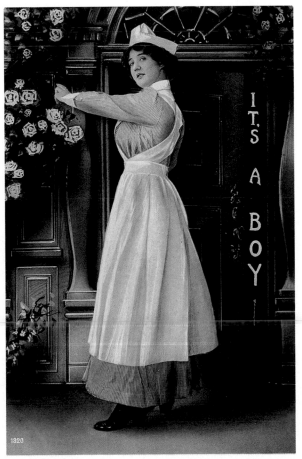

Figure 3.59.
Real photo. United States. c. 1910.

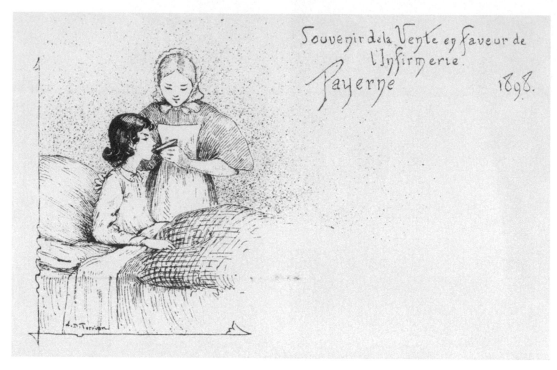

Figure 3.60. **"Souvenir of the Sale for the Payerne Infirmary."**
Switzerland. 1898. *(See note.)*

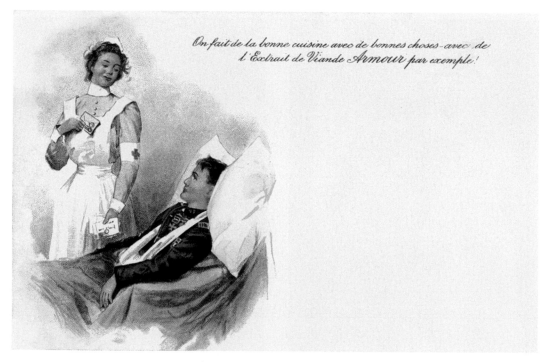

Figure 3.61. **Armour and Company, Chicago.**
France. 1899.
"One makes good cuisine with good ingredients. . . . with Armour Meat Extract, for
example." Spanish American War. *(See note.)*

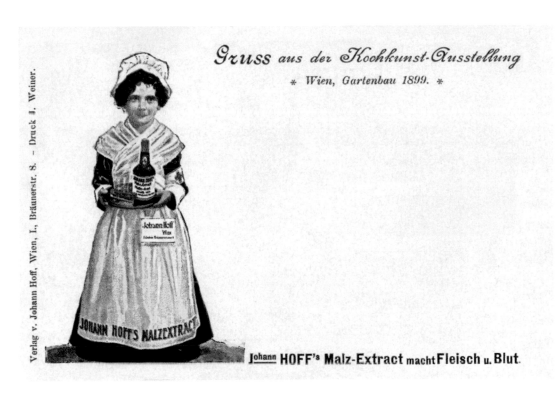

Figure 3.62. **"Johan Hoff's Malt Extract, Made with Flesh and Blood."**
"Greetings from the Cooking Arts Exposition."
Vienna, Austria.

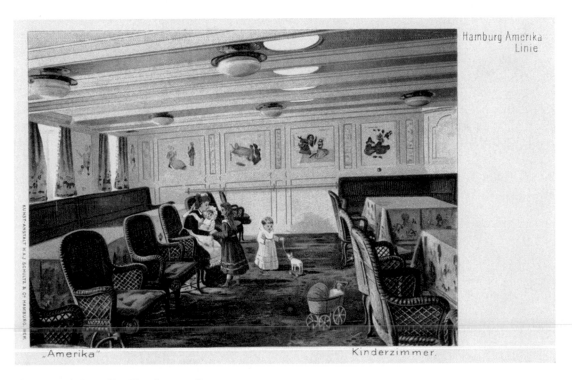

Figure 3.63. **"Amerika. The Playroom."**
Hamburg-Amerika Line. 1905. *(See note.)*

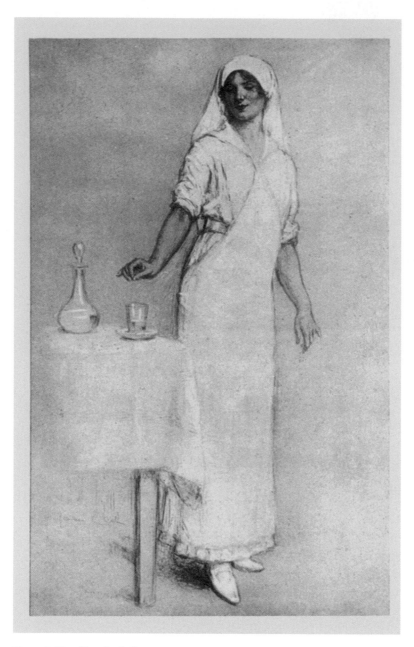

Figure 3.64. "Saccharin."
France. c. 1912.
Saccharin was the world's first artificial sweetener. *(See note.)*

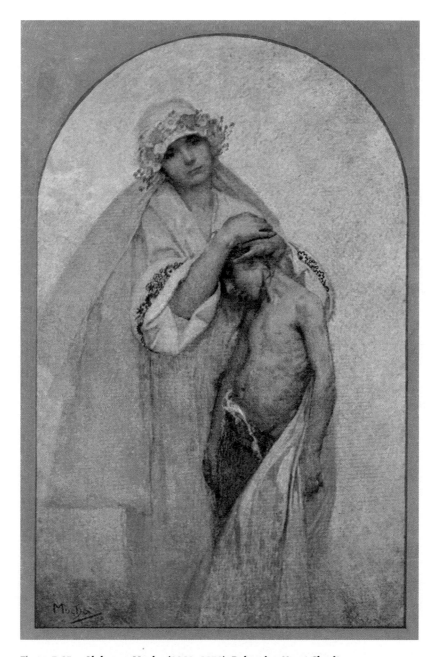

Figure 3.65. **Alphonse Mucha (1860–1939). Bohemian Heart Charity.**
Prague, Czechoslovakia. 1912. *(See note.)*

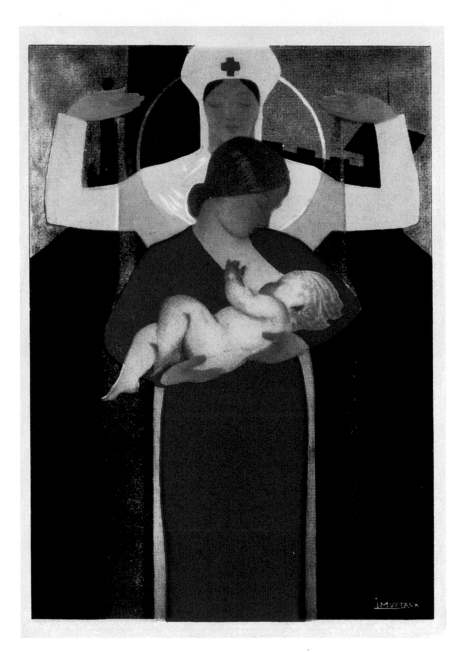

Figure 3.66. **"The mother breast-feeds her child. . . ."**
Spain. c. 1930. *(See note.)*

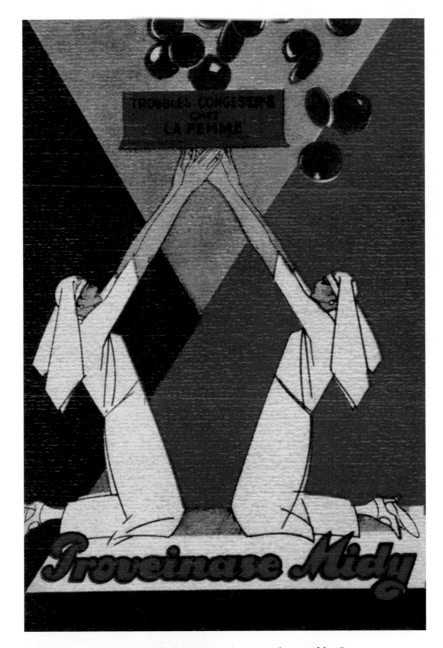

Figure 3.67. **Proveinase Midy. "For Women's Congestive Troubles."**
France. 1927. Futurism. *(See note.)*

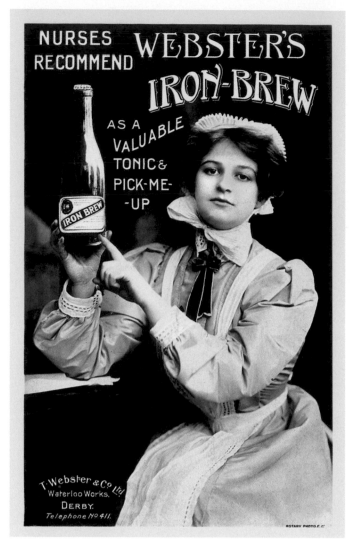

Figure 3.68. **Webster's Iron Brew.**
England. c. 1910.

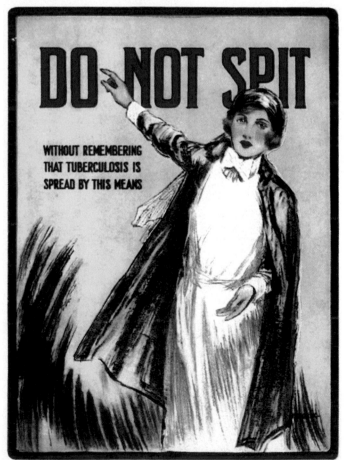

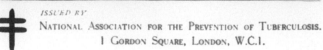

Figure 3.69. **National Association for the Prevention of Tuberculosis.**
England. c. 1910.

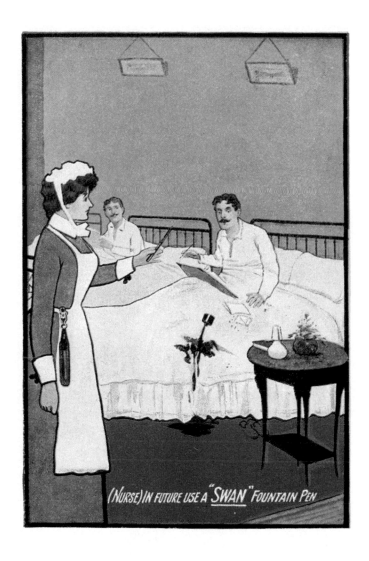

Figure 3.70. **Swan Fountain Pen Company, Ltd.**
England. 1914. *(See note.)*

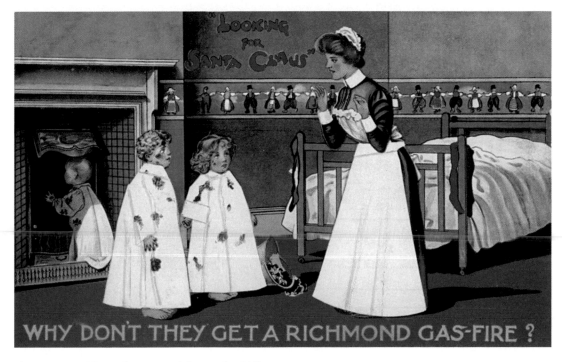

Figure 3.71. **Richmond Stoves and the North Middlesex Gas Company.**
England. 1912.

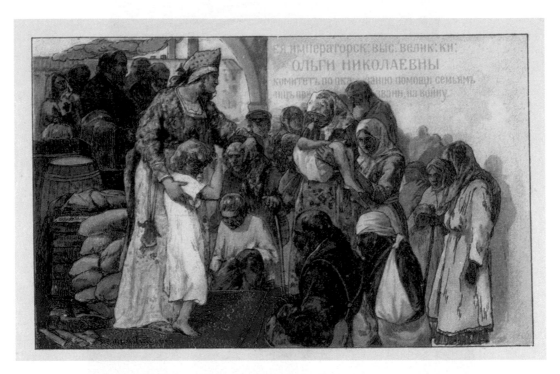

Figure 3.75.   "Her Imperial Highness, the Grand Duchess Olga Nikolaevna's Committee to Provide Assistance to Families of Soldiers Injured in the War." Russia. c. 1914. (See Fig. 4.88). *(See note.)*

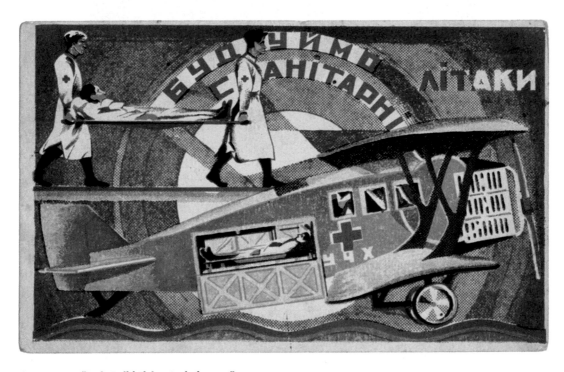

Figure 3.76.   "Let's Build Flying Ambulances." Ukraine, U.S.S.R. c. 1927. Constructivism. *(See note.)*

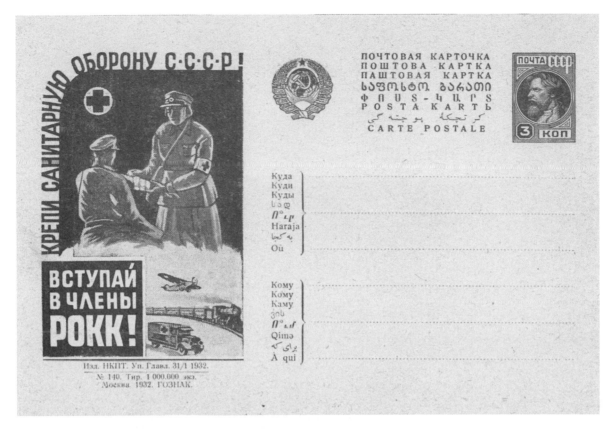

Figure 3.77. Russian Society of the Red Cross. "Strengthen the medical defense of the USSR. Become a member of the Russian Society of the Red Cross."
Moscow. 1932. *(See note.)*

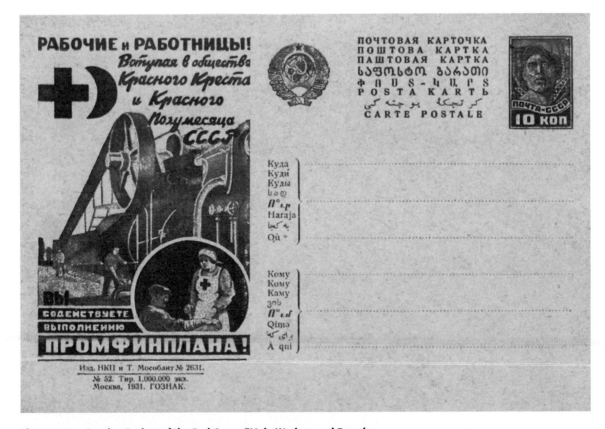

Figure 3.78. Russian Society of the Red Cross. "Male Workers and Female Workers! By becoming a member of the Red Cross and Red Crescent Societies of the USSR, you will participate in fulfilling the Industrial and Financial Plan."
Moscow. 1931. *(See note.)*

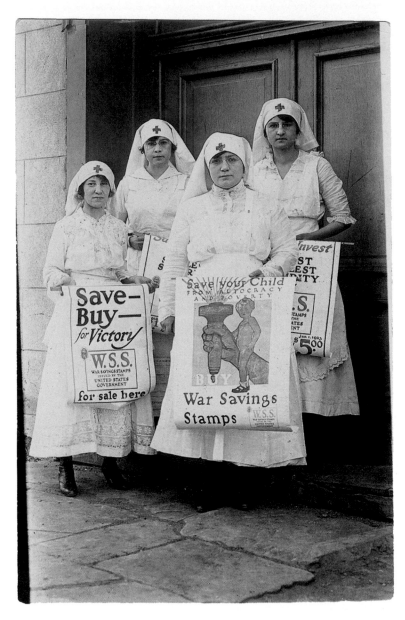

Figure 3.79.
Real photo. United States. 1917. *(See note.)*

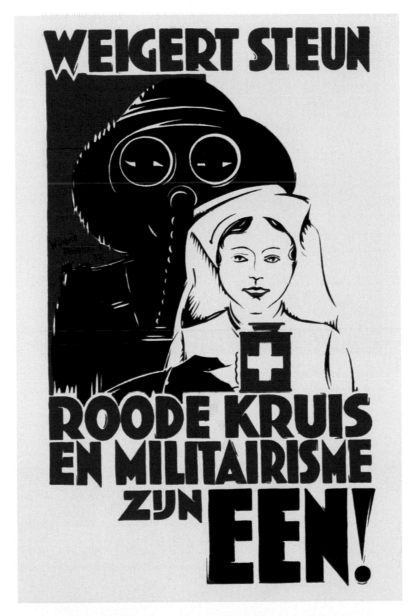

Figure 3.80.   Dutch Office of Youth Against War Campaign. "Withhold Support. The Red Cross and the Military are One!"
The Netherlands. 1932. *(See note.)*

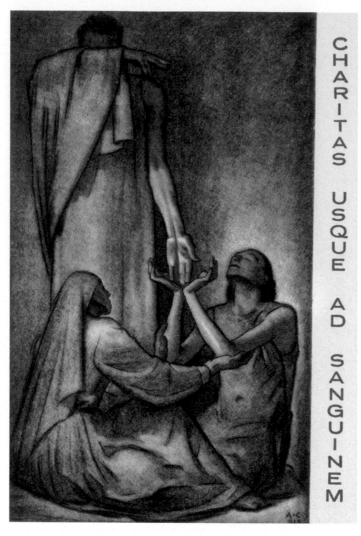

Figure 3.81. **"Charity, even unto blood."** (Latin).
Associazione Voluntari Italiani del Sangue (AVIS). Italian Association of Voluntary
Blood Donors. Italy. c. 1925. *(See note.)*

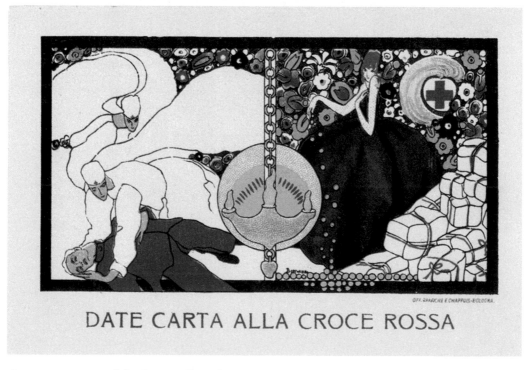

DATE CARTA ALLA CROCE ROSSA

Figure 3.82. **E. Bonazzi. "Red Cross Gift Card."**
Art Deco. Italy. c. 1930. *(See note.)*

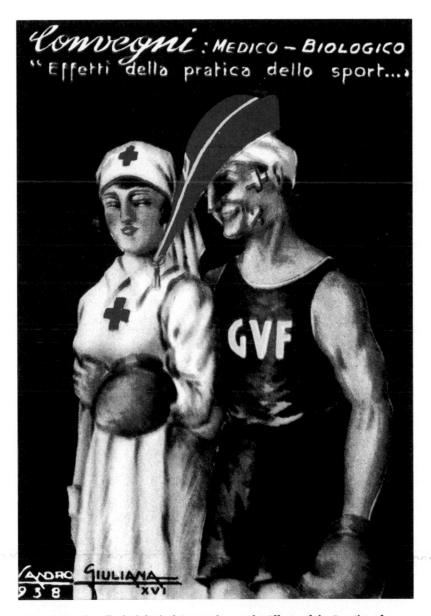

Figure 3.83. **"Medical-Biological Convention on the Effects of the Practice of Sports." Littoriali della Cultura e dell'Arte.**
Italy. 1938. *(See note.)*

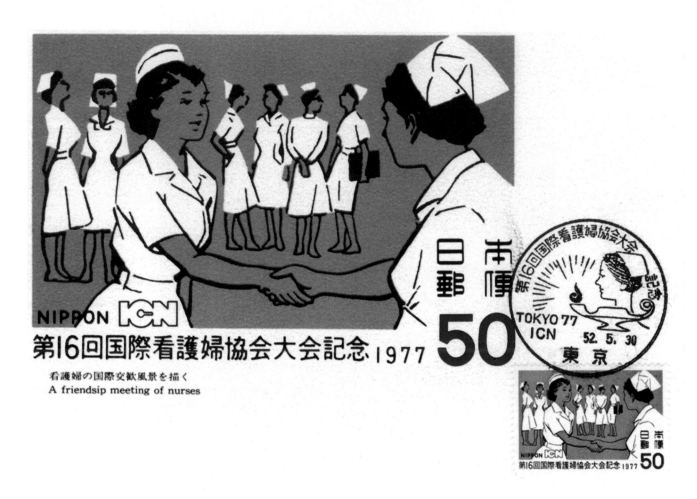

Figure 3.84.   **16th Meeting of the International Congress of Nurses in Tokyo, 1977. Japan Stamp Publicity Association.**
Japan. 1977. *(See note.)*

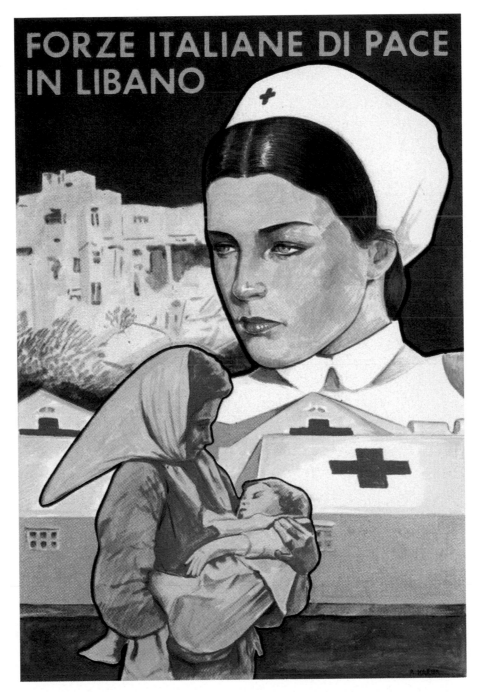

Figure 3.85. **Italian Peace Keeping Force in Lebanon.**
Italy. 1982. *(See note.)*

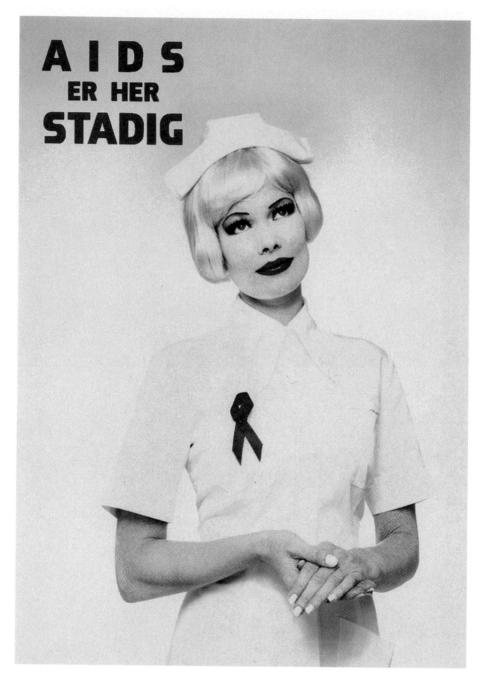

Figure 3.86. **"AIDS is Still Here."**
World AIDS Day, December, 1997. Denmark. *(See note.)*

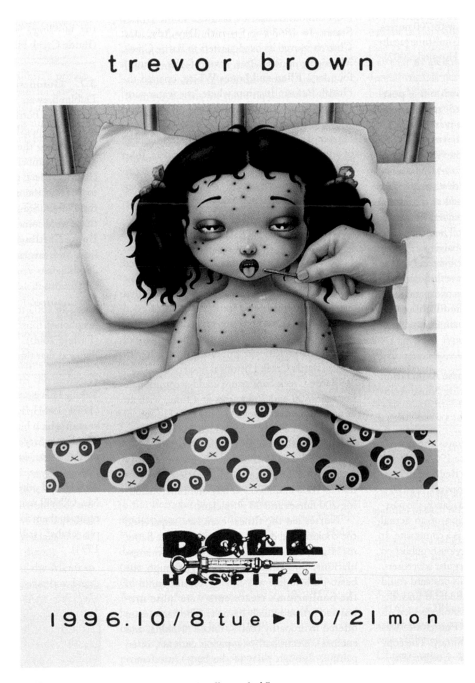

Figure 3.97. Trevor Brown (1959–), "Doll Hospital."
Japan. 1996. *(See note.)*

The Illinois Training School for Nurses opened in 1881. Its first class of eight pupils graduated in 1883. In 1914, when these postcards were issued, the school had an enrollment of 160 pupils, including 17 postgraduate students. The school continued until 1929, but had to be disbanded in 1930 due to financial difficulties at the school and county levels. The school's assets were transferred to the University of Chicago.

Isabel Hampton Robb (1860–1910). In 1886 the Illinois Training School for Nurses hired Isabel Hampton as its Superintendent of Nursing. Then 26 years old, she was a graduate of the Bellevue Training School for Nurses. She transformed the Illinois Training School into one of the finest professional nursing schools of the time. Miss Hampton placed the school on a graded system of teaching, replaced lectures with textbooks as the primary method of instruction, and secured specialty experience for the pupils through an affiliation with nearby Presbyterian Hospital (which opened its own school of School of Nursing in 1903).

Isabel Hampton left the Illinois Training School in 1889 to organize the Johns Hopkins School for Nursing in Baltimore. In 1894, in London, Hampton, carrying a bouquet sent to her by Florence Nightingale, married Dr. Hunter Robb. In 1896 Mrs. Robb organized the Nurses' Associated Alumnae of the United States and Canada, which in 1911 became known as the **American Nurses Association** (ANA). Robb was also instrumental in organizing what today is the **National League for Nursing Education** (Schriver, 1930). In 1976, among the first nurses so honored, she was inducted into the ANA Nursing Hall of Fame (American Nurses Association, 2002).

3.22. This card, postmarked "Port Angeles, Wash., May 11, 1937," was issued during the Great Depression. At the time, 6,500,000 individuals (15% of the work force) were still unemployed. Nurses and hospitals, however, were starting to recover, in part thanks to the Works Progress Administration, Social Security Act, and other federal programs.

From reverse: "**National Hospital Day,** inaugurated May 13, 1921, has become an occasion when hundreds of thousands of people visit the hospitals. It is an opportunity for the public to visit the community institution, to learn something of its services, facilities, purposes and problems. The hospital has become an important factor in community life. It is a place, not only for the sick, but for teaching and research. It is, in fact, a health center. You are cordially invited to visit us. You will have an interesting and profitable time."

Christopher Gregg Parnall, M.D. (1880–1960), Professor of Administrative Medicine at the University of Michigan School of Medicine and Director of the University Hospital, is acknowledged as the planner and initiator of National Hospital Day. It was presided over by the **American Hospital Association** (AHA), which set the annual date as May 12, the anniversary of the birthday of Florence Nightingale. National Hospital Day was first observed in 1921 (ViaHealth, 2002). For more on Florence Nightingale, see Figure 5.11.

National Hospital Day has become National Hospital Week, which occurs in May, with the exact dates set each year by the AHA. National Nurses Week, also held in May, is presided over by the American Nurses Association. In 1994, the permanent dates for National Nurses Week were set as May 6–12.

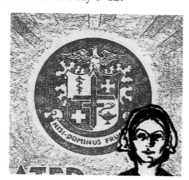

Detail of Figure 3.22.

The seal on the card is the seal of the AHA. From the American Hospital Association (2002): "The seal was adopted in 1927. In the center is the Lorraine Cross, which has been the emblem of relief to the unfortunate since medieval times. The caduceus, or the Wand of Mercury and Serpent of Aesculapius, has symbolized the healing art for many thousands of years. [In fact, the Wand of Mercury is not shown in the seal. See introduction to Chapter 1, Hygeia, for the history of the caduceus.] The Maltese Cross has been the emblem of the Knights of Saint John of Jerusalem since 1092 A.D., and for several hundred years has also been used by the St. John Ambulance service. The international emblem for the relief of sick and wounded is the Geneva, or Greek, Cross. The urn lamp is universally accepted as symbolic of knowledge and is the official emblem of the **Florence Nightingale Nurses.** The American eagle symbolizes the United States of America; the maple leaves the Dominion of Canada; and the whole is supported by the Latin motto *Nisi Dominus Frustra* (Without God we can do nothing)."

3.23. At the beginning of the 20th century, **James Montgomery Flagg** (1877–1960) was one of America's leading illustrators. Magazines that published his work included *McClure's, Collier's Weekly, Ladies' Home Journal, Cosmopolitan, Saturday Evening Post,* and *Harper's Weekly.* During World War I, Flagg designed 46 posters for the government, including the famous Uncle Sam recruitment poster for which he is best known, captioned, "I Want You for the U.S. Army."

The **Stage Women's War Relief** is now known as the American Theatre Wing. The Wing collaborates with the League of American Theatres and Producers on the governance of the Tony Awards. The Wing's history dates back to 1917 when Rachel Crothers and six other prominent women in the American theater formed the Stage Women's War Relief. Through their efforts during World War I, the group expanded into one of the most active relief organizations in the world. Antoinette Perry, a former actress and director, succeeded Rachel Crothers at the Wing. **The Tony Awards,** first handed out April 7, 1947, presented each year for outstanding contribution to U.S. theater, are affectionately named for Perry (American Theater Wing, 2002).

3.24 to 3.25. **The White Angel Jungle** was a soup kitchen for the jobless in San Francisco during the **Great Depression.** Just over 250 men, most (in spite of their poverty) wearing sports jackets, and about 20 women can be counted in the photograph. The nurse in the inset of Figure 3.24 also appears in Figure 3.25. Figure 3.24 was produced as an advertisement to alert the residents of the city to the Jungle's existence and to announce that it was operated under the guidance of nurses. The words "White Angel Jungle San Francisco" are not actually on the wall but were added by the photographer. (The right edge of the flagpole isn't quite straight where the pole seems to pass in front of the sign, because a small amount of ink got onto the image of the pole during the retouching.) "White Angel" on the bow of the "ship" and on the banner strung between the masts is actual signage.

3.26 to 3.28. The stewardesses are registered nurses.

The following, by Don Preziosi, is reprinted from Postcard Collector magazine with permission of the author (Preziosi, 2002). All rights reserved.

"The Origin of the Airline Stewardess"
One of my main postcard collecting interests has been early U.S. commercial aviation. In pursuing this interest, I have collected many stewardess (and steward!) cards. While I was aware that the earliest stewardesses were also registered nurses (on the back of early aviation postcards with stewardesses this asset is usually mentioned), I was not aware of the origin of this concept. Recently, I came across a copy of a 1930 memo written by S. A. Simpson, a district manager for **Boeing Air Transport,**

to **W. A. Patterson,** then the assistant to the president of Boeing, and subsequently the board chairman of United Air Lines. Apparently Simpson was on a flight from Reno when he had to serve lunch to the passengers because the co-pilot, who normally assumed this duty, was occupied at the controls. Simpson recognized that a third crew member—a steward—would be very useful during a flight.

At about that time, a young nurse named **Ellen Church*** [see below] called Simpson with a similar proposal. She had been fascinated with aviation since she was a child, and wanted to combine her two interests. Instead of a steward, Ellen suggested a stewardess who would have the advantage of being a registered nurse.

Simpson's 1930 memo is reproduced below. I have only edited it slightly for length.

"As a suggestion—I was just wondering if you had ever given any serious thought to the subject of young women as couriers. It strikes me that there would be a great psychological punch to having young women stewardesses or couriers, or whatever you want to call them . . . I have in mind a couple of graduate nurses that would make exceptional stewardesses. Of course it would be distinctly understood that there would be no reference made to their hospital training or nursing experience, but it would be a mighty fine thing to have this available, sub rosa, if necessary either for air sickness or perhaps something else worse.

"Imagine the psychology of having young women as regular members of the crew. Imagine the national publicity we could get from it, and the tremendous effect it would have on the traveling public. Also imagine the value that they would be to us not only in the neater and nicer method of serving food and looking out for the passengers' welfare, but also in an emergency.

"I am not suggesting at all the flapper type of girl, or one that would go haywire. You know nurses as well as I do, and you know that they are not given to flightiness—I mean in the head. The average graduate nurse is a girl with some horse sense and is very practical and has seen enough of men to not be inclined to chase them around the block at every opportunity.

"Further, as a general rule nurses are not of the 'pretty' type which lends to their usefulness in this case.

"The young women that we would select would naturally be intelligent and could handle what traffic work aboard was necessary, such as keeping of records, filling out reports, issuing tickets, etc. They would probably do this as well or better than the average young fellow . . .

"As to the qualifications of the proposed young women couriers, their first paramount qualification would be that of a graduate nurse (although this would never be brought into the foreground in advertising . . . as it sort of sounds as though they are necessary); and, secondly, young women who have been around and are familiar with general travel—rail, steamer and air . . ."

The requirement for stewardesses to be registered nurses was phased out in the 1940s. Please note, the words in the memo are Simpson's, not mine.

***Ellen (Marshall) Church** (1904–1965) was the world's first airline stewardess. Employed in 1930 by United Airlines, she organized the pioneer group Sky Girls. As a young nurse in San Francisco, Miss Church approached officials of Boeing Air Transport, a parent company of United, and proposed that stewardesses be added to flight crews. Her idea was accepted: she and seven other nurses began flying between Chicago and San Francisco on May 15, 1930 (Iowa Division of Tourism, 2002).

3.28. **The Challenger,** operated daily between Chicago and the Pacific coast, was placed in service by the Union Pacific Railroad in August 1935. The onboard train staff included a stewardess who was also a registered nurse. Her duties were "to see to the comfort and well being of all passengers aboard with special attention to be provided to women and children." Duty hours were from 6:30 AM until 10:00 PM. Stewardess nurse service was discontinued on December 31, 1941 due to the outbreak of World War II, and restored on May 14, 1947. Stewardess nurses worked the Challenger until the train was discontinued in 1971 (*The Streamliner*, 1994).

3.29 to 3.32. These postcards are part of a series that includes Figure 3.39. They were reproduced from full-color posters issued by the Red Cross for its annual enrollment drives.

Figure 3.32 was painted by **Lawrence Wilbur** (1897–1988), a noted American artist who specialized in Red Cross poster design. His pictures of nurses appear on Red Cross posters as early as 1917 and as late as 1954.

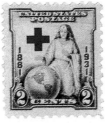

2-cent stamp.

One of his posters, the 1930 Red Cross Roll Call poster, "The Greatest Mother," became the basis for the 1931 2¢ U.S. postage stamp commemorating the 50th anniversary of the American Red Cross.

3.35. **Harry-Anna Crippled Children's Home** in Umatilla, Florida was founded in 1933 by the Benevolent and Protective Order of the Elks (a fraternal order) as a facility that offered free treatment to Florida children who suffered from orthopedic diseases and disabilities.

The following is reprinted with the kind permission of Richard Hill, from *The History of the British Iron Lung 1832–1995* (1995).

Polio in the 1920's affected mostly children. Patients who had "anterior" polio involving the cervical and thoracic spinal cord were unable to breathe at all. Usually only a few hours elapsed from the first signs of respiratory distress to death.

In 1926, an American, **Philip Drinker** was appointed to a commission at the Rockefeller Institute formed to develop improved methods of resuscitation. At the time Philip's brother Cecil and a young physiologist Lois Shaw were studying various aspects of respiratory physiology in cats at Harvard University. They found that if they placed an anaesthetized cat in a sealed box, with only the head exposed, they could accurately measure the amount of air the cat breathed. When the cat inhaled, its chest expanded and the pressure within the box rose because the cat was now taking up more of the volume. When the cat exhaled, the pressure fell.

After watching these experiments, Drinker reasoned that the opposite should also be true. He injected the cat with curare, which acts as a very powerful muscle relaxant, to stop its breathing. He then, having already modified the box to include a syringe to increase and lower the pressure inside, placed the cat in the device and successfully ventilated the animal for a few hours until the effects of the drug wore off.

Drinker concluded that if it worked for a cat, that it would also work for a human, which prompted him to construct an adult sized respirator, using a local tinsmith for the cabinet construction and a vacuum cleaner blower to provide the suction. The patient would be slid into the respirator on a garage mechanic's "creeper," after which the end plate was secured and a rubber collar slipped over the patient's head.

Within a few months in 1928 the first clinical trial was under way. An 8-year-old girl, comatose from lack of oxygen, was placed in the machine. Within a minute or two she regained consciousness and a little later asked for ice cream. Although this little girl died a few days later of pneumonia, the principle of External Negative Pressure Ventilation was firmly established.

Dubbed by an unknown American journalist as the "iron lung," Drinker's machine was continually improved and publicized. It finally went into commercial production and by 1931 seventy Drinker Respirators were in use throughout the USA. At least one iron lung remains in use as of this writing, at the Lane-Fox Respiratory Unit at St. Thomas' Hospital in London.

3.36. This postcard is part of series of 10 postcards issued in 1951 on the occasion of the 50th anniversary of the **Army Nurse Corps.** The Army Nurse Corps was founded as a permanent department of the Medical Department of the U.S. Army on February 2, 1901. It was a direct outcome of the nursing involvement in the Spanish American War. After World War II, the Army Medical Department was renamed the Surgeon General Corps.

At the start of U.S. involvement in World War I, there were 400 nurses on active duty, most of them assigned to posts on the Mexican Border (see also Note 2.16). By the end of the war, 21,480 nurses were in the Corps (see also 5-11). During World War II, the Army Nurse Corp increased from a peacetime strength of 7000 in 1941, to over 57,000 nurses on active duty at the time of VJ Day. They were deployed in 605 overseas and 454 mainland hospitals. During peacetime, the Army Nurse Corps staffs military hospitals, participates in worldwide relief efforts, and maintains its own nursing schools. The Army Nurse Corps celebrated its 100th anniversary on February 2, 2001. In the course of its history, over 100,000 women have served in the Corps (Zodin, 1996).

3.38. Although the postcard states that Benson's was located in Nashua, New Hampshire, it was actually just across the Merrimack River in Hudson, New Hampshire. **Benson's Wild Animal Farm** opened in 1924 as a sideline to John Benson's wild animal importing business. At the start, the display consisted of a small 4-acre pasture in which Benson placed some of the animals for the amusement of curious visitors. By 1930 Benson's Wild Animal Farm had expanded to 250 acres and boasted a wild animal circus with a live presentation of over 100 animals in various acts, including a lion tamer with his big cats, performing Liberty Horses, an elephant act, and trained chimpanzees. In 1954, the peak year, attendance reached one half million, with 17,000 customers passing through the gates on a record-setting Sunday. In the 1960s the Farm began to decline. Ultimately, high animal upkeep costs, property and machinery maintenance, and other costs proved an insurmountable barrier. After 63 years of operation, Benson's Wild Animal Park closed on October 12, 1987 (Goldsack, 1998).

3.39. This postcard is from the same series as Figures 3.29 to 3.32.

3.41. The aircraft is a Beechcraft 18 High Cabin. The ambulance is a 1958 Oldsmobile.

3.42. The aircraft is a twin-engine Piper Aztec.

3.43. Camp Tapawingo was founded in 1919 as a summer camp for girls on Lake Keyes in Sweden, Maine. It is still in operation.

3.44. The wall-mounted battery-powered cautery shown was produced by the **Bovie Corporation** from 1978–1986. Although experimental models were in use earlier, the first practical battery-powered cautery was introduced in 1852 by Mr. Robert Ellis (Ellis, 1862).

3.45. This postcard is an advertisement for a series of collectible plates done by artist **P. Buckley Moss** and produced by Anna-Perenna Porcelain.

Patricia Buckley (1933–) was born in New York City. In 1955, she married Jack Moss and moved to Waynesboro in the Shenandoah Valley of Virginia. Her art is strongly influenced by the rural Virginia countryside and the deeply religious Amish and Mennonite communities there.

3.46. Men and women of different races did not appear together on nurse postcards until the 1990s. **Maryland Suburban Hospital** was founded in 1943, and is the designated shock trauma center for Montgomery County and the surrounding area. It treats approximately 1000 trauma patients per year. Suburban employs approximately 450 nurses, sees 37,000 patients per year, and admits 12,500 of them.

3.47 to 3.59. Birth announcement postcards are not normally thought of or collected as advertising postcards, but in fact that is what they are. The most common images found on them are babies, storks, and nurses. Birth announcement postcards were very popular and were naturally produced in two versions, one for a boy and one for a girl. Since they were not bought or mailed as pairs, there wasn't much interest or opportunity to compare the boy version with the girl version. Here, the two versions are seen side by side. Examine the facial expressions of the nurses. Do you think that, in the early part of the last century, the boy baby and the girl baby were equally welcome?

3.60. Payerne is a town in western Switzerland.

3.61. The postcard, produced for the French division of the **Armour Company,** is a reproduction of the image on the United States 1899 Armour Army and Navy Calendar. It depicts a nurse and a U.S. soldier during the **Spanish-American War.** Armour distributed the calendar in the United States, but the postcards were printed and distributed in France and Germany. (See Fig. 5.78 for more Spanish American War postcards.)

3.63. All **ocean liners** had playrooms, nurseries, infirmaries, and sickbays, but few steamship companies advertised the fact. Nurses on ship advertising are rare because the possibility of sickness had to be kept far from the prospective customers' minds. Still, at least two major lines (see below) thought it was a good idea to reassure parents that the children would be well cared for.

The Hamburg-Amerika Line was started in Hamburg, Germany in 1847 as a small shipping company called *Hamburg-Amerikanische Packetfahrt-Actien-Gesellschaft* (Hamburg-American Packet Boat Joint Stock Company), or simply, Hapag AG. Hapag handled freight between Germany and the United States. In 1891, Albert Ballin, newly appointed head of the passage department, seeking another way to generate revenue, invented the concept of the "pleasure voyage," and created a new use for liners: cruise ships.

In the years between 1900 and 1914, the Hamburg-Amerika Line operated some of the most famous ships in the world. In 1905 it commissioned the Amerika, the most luxurious ship the world had ever known and, at 22,200 tons, the largest. **The Amerika** held 2662 passengers and had a crew of 577. Her passenger accommodation, far ahead of any predecessor, included suites with a private bathroom, electric elevators, a winter garden, "electrical medicinal" baths, and a Ritz-Carlton restaurant, the first a-la-carte restaurant on the North Atlantic (Landon, 1997). Hapag AG is now an international shipping conglomerate, with fleets of ships, trucks, and aircraft.

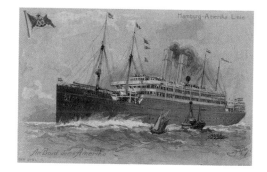

An Bord der Amerika.
Germany, 1905.

A second steamship line that advertised a nurse was the **N.Y.K. Line** (*Nippon Yusen Kaisha* or Japanese Mail Boat Company), started in 1885 and also still in existence. The postcard below, circa 1910, shows the playroom on one of its England Division cruise ships. (N.Y.K. Line, 2002).

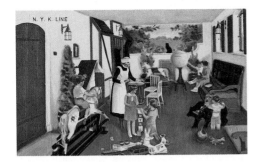

Nippon Yusen Kaisha playroom.
1910.

3.64. Issued by the Rhone-Poulenc Society of Pharmaceutical Manufacturers.

Saccharin is the world's oldest low-calorie sweetener. It was discovered accidentally in 1879 by **Constantine Fahlberg,** a chemistry researcher at Johns Hopkins University. Fahlberg was working on new food preservatives when he accidentally spilled some of the compound he had synthesized on his hands. When he went home that night and ate his dinner, he noticed the intense sweetness of the compound. (Apparently he went home from the lab and ate without washing his hands!) Fahlberg named the compound "saccharin" after *saccharum,* the Latin word for sugar (Hodgin, 2002).

3.65. Alphonse Mucha (1860–1939) is the most famous artist of the Art Nouveau movement. Mucha became so associated with **Art Nouveau** that it was often referred to as "*Style Mucha.*" In 1912, Mucha departed the Art Nou-

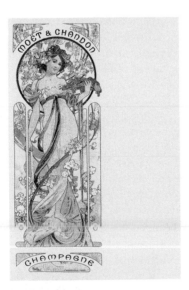

Alphonse Mucha. (Postcard courtesy of www.vintagepostcards.com)

veau style and began the first in a series of 20 large historical paintings illustrating the "Epic of the Slavic People." Although the Heart Charity postcard was produced during that latter period, Art Nouveau elements are still there, though subdued. Compare the later work with his classic Art Nouveau advertising shown here.

3.66. From reverse: "The mother breast-feeds her child, fulfilling the sacred duty which motherhood imposes on her." Women's Social Action Program Savings Pension Plan (same series as Fig. 2.41).

3.67. From reverse: "Various conditions can immobilize a large part of our blood. It is a step toward death if blood does not circulate. *Proveinase Midy* restores the circulation."

Futurism was an international art movement founded in Italy in 1909. It originated with a manifesto, issued by F. T. Marinetti. Speaking for a small group of anarchists, Marinetti proclaimed, "It is from Italy that we launch through the world this violently upsetting incendiary manifesto of ours. With it, today, we establish Futurism, because we want to free this land from its smelly gangrene of professors, archaeologists, ciceroni and antiquarians. For too long has Italy been a dealer in second-hand clothes. We mean to free her from the numberless museums that cover her like so many graveyards."

And, "We will glorify war—the world's only hygiene—militarism, patriotism, the destructive gesture of freedom-bringers, beautiful ideas worth dying for, and scorn for woman. We will destroy the museums, libraries, academies of every kind, will fight moralism, feminism, [and] every opportunistic or utilitarian cowardice" (Marinetti, 1909).

The art is identified by its triangular and trapezoidal forms, its typical use of red and black, and its dynamic typeface. Originally Futurism's thematic elements celebrated machines, war, and misogyny. How ironic that only two decades after its inception, the style appears on an advertisement for relief of "female troubles."

3.70. The fountain pen was invented in 1884 by Lewis Waterman, an insurance broker.

3.73 to **3.74.** **Art Deco** takes its name from the *Exposition Internationale des Arts Décoratifs et Industrials Modernes* held in Paris in 1925. It represented a movement away from the organic forms of Art Nouveau. Although historians consider the Exposition to be the dividing line between the Art Nouveau and Art Deco periods, Art Deco was fully formed in the pre-war period. The exposition itself had originally been sched-

uled for 1915, but the war delayed it for a full decade. The graphic style is characterized by bold use of color, flat broad geometric shapes, and sharply defined outlines.

You can trace the forms as they become more stylized. Start with Figure 3.72, which, although French, is very similar to Italian design before the war. The style is moving toward Deco, but still presents relatively realistic facial features. Figure 3.73 is pure, unmistakable Art Deco, exactly as defined above (see also Figs 3.33 and 3.34). Finally, Figure 3.74 demonstrates Deco's movement toward a more stylized **Modernism.** The difference between Figure 3.74 and Modernism is really a matter of what the art portrays, not how it is drawn. Deco and Modernism were both "legitimized" by, and more or less sprang from Cubism, which was introduced between 1906 and 1916. Modernism, which included Futurism and Constructivism, emphasized technological themes and supported an economic revolution. Art Deco, in contrast, was seen by the Modernists as superficial in content, too eclectic in form and too feminine. To the Modernists, Art Deco was a holdover from a pre-war past that was aristocratic, frivolous, and ultimately disastrous. Both schools had strong influence on the forms that emerged after World War II.

3.75 to 3.78 show a progression through three periods in Russian history.

3.75. This postcard was issued in the final years of the reign of Russian royalty. The **Tsarina Alexandra Fedorovna** and two of her daughters, **Olga Nikolaevna** and **Tatiana Nikolaevna,** served as nurses during World War I. (See also Notes 4.87 to 4.90.) Note the Red Cross nurse standing at the extreme left.

3.76. When the Tsar was overthrown in the Revolution of 1918, the independent **Ukrainian People's Republic** was proclaimed, allying itself with the Central Powers (Germany, Austro-Hungary, and Italy). After the capitulation of the Central Powers, and after a 2-year Soviet civil war, most of the Ukraine came under Soviet control and in 1922 became a constituent republic of the USSR. Now it is an independent sovereign nation.

The art on the postcard is in a style known as **Constructivism** (see also Notes 3.73 and 3.74). Constructivism was begun by Russian avant-garde artists just prior to World War I, having taken shape during the late flowering of the Art Nouveau movement. After the war, there was almost total economic collapse, famine, and bitter discontent in Russia. In desperation, Lenin introduced the **New Economic Policy** (NEP), which allowed some private enterprise to return. Small farms and businesses flourished, while the state kept control of heavy industry, transport, and foreign trade. This relatively free period featured experimentation in all fields; in the arts, the Constructivist movement became dominant.

The name "Constructivism" comes from the manifesto published by the movement's founders in 1920. This group wanted to design and build objects that reflected a wholehearted acceptance of modernity. In that way, art would contribute to the "construction" of a new communist society. The motifs reflect the rise of commerce and technology. The style is one of abstraction with a focus on geometric shapes, especially circles and sectors.

3.77 to **3.78.** Constructivism in the USSR lasted roughly until 1928. In that year Stalin, who had by then assumed complete control of the government, put an end to the NEP and forced the country into his **Five Year Plan.** Intended to turn the USSR rapidly into a powerful industrial nation, it called for vast production increases and massive construction throughout the country. The Plan was unrealistic and irrational, and caused the deaths of millions. A major aspect of the Plan was the destruction of private farming and the creation of collectives where the peasants worked for the state. Used to working their own land, the peasants were not eager to relocate to the giant collective farms. In spite of widespread resistance, however, the intended goals were achieved through brutal enforcement. Collective farming brought about the famine of 1932–1933. It is estimated that over 25 million peasants were relocated, and 7 million perished during that period.

The 1930s saw mass purges of intellectuals, artists, rich farmers, and clergy. The Church was seen to be in opposition to the state, and worship was deemed shameful. Experiments in society ended, and all forms of expression were mobilized to serve the state. In 1932, Stalin decreed that all art must be "realistic" portrayals of Soviet life and Communist values. Figures 3.77 and 3.78 are examples of this style of art. Both are postal cards, a specialized form of postcard issued by the government with the stamp preprinted as part of the design.

To the left of the stamp, the word "Post Card" is printed in eight languages: Russian, Ukrainian, Belorussian, Georgian, Armenian, Turkmen, Uzbek, and French. French is there to conform to International Postal Regulations at the time. The others were the major languages spoken in the Soviet Republic, which, in 1931–1932, consisted of the Russian Federation, Ukraine, Belorussia, Transcaucasian Federation, Turkmenistan, and Uzbekistan. Note that in Figure 3.78 the Red Cross emblem employs both the cross and the crescent, accommodating Christianity and Islam, the two major religions of the USSR.

3.79 and **3.80.** Figure 3.80 is one of only two postcards I have seen that show the nurse in a politically negative light. (See Figure 5.17 for the other.) Here she represents the **Red Cross as a capitalistic military organization.** This stance is typical of postwar Socialism, which bases its argument as follows: The Red Cross has relied on national governments for patronage and, in fact, is interfaced with political entities at all levels: local, national, and international. The national governments of the westernized world are involved with defense, war readiness (some engaged in active combat), and large corporate military suppliers. Therefore, one could argue that the military industries, the government, and the Red Cross are all tied together.

Whatever the merits of the argument, **Socialists** take the position that war is a method to resolve capitalistic quarrel, waged for economic gain. Any national body associated with the military is itself seen as a militaristic organization. It is not altogether surprising, then, that a socialist artist would equate an established national military with the Red Cross and be opposed to both. The postcard is done in socialist colors (red and black).

The real photo, taken during World War I, 15 years before the postcard in Figure 3.80, can be seen to support the Socialist argument. Here, the Red Cross is acting more or less like a government agency (which it is not), by selling war stamps and turning over the proceeds to the U.S. government for military purposes. The posters in the photo declare that savings stamps must be purchased to ensure victory. The good citizen is given the choice of supporting either poverty and autocracy or the war effort. The safety of the children depends on making the correct decision. In the foremost poster, a little girl is leaning on a giant arm whose strong fist is holding the Torch of Victory. The Torch is anchored in the word "BUY."

Continuing the argument for the Red Cross as a military organization, since the Red Cross has recruited thousands of women for the Army Nurse Corps, some of its poster art can be construed as a form of military enlistment propaganda. In 1917, the American Red Cross became so identified with the war effort that Louis Nagler, the assistant Secretary of State for Wisconsin, was jailed for obstructing military efforts in wartime after making disparaging remarks about the Red Cross, accusing it of being a "bunch of grafters" working for war-mongering capitalists (Hutchinson, 1998, p. 268–275).

Even **Florence Nightingale** on at least one occasion had misgivings concerning the Red Cross Society's potential for facilitating war. In reply to one of Henry Dunant's first letters to her, in 1864, she wrote "such a society would take upon itself duties which ought to be performed by the government of each country and so would relieve them of responsibilities which really belong to them and which they can properly discharge and being relieved of which would render war more easy," (Nightingale, F., 1864, in Hutchinson, 1998, p. 350).

3.81. *Associazione Voluntari Italiani del Sangue* (AVIS), the Italian Voluntary Blood Donors Association, is a national-level association with branches all over Italy. It was begun in the 1920s on the initiative of a physician, Dr. Vittorio Formentano, and it subsequently became the largest blood donors' association in Italy (AVIS, 2000).

3.82. The right panel is typical of a good **Italian glamour** card. The design on the left is also Deco, unique and very well done.

3.83. *Littoriali della Cultura e dell'Arte* was a Fascist organization, basically a debating society on cultural and art topics. The *littore* was a Roman junior official who carried around the fasces. In Mussolini's time, you were named a *littore* if you won a series of competitive contests. The Littoriali belonged to the GVF (*Gruppi Universitari Fascisti*—Fascist University Groups) and sponsored the sports medicine convention (Merriam, 2002).

3.84. Founded in 1899, the **International Council of Nurses** (ICN) is a federation of national nurses' associations representing nurses in more than 120 countries. Operated by nurses for nurses, ICN works "to ensure quality nursing care for all, sound health policies globally, the advancement of nursing knowledge, and the presence worldwide of a respected nursing profession and a competent and satisfied nursing workforce (ICN, 2002)." The ICN, headquartered in Geneva, Switzerland, holds an International Congress annually. The host organization for the convention commemorated on the postcard was the **Japanese Nursing Association.** The convention, the first ICN Congress in Asia, was held from May 30 to June 3, 1977, and had 11,470 participants (Santos, 2002).

3.85. In 1968, **Palestinians** began using **Lebanon** as a base for activities against Israel. The first **Israeli retaliatory raid of Beirut** by Israeli forces took place in December of that year. Since then, Israel has mounted several incursions into Lebanon. On June 7, 1982, during the

Lebanese Civil War (1975–1990), following an attempted assassination of the Israeli ambassador to the United Kingdom, Israel launched a full-scale invasion of Lebanon.

On September 14, 1982, Lebanese president-elect Bashir Gemayel, leader of the right wing Phalangist movement, was assassinated by a bomb for which the Palestinians were initially blamed. (Actual responsibility for the bombing has never been established.) The following day, Israeli forces moved into West Beirut. On September 16–18, in the worst atrocity of the 15-year civil war, the Phalangist (Arab) Christian militia, commanded by Elie Hobeika, was allowed into the Sabra and Chatila refugee camps by the Israelis. The militia then proceeded to massacre more than 1000 Palestinian refugees. The first contingent of a mainly U.S., French,

and Italian peacekeeping force, requested by Lebanon, arrived in Beirut on September 24, 1982. The postcard was issued in 1983 to commemorate the arrival in Lebanon of the Italian contingent of that force.

In 1983 an official Israeli inquiry found that the defense minister, **Ariel Sharon,** bore "personal responsibility." He was forced to resign his portfolio. The inquiry said the massacre was carried out by a Phalangist unit acting on its own, but Israel had allowed it to enter the refugee camps. In 2001, Ariel Sharon was elected Prime Minister of Israel (Guardian Newspapers, U.K., 2002).

3.86. **The first World AIDS** day was held in 1988, sponsored by the **World Health Orga-**

nization. The event is now organized by the Joint United Nations Program on HIV/AIDS (UNAIDS), which was formed in 1996. Since the epidemic began, more than 60 million people have been infected with the virus and over 23 million people have died from causes directly related to it. At the end of 2001, an estimated 40 million people globally were HIV positive (UK National AIDS Trust, 2002).

3.87. **Trevor Brown** (1959–). This postcard is an advertisement for an exhibition of Brown's work at Art Box Keibunsha, a gallery in Kyoto, Japan. Only the nurse's arm and hand appear in the picture. (See also Figs. 2.52 to 2.55.)

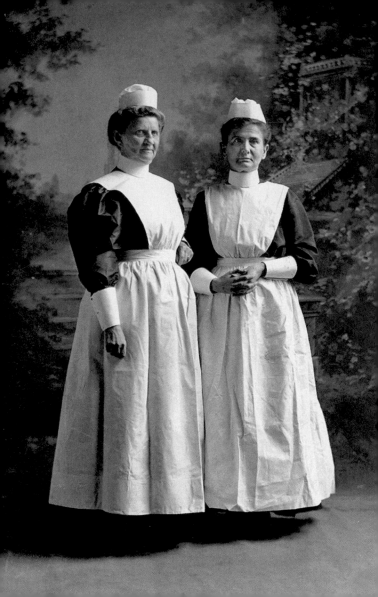

Portraits

*T*his chapter is divided into three segments: ordinary nurses (Figs. 4.1 to 4.56), performers (Figs. 4.57 to 4.75), and royalty (Figs. 4.76 to 4.125).

Black and white portraits of early 20th century nurses are interesting studies in contrasts. Until quite recently, nurses wore starched white caps; not long before caps were phased out, nurses also wore white aprons, skirts, and blouses with highly starched (and often chafing) white collars and cuffs. The shapes and sizes of the cap were quite varied, as were the uniforms themselves. Dozens of styles can be found in any illustrated nursing history book, but not usually in a way that allows direct comparisons. When caps and uniforms are viewed in groups, interesting variations and subtleties appear that are not apparent in single portraits.*

Because the white uniform on a dark ground is so visually compelling, it is easy to overlook the nurse herself. However, if we look beyond the uniform and the (possibly) outdated hairstyle, we see a person who had many of the same concerns we do. She was striving to become better at nursing. She had difficult and trying days, and personally fulfilling days. She was dedicated to her patients and concerned about the state of the health care system. The companions on our professional path are across time, as well as across geography.

This chapter has some conspicuous absences. For one thing, only a few sovereign states are represented. Since the United Kingdom and the United States produced more nursing portrait postcards than other countries, a large proportion of the images are from there. Also, there are no portraits representing the two most significant minority groups in U.S. nursing: African American nurses and male nurses. The contribution made (and being made) by these nurses is unquestionably significant, but, sadly, very few postcard portraits represent them. (Because such postcards are so rare, I have chosen to place them together, starting with Figure 6-25.)

Performers

Nurses portrayed on stage, in the movies, and on television have contributed to the public perception of nursing as much as, if not more than, actual nurses. The presentations, for the most part, have not been favorable. The vast majority of actresses who played nurses in roles other than extras in the movies, both silent and talkie, were cast as love interests. They fell in love with the doctors or vice versa, or they fell in love with the patient or vice versa.

Several excellent early films about nurses showed depth of character, including *Night Nurse* (1931), *Nurse Edith Cavell* (1939), and *So Proudly We Hail* (1943). For the most part, however, the nurse's character has been shallow, limited to a few endearing or not-so-endearing traits. If they were not involved in romance, the nurses provided laughs, were victims of criminals, or, in some cases, were criminals themselves.

During both world wars, and in movies about those wars, nurses were shown as sacrificing heroines, angels of mercy, and occasionally as substitute mothers for the boys overseas. Nevertheless, for the most part, they continued to provide the romantic interest. This trend has continued into the 21st century. The first movie of the 21st century about nurses was *Pearl Harbor* (2001), in which nurse Evelyn Stuart, played by Kate Beckinsale, is the woman in a love triangle involving both the male co-stars.

*NOTE: The portraits in Figures 4.1 to 4.21 are all of United States nurses. Figures 4.22 to 4.48 are of nurses worldwide. See if you can guess the country by the uniform before looking at the key below the images.

Following World War II, nurses were shown as maternal, unassertive, submissive, and domestic. Postwar society did not support autonomous women. In the 1960s, as sexual content in the movies became more explicit, nurses became sex objects. (Nurses had been sex objects before, of course, since the days of vaudeville and slapstick, when they played lewd or scantily dressed assistants opposite lecherous doctors.)

The role of nurses in movies has not changed much since movies were introduced. Nurses are more realistically depicted in television drama, but even there one finds a fine line between soap opera and prime-time nurse behavior. Even in the somewhat more realistic shows such as *ER,* the interactions are distorted. It is impossible to demonstrate in the media what the average nurse, even the average emergency room nurse, does on the job from day to day. Still, the public will most likely continue to form impressions from what they see on the screen for quite some time to come. (See general note for "Performers" in the notes section.)

Royalty and Aristocracy

The story of royal families reads like the drama in any family history: who was feuding with whom, who absconded with what, who was compassionate and giving, who was insane, and who was honorable. However, the aristocratic houses, in dynasties unbroken for centuries, controlled the land, wealth, and fates of the populace in most of the Western world. The consequences of their acts were potent during the entire 20th century. They affect us still.

The contribution of royalty during the late 19th and early 20th century to nursing cannot be overstated. Royals founded nursing services. They patronized and donated enormous sums from their private wealth to hospitals and nursing schools. They visited and subsidized the poor and the sick and, in not a few cases, trained as nurses themselves. They did so out of genuine caring. They were not subject to re-election; their activities were not calculated to improve their public image.

Queen Eleonore of Bulgaria engaged nurses from Lillian Wald's Henry Street Settlement to teach principles of community nursing to the royal family. The sister of the Tsarina of Russia gave all of her wealth to found a nursing order. Her devotion to that order was so great that she was canonized by the Russian Orthodox Church. She died in a mineshaft where she had been thrown with her relatives by the Bolsheviks, who then dynamited the shaft. She was tending the wounded to the end.

During World War I, many of the royals served as nurses, not just in name, but actually working among the wounded. They changed bloody bandages, carried supplies, and received the last words of the dying. The Empress of Russia and her daughters, and the Queen of Romania and her daughters, all received formal training as nurses and served in their country's hospitals. Princess Mary of England, who was so painfully shy that public appearances actually made her ill, overcame this trait to be a nurse's aide, at age 17, in a war hospital. These are only a few examples of a more widespread trend of the aristocracy's involvement in patient care.

The noble and royal houses of Europe are intricately, and often confusingly, interrelated. Marriages were often arranged to gain influence in a particular court; thus a noble from one house or court might hold a title in several others. I have presented the House of Saxe-Coburn-Gotha, with Queen Victoria as the focal point, as a key to understanding royal descent. Because so much of European royalty is related to them, the notes on Victoria and the mini-biographies of her children provide a good reference for the section on royalty.

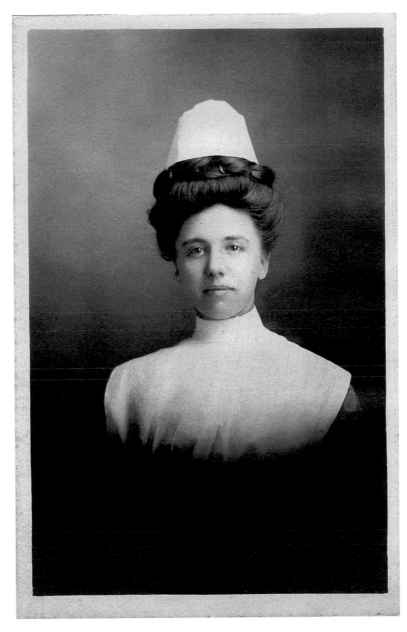

Figure 4.2.

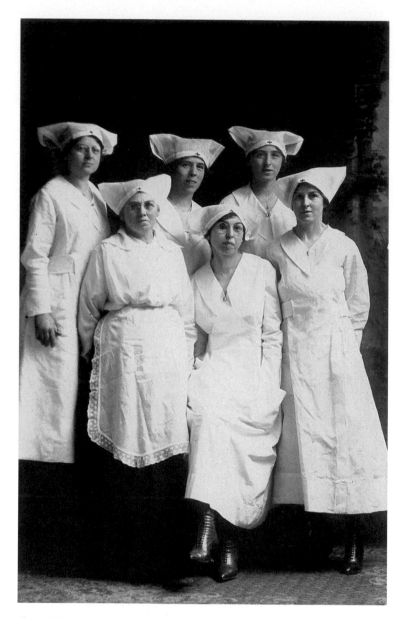

Figure 4.3.

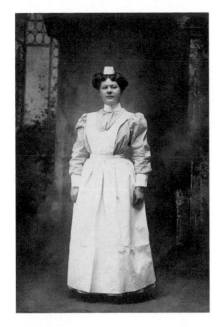

Figure 4.4.

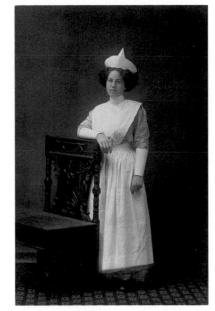

Figure 4.5.

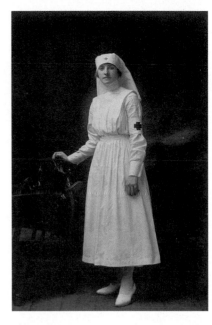

Figure 4.6.

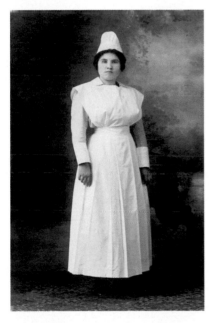

Figure 4.7.

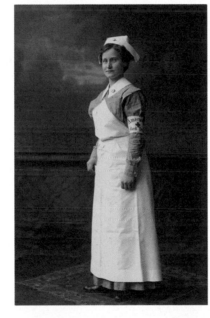

Figure 4.8.

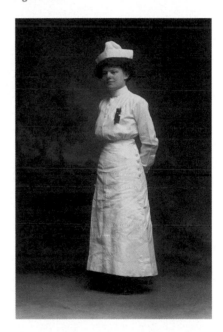

Figure 4.9.

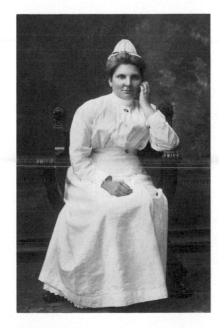

Figure 4.10.

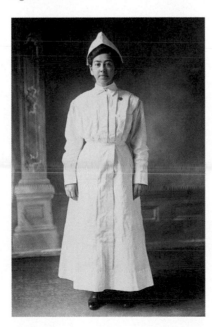

Figure 4.11.

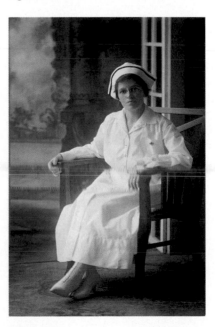

Figure 4.12.

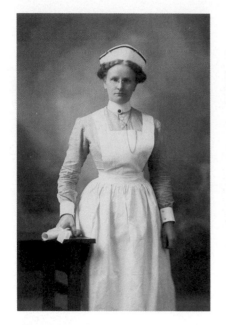

Figure 4.13.

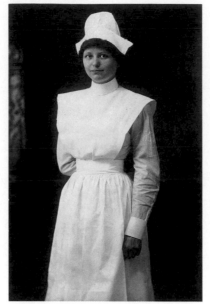

Figure 4.14.

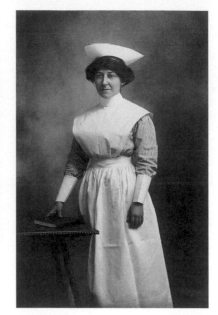

Figure 4.15.

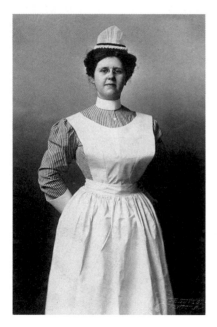

Figure 4.16.

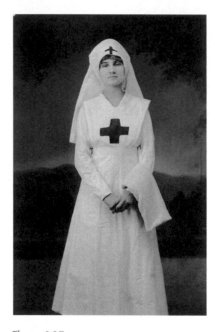

Figure 4.17.

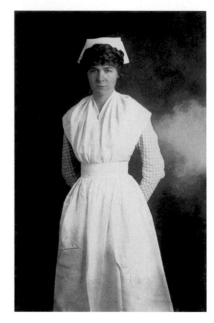

Figure 4.18.

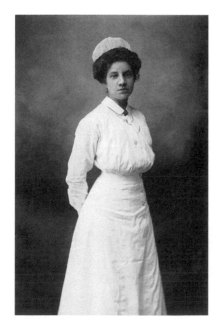

Figure 4.19.

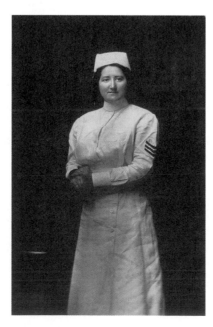

Figure 4.20.

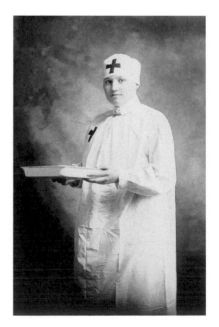

Figure 4.21.

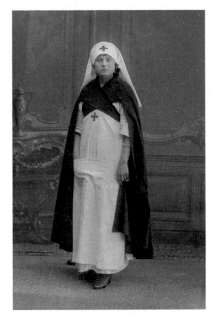

Figure 4.22.

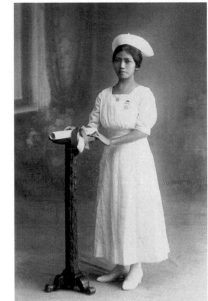

Figure 4.23.

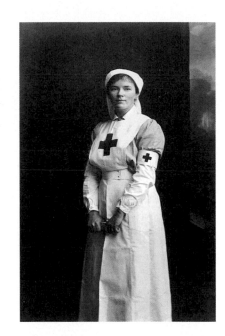

Figure 4.24.

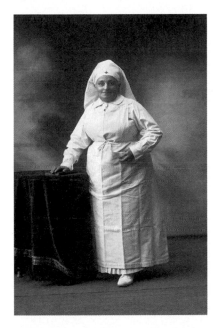

Figure 4.25.

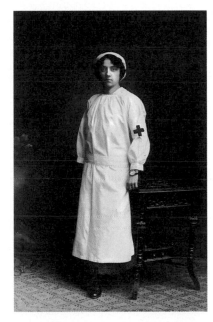

Figure 4.26.

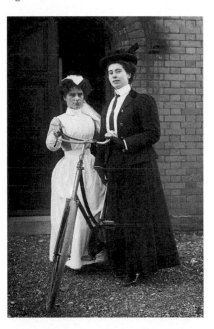

Figure 4.27.

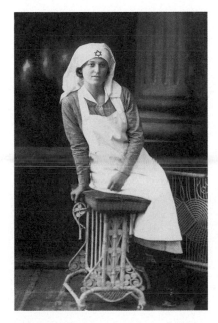

Figure 4.28.

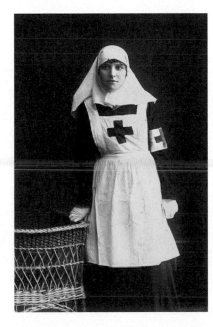

Figure 4.29.

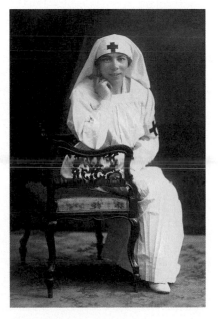

Figure 4.30.

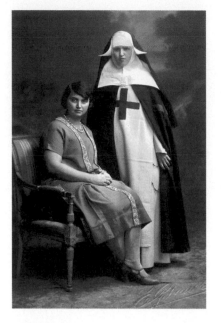

Figure 4.31.

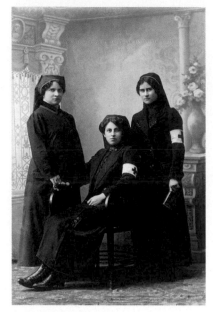

Figure 4.32.

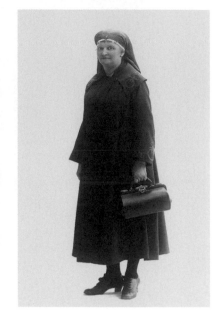

Figure 4.33.

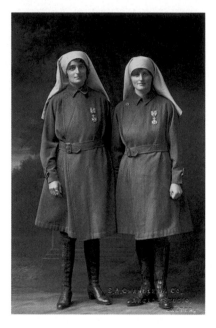

Figure 4.34.

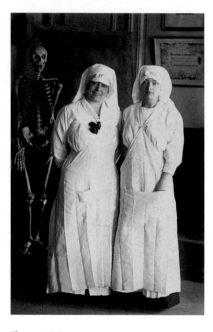

Figure 4.35.

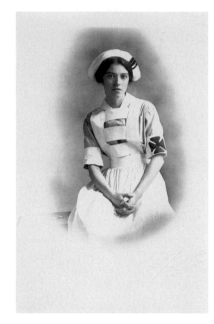

Figure 4.36.

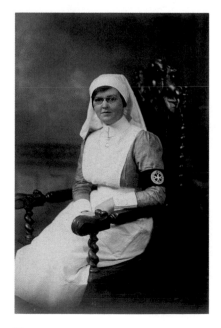

Figure 4.37.

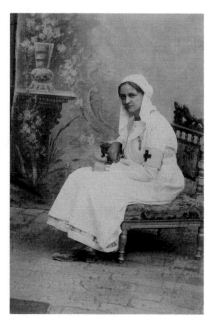

Figure 4.38.

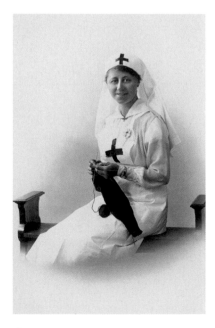

Figure 4.39.

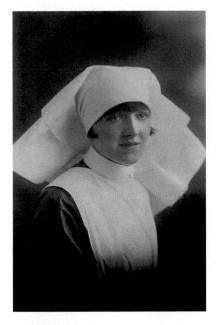

Figure 4.40.

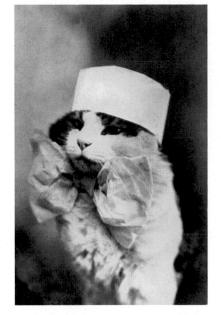

Figure 4.41.

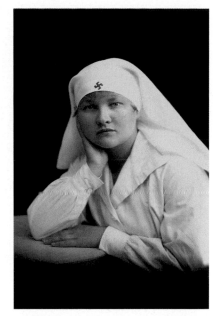

Figure 4.42.

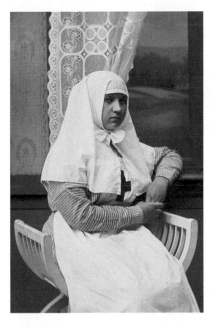

Figure 4.43.

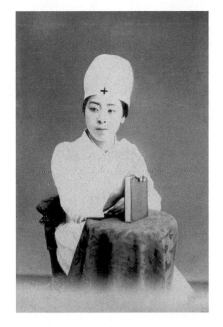

Figure 4.44.

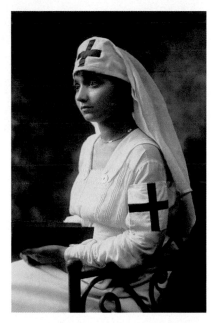

Figure 4.45.

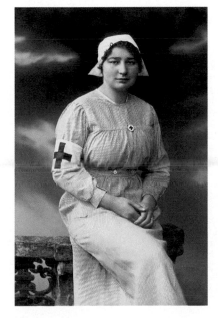

Figure 4.46.

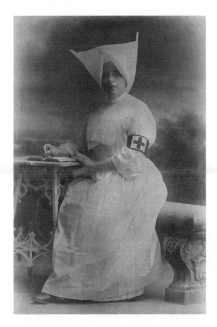

Figure 4.47.

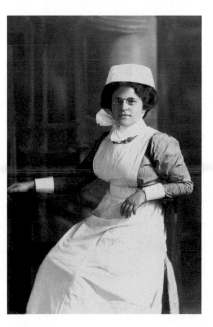

Figure 4.48.

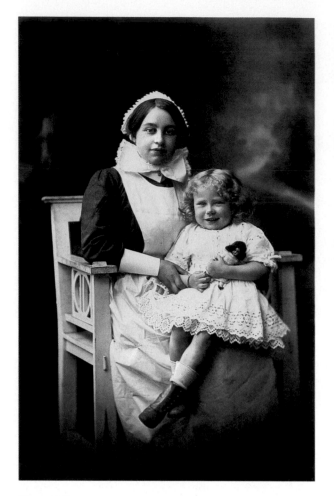

Figure 4.49.
England.

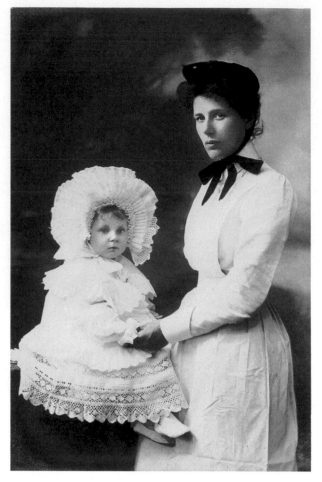

Figure 4.50.
England.

United States 1910–1920

4.1. Unidentified.
4.2. Unidentified.
4.3. Unidentified.
4.4. Unidentified.
4.5. Unidentified.
4.6. Unidentified.
4.7. Unidentified.
4.8. Louise Hoelderlin.
4.9. Mary B. Christie, New York, New York.
4.10. Telluride, Colorado.
4.11. Elizabeth Brownfield, Antioch, Ohio.
4.12. Biddeford, Maine.
4.13. Unidentified.
4.14. Aberdeen, South Dakota.
4.15. Unidentified.
4.16. Harriet E. Mathews, Trenton, New Jersey.
4.17. Unidentified.
4.18. Unidentified.
4.19. Unidentified.
4.20. Unidentified.
4.21. Unidentified.

Worldwide 1910–1924

4.22. France.
4.23. Philippines.
4.24. England.
4.25. England.
4.26. Portugal.
4.27. England. Queen's Nurse.
4.28. Palestine.
4.29. Latvia.
4.30. Belgium.
4.31. France.
4.32. Germany.
4.33. Belgium.
4.34. England.
4.35. France.
4.36. United States.
4.37. England. St. John's Ambulance.
4.38. Yugoslavia.
4.39. United States.
4.40. Matron. England.
4.41. England.
4.42. Latvia.
4.43. Estonia.
4.44. Japan.
4.45. United States.
4.46. Germany.
4.47. France.
4.48. England.

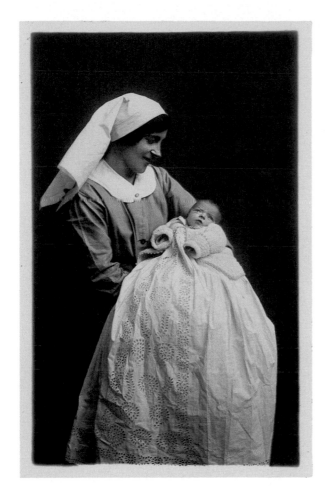

Figure 4.51.
England. 1924.

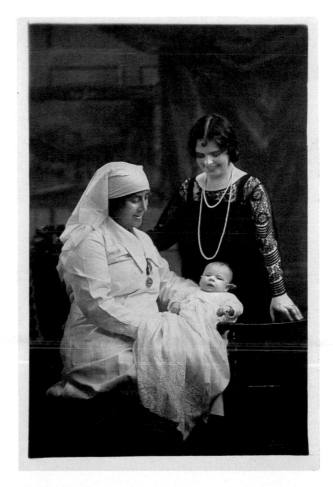

Figure 4.52.
England. c. 1915.

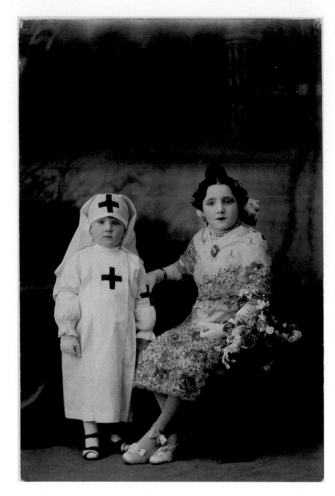

Figure 4.53. Mother and Daughter.
Unidentified European.

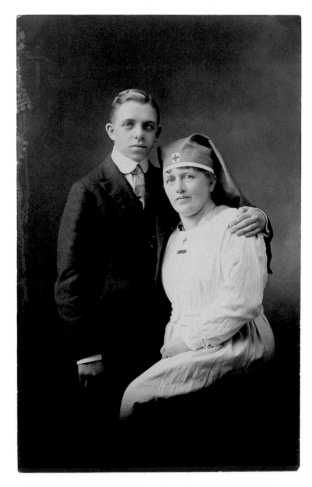

Figure 4.54. "Nurse Brenton with her son Ray Brenton."
United States. c. 1910.

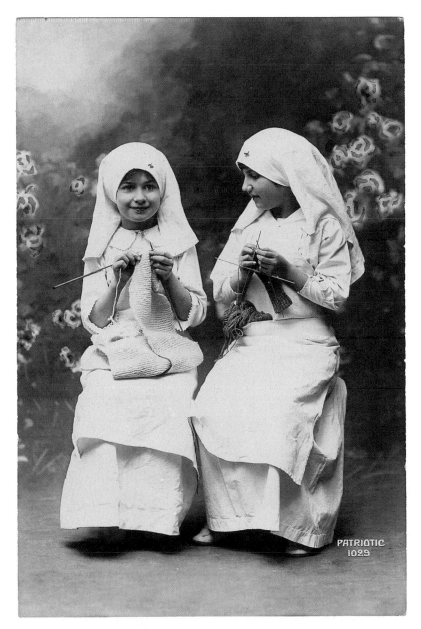

Figure 4.55.
France. c. 1915 *(See note.)*

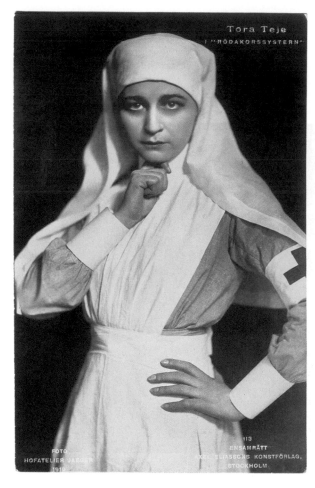

Figure 4.59. Tora Teje. "The Red Cross Nurse."
Sweden. 1919. *(See note.)*

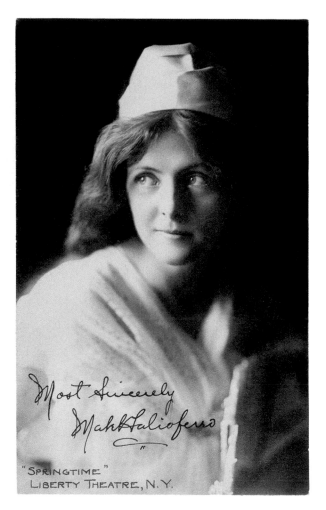

Figure 4.60. Mabel Taliaferro. "Springtime," Liberty Theater, New York.
United States. c. 1917. *(See note.)*

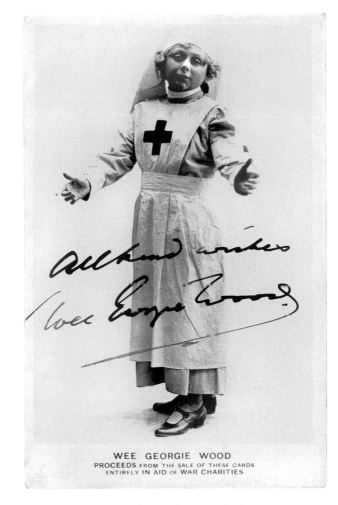

Figure 4.61. **Wee Georgie Wood.** Autographed. England. c. 1916. *(See note.)*

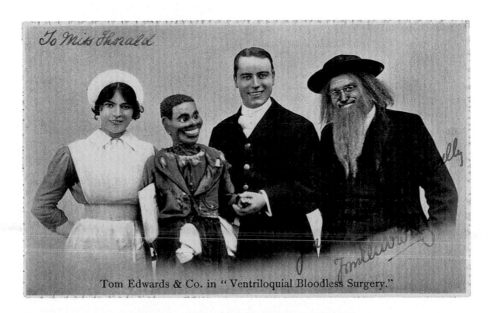

Figure 4.62. **"Tom Edwards & Co. in 'Ventriloquial Bloodless Surgery.'"** United States. 1919. *(See note.)*

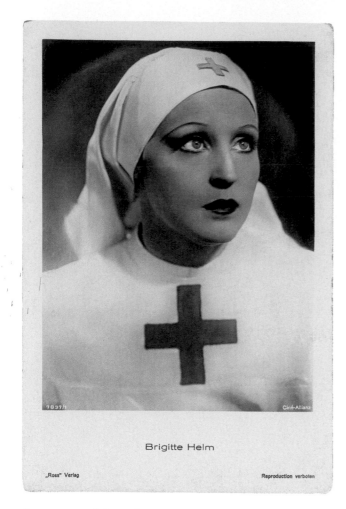

Figure 4.63. **Brigitte Helm.**
Germany. c. 1930. *(See note.)*

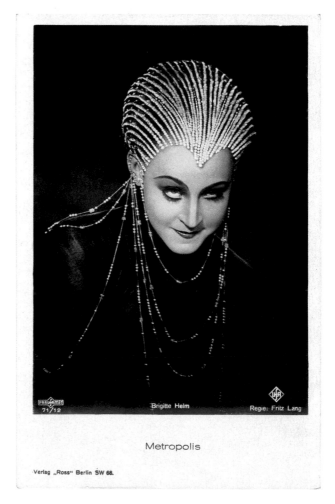

Figure 4.64. **Brigitte Helm. "Metropolis. "**
Germany. 1927. *(See note.)*

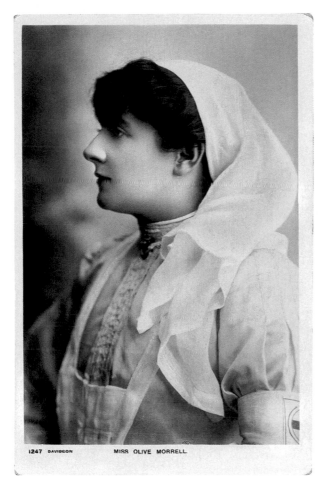

Figure 4.65. **Olive Morrell.**
England. 1908.

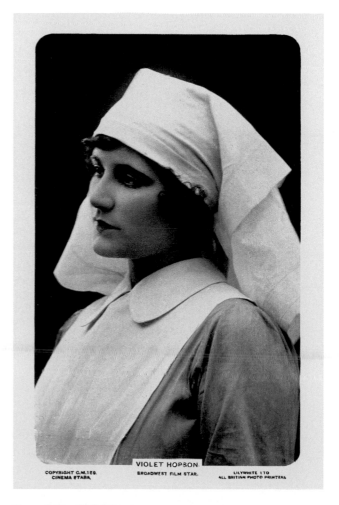

Figure 4.66. **Violet Hopson.**
England. c. 1920. *(See note.)*

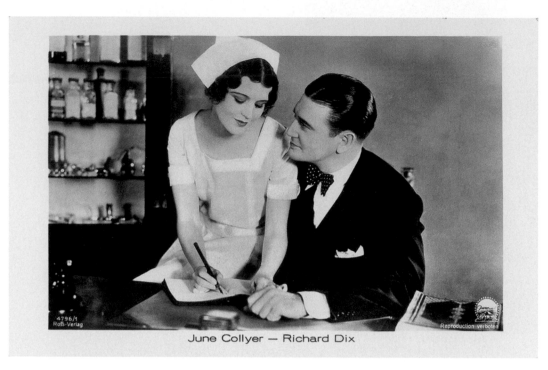

June Collyer — Richard Dix

Figure 4.67. **June Collyer with Richard Dix in "The Love Doctor."**
Germany. 1929. *(See note.)*

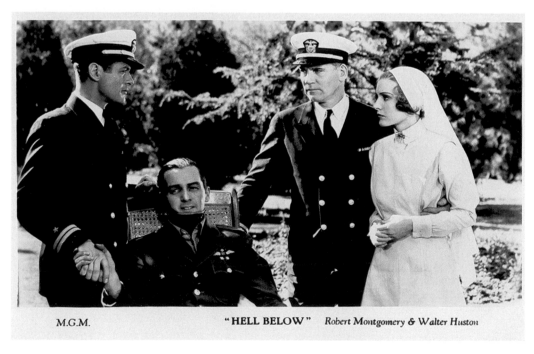

M.G.M.   "HELL BELOW"   *Robert Montgomery & Walter Huston*

Figure 4.68. **Madge Evans in "Hell Below."**
United States. 1933. *(See note.)*

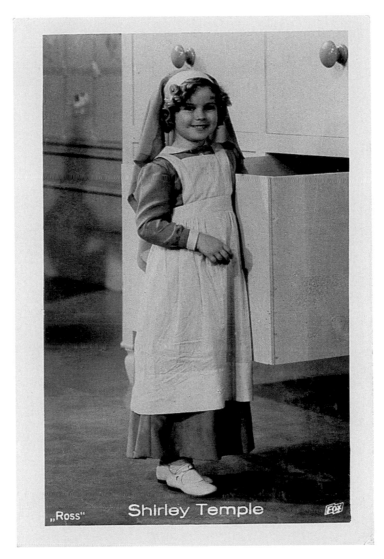

Figure 4.69. **Shirley Temple.**
United States. c. 1935. *(See note.)*

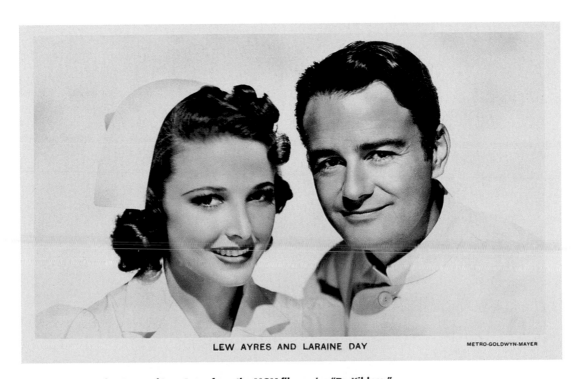

Figure 4.70. **Laraine Day and Lew Ayres from the MGM film series "Dr. Kildare."**
United States. c. 1940. *(See note.)*

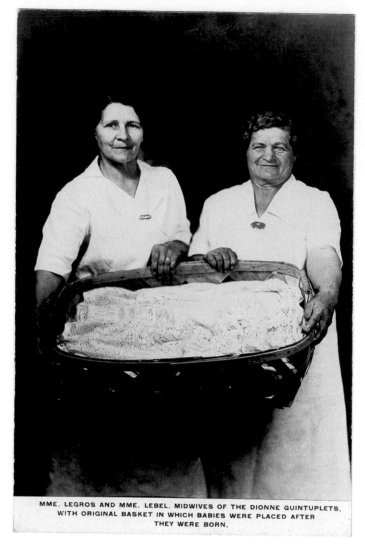

MME. LEGROS AND MME. LEBEL, MIDWIVES OF THE DIONNE QUINTUPLETS, WITH ORIGINAL BASKET IN WHICH BABIES WERE PLACED AFTER THEY WERE BORN.

Figure 4.71. **"Madame Legros and Madame Lebel."**
Canada. 1937. *(See note.)*

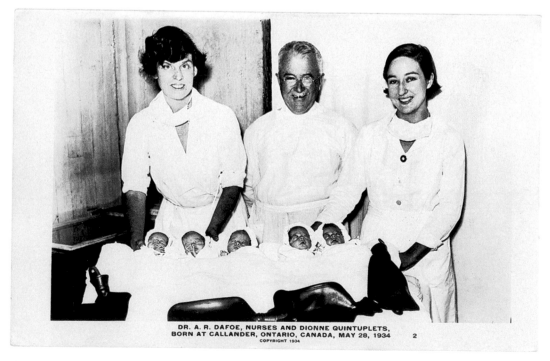

DR. A. R. DAFOE, NURSES AND DIONNE QUINTUPLETS, BORN AT CALLANDER, ONTARIO, CANADA, MAY 28, 1934   2
COPYRIGHT 1934

Figure 4.72. **"Dr. A. Dafoe, nurses and Dionne Quintuplets."**
Canada. 1934. *(See note.)*

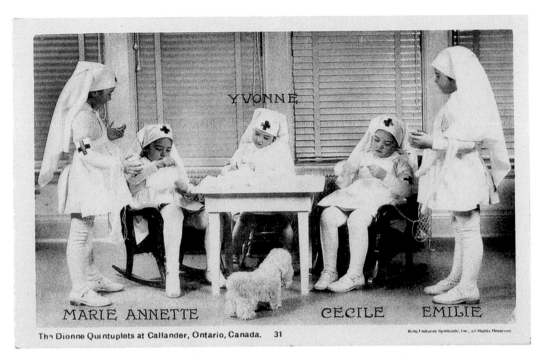

Figure 4.73. **"The Dionne Quintuplets."**
Canada. c. 1942. *(See note.)*

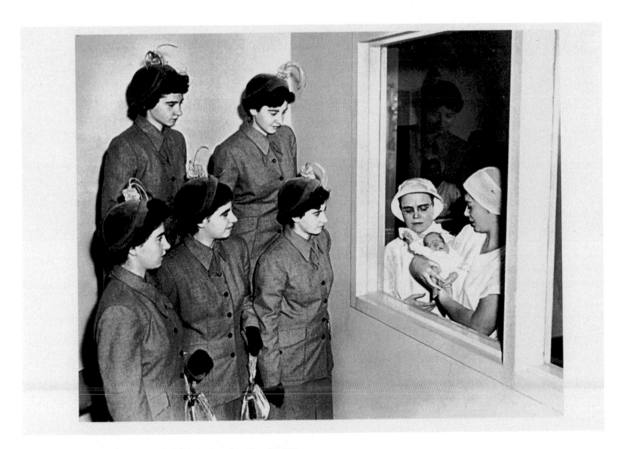

Figure 4.74. **"Quintuplets visit infants ward at Hospital."**
United States. 1996. *(See note.)* Photograph by Ernie Sisto, October 20, 1950.
© The New York Times, used with permission, all rights reserved.

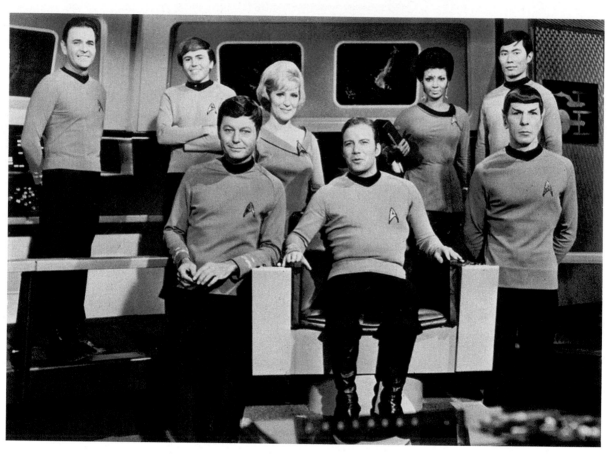

Figure 4.75. **Majel Barrett Roddenberry as Head Nurse Christine Chapel and other officers on the bridge of Federation starship U.S.S. Enterprise NCC-1701.** *(See note.)*

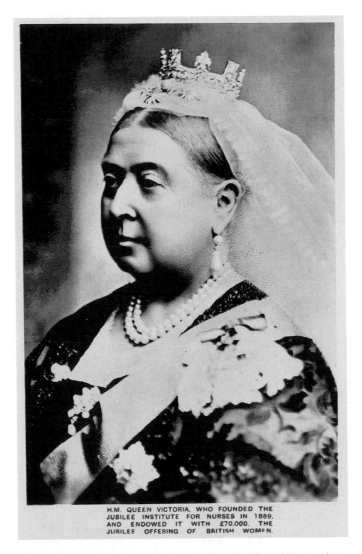

H.M. QUEEN VICTORIA, WHO FOUNDED THE
JUBILEE INSTITUTE FOR NURSES IN 1889,
AND ENDOWED IT WITH £70,000. THE
JUBILEE OFFERING OF BRITISH WOMEN.

Figure 4.76. **"H.M. Queen Victoria, who founded the Jubilee Institute for Nurses in 1889 and endowed it with £70,000. The Jubilee Offering of British Women."**
England. 1927. *(See note.)*

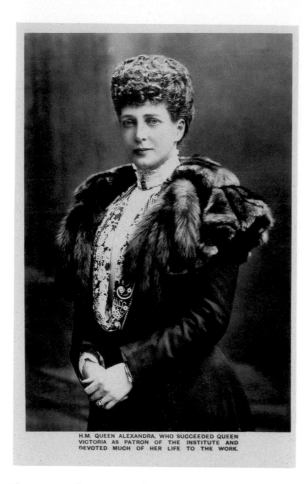

Figure 4.77. "H.M. Queen Alexandra, who succeeded Queen Victoria as Patron of the Institute and devoted much of her life to the work."
England. 1927. *(See note.)*

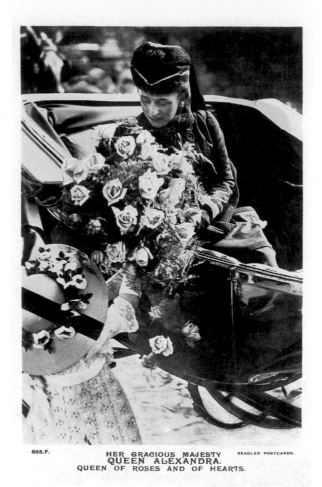

Figure 4.78. "Her Gracious Majesty, Queen Alexandra, Queen of Roses and of Hearts."
England. 1927. *(See note.)*

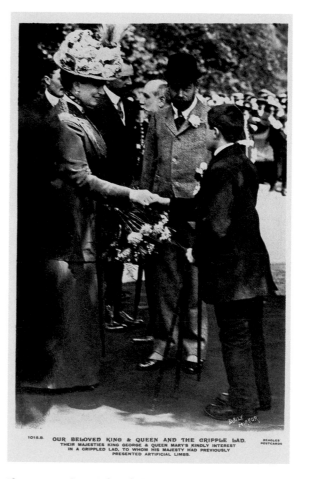

Figure 4.79. "H.M. Queen Mary, now patron of the Institute for Nurses. Her Majesty, together with the King, has approved the present National Memorial Scheme."
England. 1927. *(See note.)*

Figure 4.80. "Our Beloved King and Queen and the Cripple Lad. Their Majesties King George and Queen Mary's kindly interest in a crippled lad to whom His Majesty had previously presented artificial limbs."
England. c. 1919. *(See note.)*

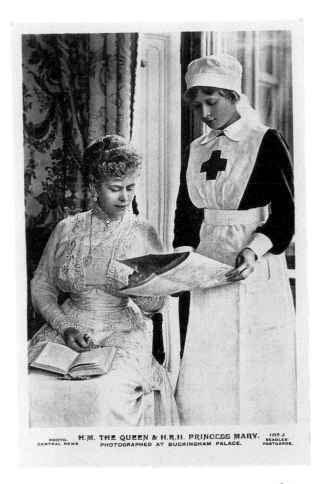

Figure 4.81. "H.M. the Queen & H.R.H. Princess Mary photographed at Buckingham Palace."
England. c. 1915.

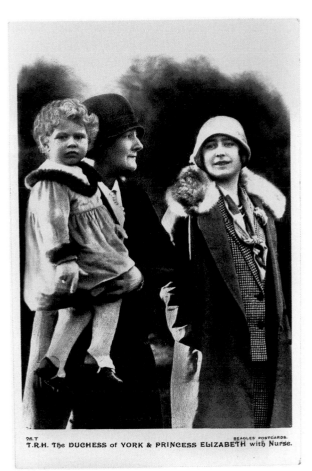

Figure 4.82. The Duchess of York [The Queen Mother to Queen Elizabeth II] and Princess Elizabeth [Queen Elizabeth II] with Nurse [Mrs. Clara Knight].
England. 1936. *(See note.)*

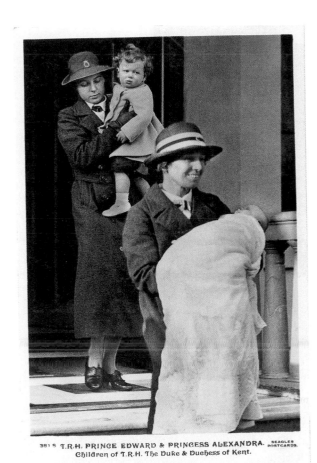

Figure 4.83. T.R.H. Prince Edward and Princess Alexandra [grandchildren of King George V].
England. 1936. The woman carrying the Prince is a nanny; the woman carrying the Princess is a nurse. *(See note.)*

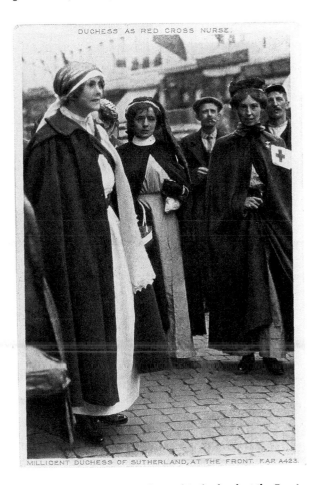

Figure 4.84. Millicent, Duchess of Sutherland, at the Front.
1914. *(See note.)*

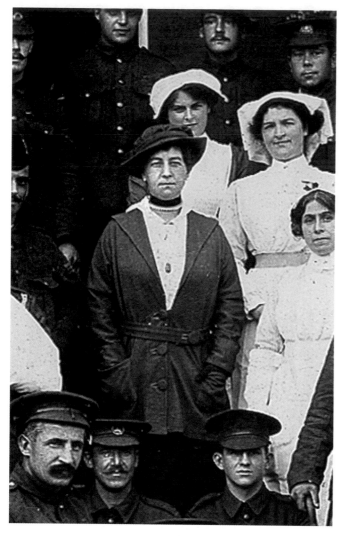

Figure 4.93. **Her Imperial Highness Grand Duchess George of Russia. Detail of Fig. 4.94.**
England. c. 1915. *(See note.)*

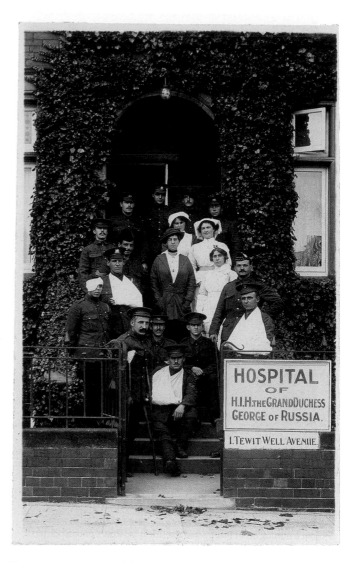

Figure 4.94. **Her Imperial Highness Grand Duchess George of Russia.**
England. c. 1915. *(See note.)*

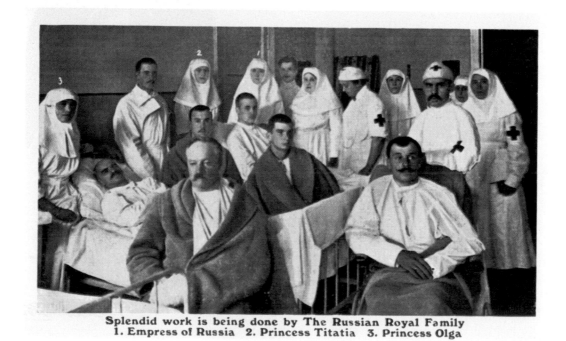

Figure 4.95. **Tsarina Alexandra with daughters Olga and Tatiana**
(spelled incorrectly on the postcard).
Russia. 1914.

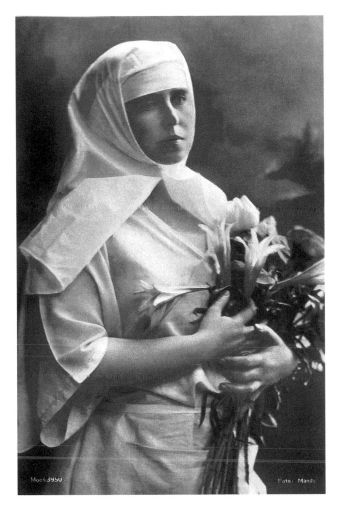

Figure 4.96. **Queen Marie of Romania.**
Romania. c. 1914. *(See note.)*

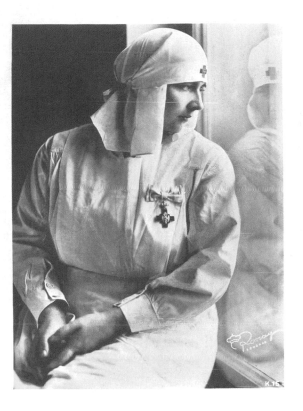

НЬ. В. КРАЉИЦА МАРИЈА.
NJ. V. KRALJICA MARIJA.

Figure 4.97. **Princess Marie.**
Queen Marie of Romania's daughter, here as Queen of Yugoslavia.
Yugoslavia. c. 1926. *(See note.)*

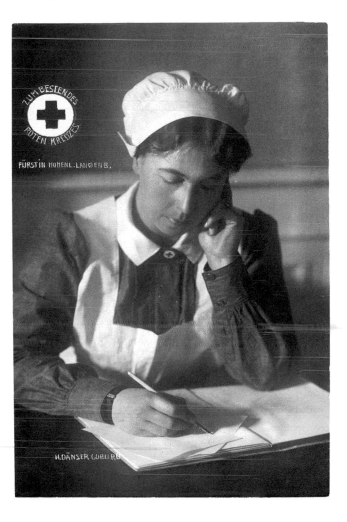

Figure 4.98. **Princess Alexandra of Saxe-Coburg-Gotha.**
Queen Marie of Romania's sister.
Romania. Germany. c. 1915.

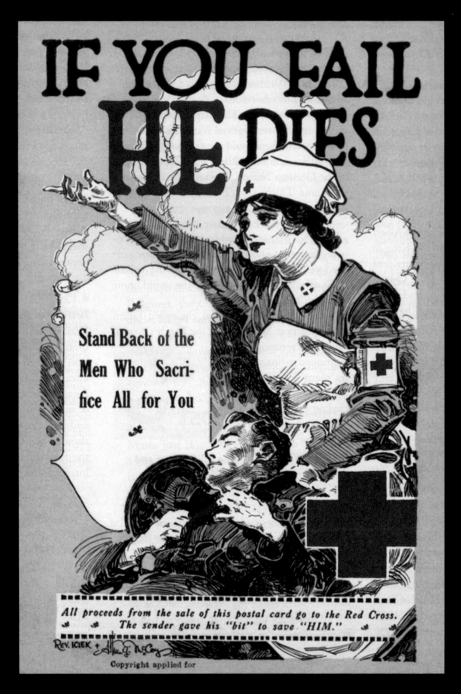

Figure 5.1.
United States. 1917. *(See note.)*

War!

Nursing is depicted on postcards from these 20th-century wars:

Boer War (1899–1902)
Spanish American War (1898)
Russo-Japanese War (1904–1905)
Balkan Wars (1912–1913)
Mexican Incursion (1914–1917)
Russian Civil War (1917–1922)
World War I (1914–1918)
Spanish Civil War (1936–1939)
Sino-Japanese Wars (1937–1945)
World War II (1939–1945)
Korean War (1950–1953)
Vietnam War (1964–1973)
Middle East Conflicts (1970s–1980s)

Not all the above conflicts are represented in this chapter, for various reasons. Postcards of the Balkan War have such inferior graphics that they are not worth including. The Mexican Incursion is included in Chapter 3 because the best nursing postcard that emerged from it is an advertising postcard. The Sino-Japanese war is represented in Chapter 7. Postcards from the later wars are excluded because the art and photography associated with those wars were better represented in other media (eg, newspapers, weekly magazines, and television). The one major exception is postcards from Germany during World War II, because the Nazis exploited every means of propaganda available.

Nursing postcards of World War I are another matter altogether. More nurse-related postcards were issued during World War I than during any other 4-year period in history. In fact, it is likely that the number of nursing postcards issued during World War I is equal to the sum of all other nursing postcards combined.

The experience of war often summons extraordinary bravery and sacrifice, willing or compelled, from its participants. Whenever possible, this section attempts to present those aspects. However, certain images of war, while fascinating in many respects, contain a dangerous deceit. The fear and suffering of tormented victims is abstracted, kept cosmetic, even when the scenes depict the wounded and the dead. One can even admire the quality of the image: this photograph has excellent clarity, that painting captures a subtle emotion, and so forth.

War is not a romantic heroic fantasy, as expressed in Rupert Brooke's well-known lines, "If I should die, think only this of me: That there's some corner of a foreign field, That is for ever England. . . ." War is grotesque, not picturesque. We must be careful not to fall into the delusion of thinking otherwise, all the more so since the conditions and ideologies that have fomented war in the past are remarkably similar to those in the present.

World War I

World War I began as a European conflict with Austria-Hungary's declaration of war against the Kingdom of Serbia on July 28, 1914 and escalated within a matter of days to global warfare. Russia mobilized its army in response to Austria's mobilization. Germany demanded that

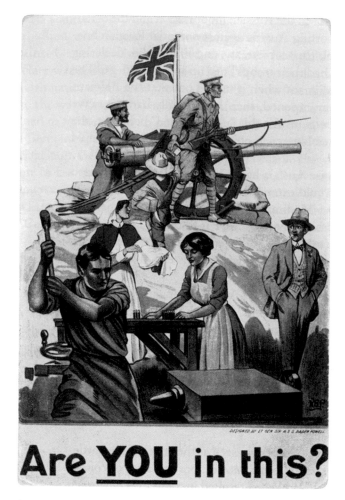

**Figure 5.2. General Sir Robert Baden-Powell (1857–1941).
"Are YOU in This?"**
England. 1914. (See note.)

Baden-Powell was the founder of the Boy Scouts.

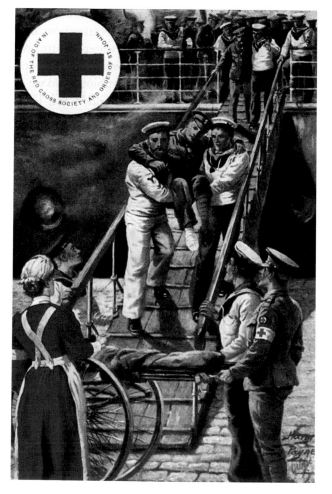

Figure 5.3. Harry Payne (1858–1927).
England. 1915. (See note.)

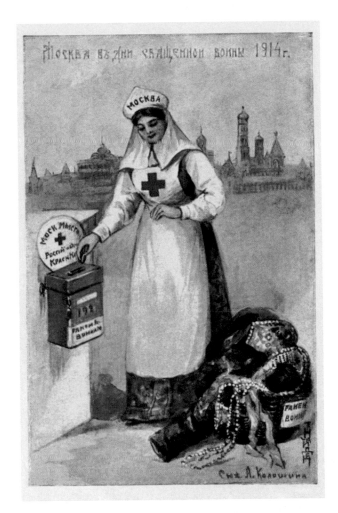

Figure 5.4. **"Moscow. The Holy War of 1914."**
Russia. 1914. *(See note.)*

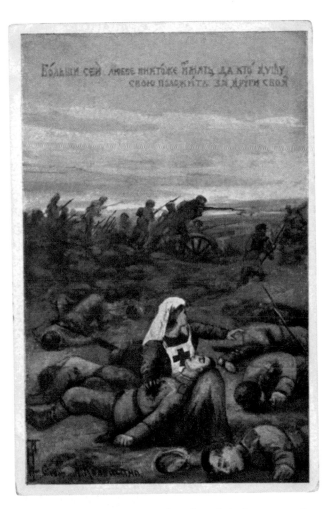

Figure 5.5. **"There is no greater love than that of someone who lays down her life for her friends."**
Russia. 1914. *(See note.)*

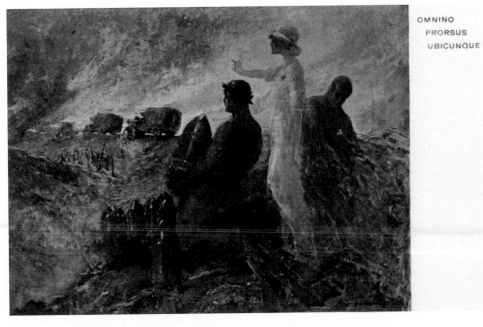

Figure 5.6. **2nd Motor Transport Corps. "Always Forward, Always Ready."**
Italy. 1916.

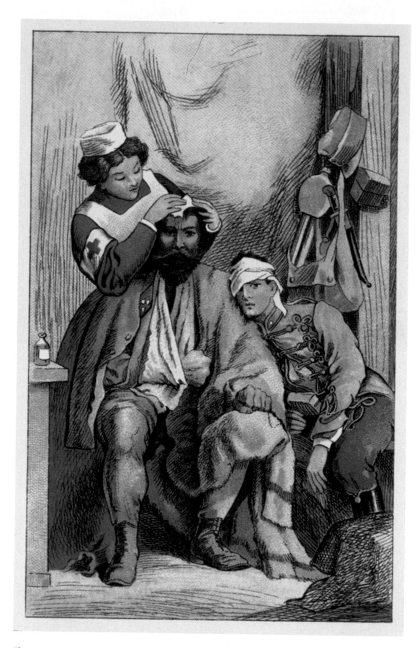

Figure 5.7.
Austria. 1914. *(See note.)*

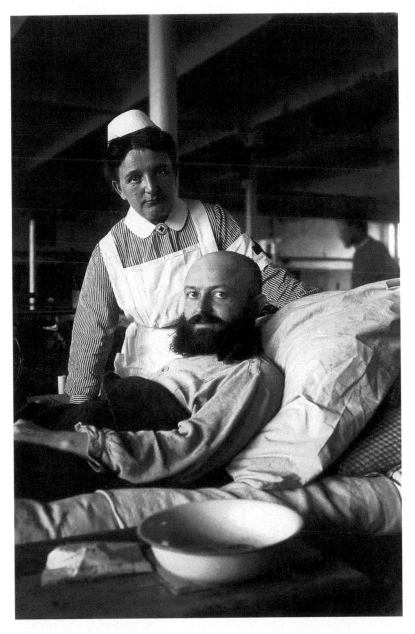

Figure 5.8.
Germany. 1915.

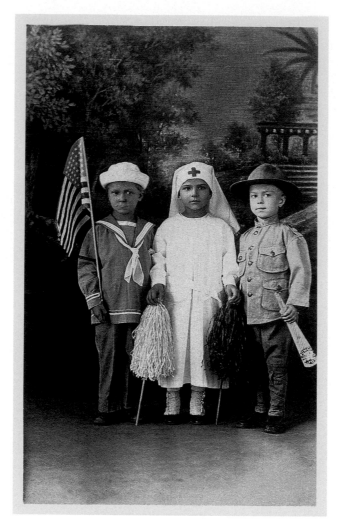

Figure 5.9.
United States. 1917.

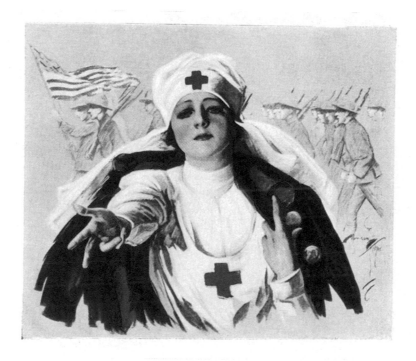

Figure 5.10.   Harrison Fisher (1877–1934). "Have you Answered the Red Cross Christmas Roll Call?"
France. 1920. *(See note.)*

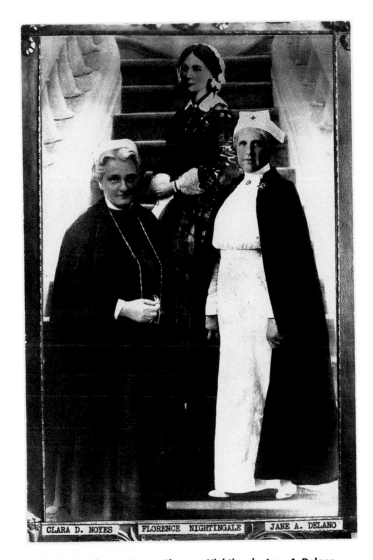

CLARA D. NOYES   FLORENCE NIGHTINGALE   JANE A. DELANO

Figure 5.11.   Clara D. Noyes, Florence Nightingale, Jane A. Delano.
Photo montage.
United States. 1918. *(See note.)*

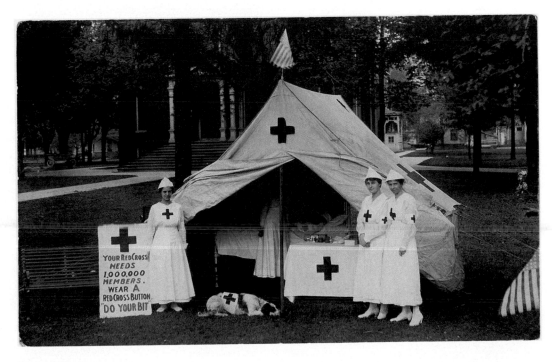

YOUR RED CROSS NEEDS 1,000,000 MEMBERS. WEAR A RED CROSS BUTTON "DO YOUR BIT"

Figure 5.12.
United States. 1917. *(See note.)*

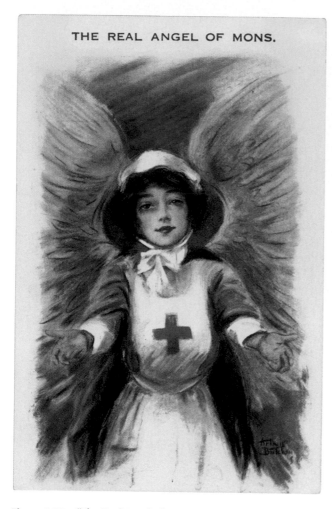

THE REAL ANGEL OF MONS.

Figure 5.13. **"The Real Angel of Mons."**
England. 1915. *(See note.)*

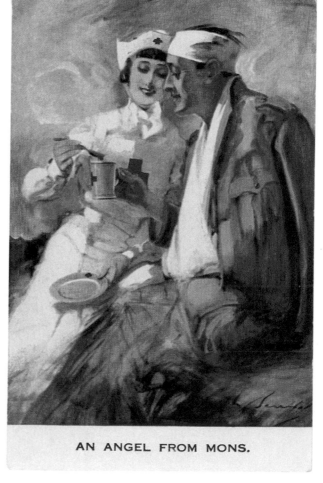

AN ANGEL FROM MONS.

Figure 5.14. **William Barribal (1873–1956). "An Angel from Mons."**
England. 1916. *(See note.)*

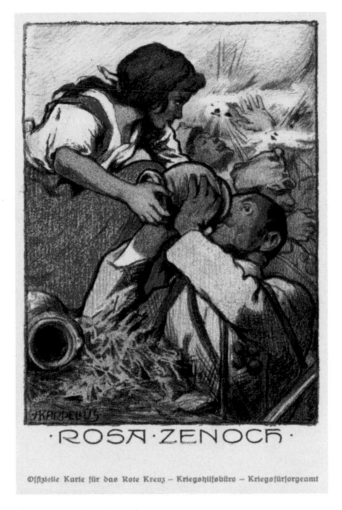

Figure 5.15.   **Rosa Zenoch.**
Austria. 1916. *(See note.)*

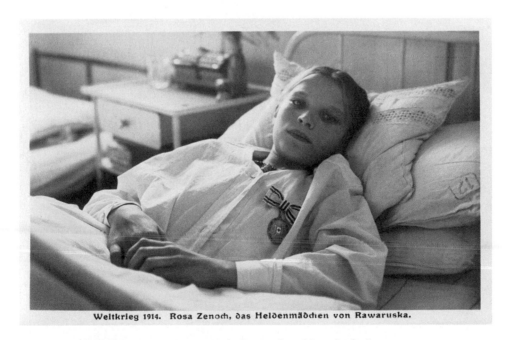

Figure 5.16.   **"World War, 1914. Rosa Zenoch, the Heroine of Rava Ruska."**
Austria. 1914. *(See note.)*

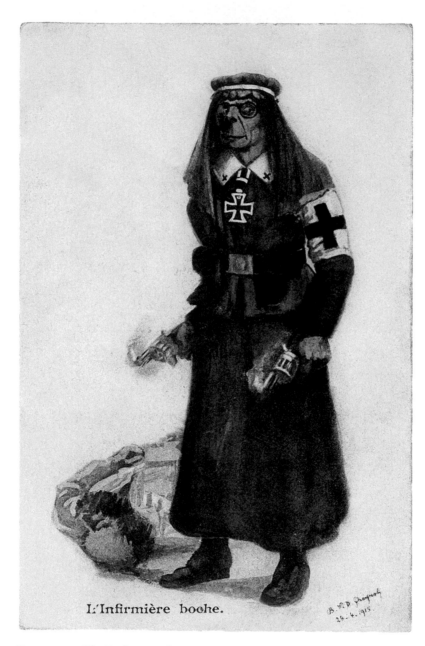

L'Infirmière boche.

Figure 5.17. **"The Boche nurse."**
France. 1915. *(See note.)*

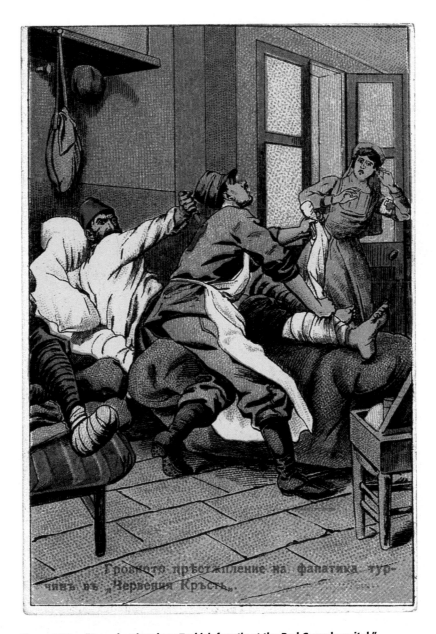

Figure 5.18. **"An ugly crime by a Turkish fanatic at the Red Cross hospital."**
Bulgaria. c. 1915.

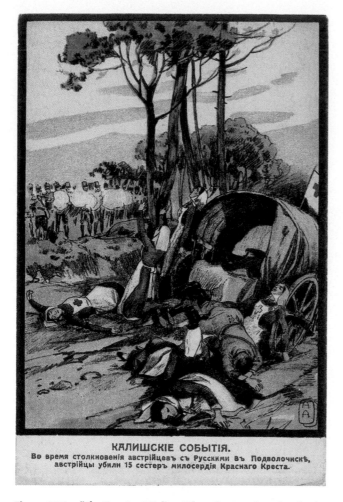

Figure 5.19. **"The Events at Kalisz. When the Austrians fought the Russians at Podvolochisk, the Austrians killed fifteen Sisters of Mercy of the Red Cross."**
Russia. 1914. *(See note.)*

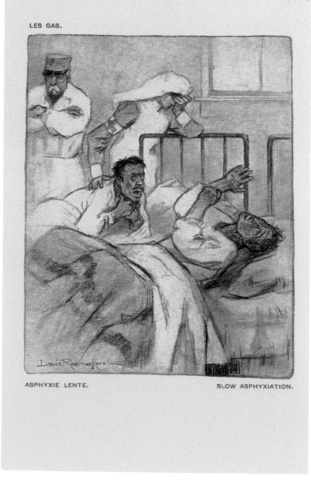

Figure 5.20. **"Gas. Slow Asphyxiation."**
France. c. 1918. *(See note.)*

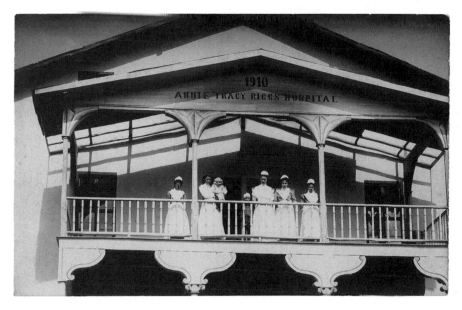

Figure 5.21. **Annie Tracy Riggs Memorial Hospital.** This postcard relates to the Armenian genocide.
Harpoot, Turkey. 1915. *(See note.)*

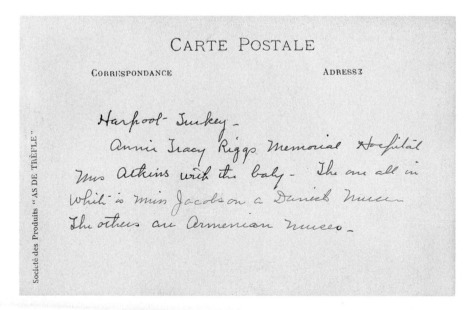

CARTE POSTALE

CORRESPONDANCE   ADRESSE

Harpool- Turkey-
Annie Tracy Riggs Memorial Hospital
Mrs Atkins with the baby- The one all in
white is miss Jacobson a Danish nurse
The others are Armenian nurses-

Société des Produits "AS DE TRÈFLE"

Figure 5.22. **Reverse of Fig. 5.21.**

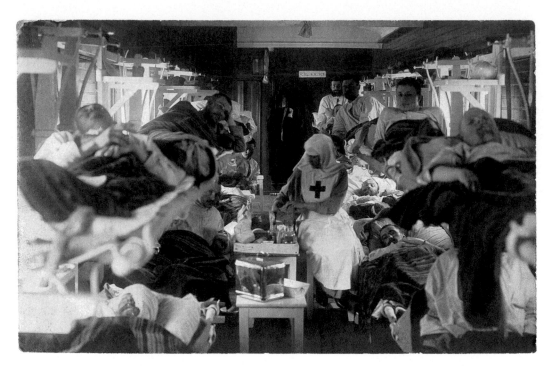

Figure 5.23. **Russian hospital train.**
Russia. c. 1915.

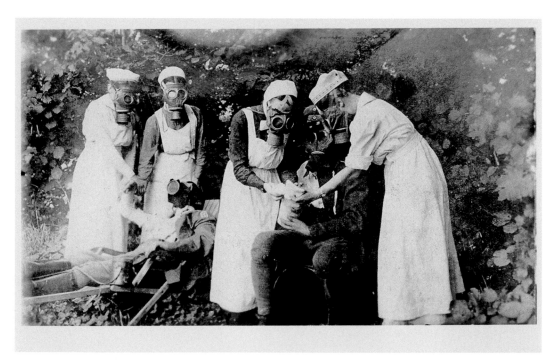

Figure 5.24.
Germany. 1916. *(See note.)*

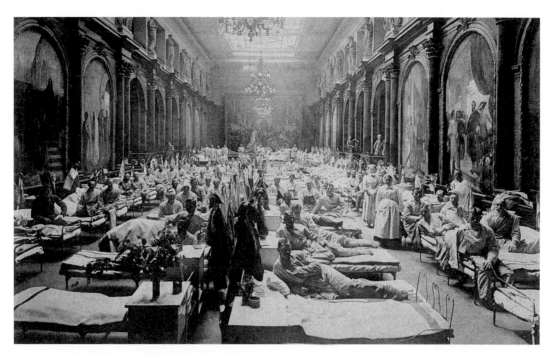

Figure 5.25. *Kriegslazarett II* **(War Hospital), Brussels.**
Palais des Académies. Belgium. c. 1915.

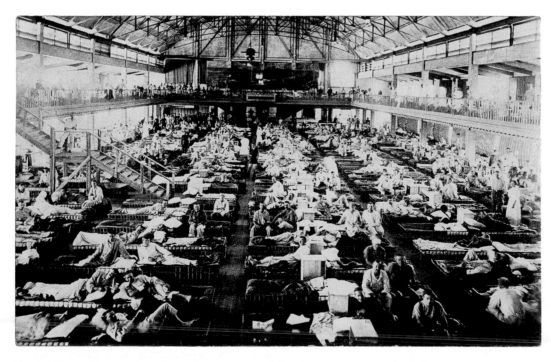

Figure 5.26.
France. c. 1916.

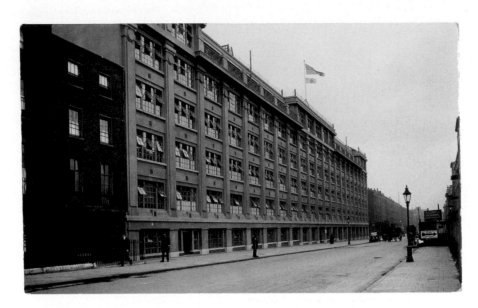

Figure 5.27. **King George Military Hospital. Exterior view of the hospital along Stamford Street.** *(See note.)*

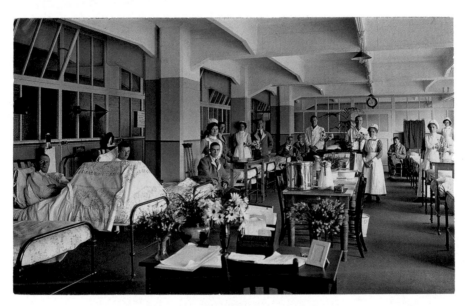

Figure 5.28. **King George Military Hospital. C2 Ward.** *(See note.)*

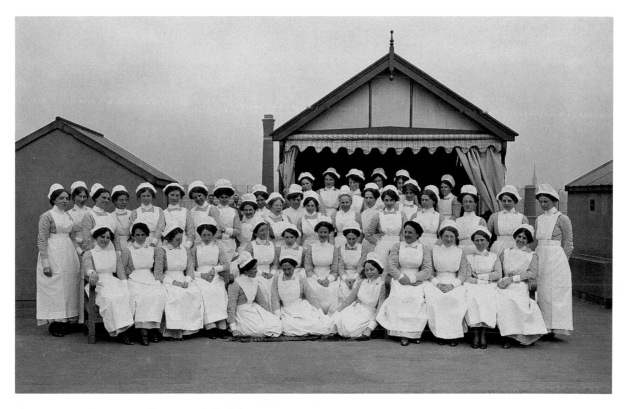

Figure 5.29. **King George Military Hospital. Night nurses.** *(See note.)*

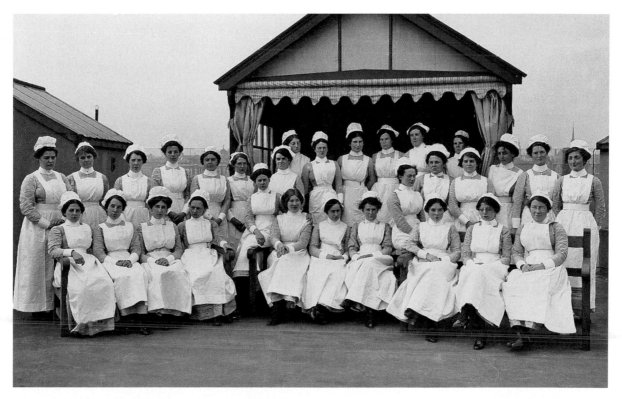

Figure 5.30. **King George Military Hospital. Day nurses.** *(See note.)*

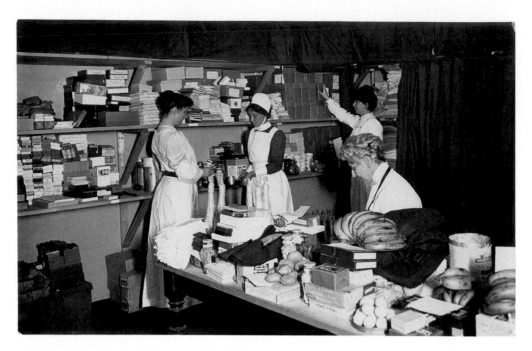

Figure 5.31.   **King George Military Hospital. The Marchioness of Ripon in the receiving commissary.** *(See note.)*

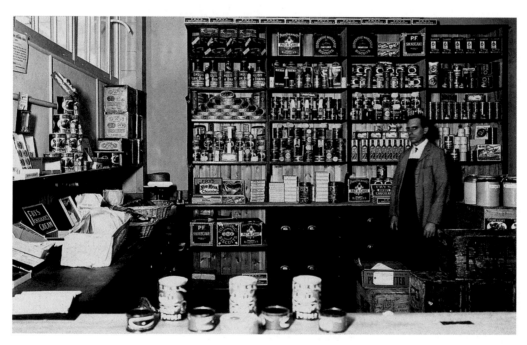

Figure 5.32.   **King George Military Hospital. Hospital gift shop.** *(See note.)*

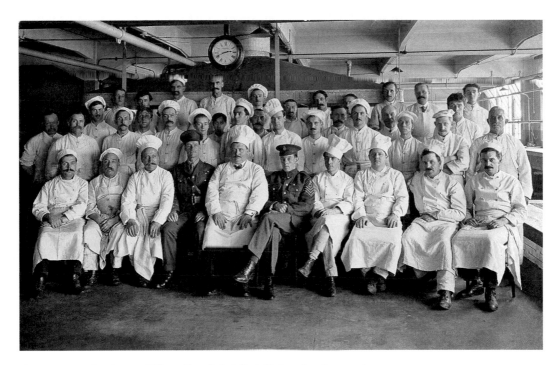

Figure 5.33.   **King George Military Hospital. Full staff of cooks.** *(See note.)*

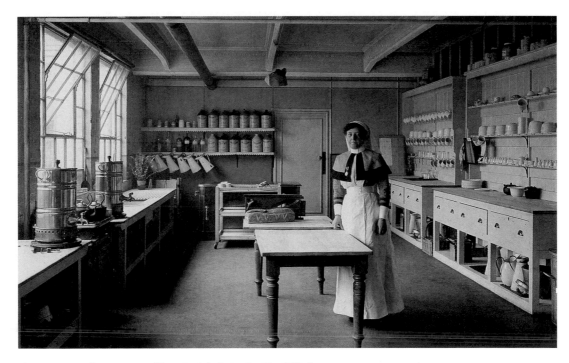

Figure 5.34.   **King George Military Hospital. A5–B5 Ward Kitchen.**
Sister Chapman. *(See note.)*

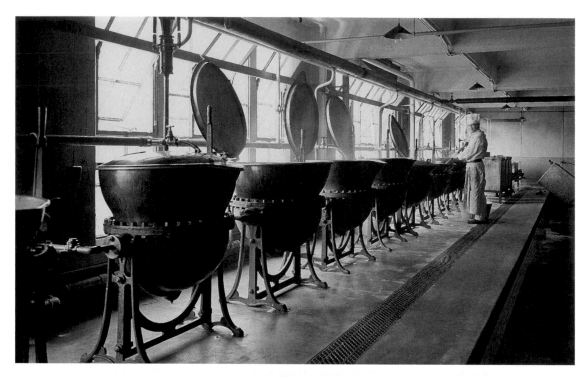

Figure 5.39. **King George Military Hospital. Kitchen coppers.** *(See note.)*

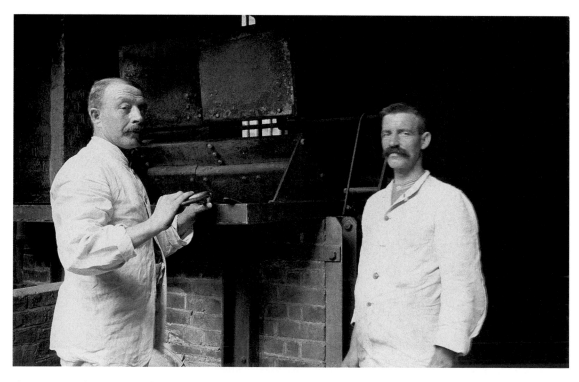

Figure 5.40. **King George Military Hospital. Destructor and staff.** *(See note.)*

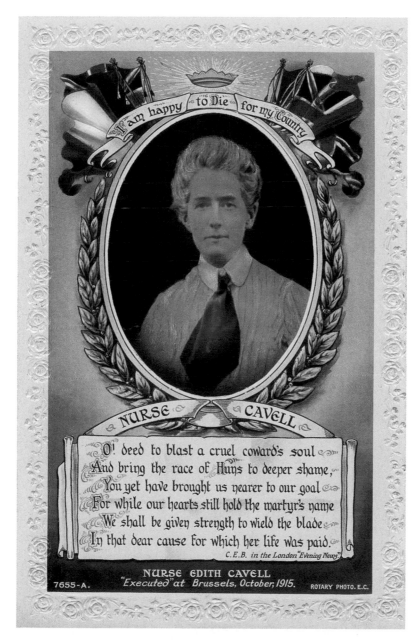

Figure 5.42. **Nurse Edith Cavell.** *(See note.)*

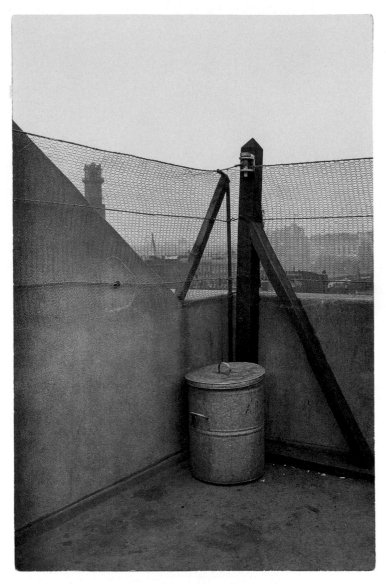

Figure 5.41. **King George Military Hospital. Accident 13-9-15.**
Photo 14-9-15. Temporary restraint. *(See note.)*

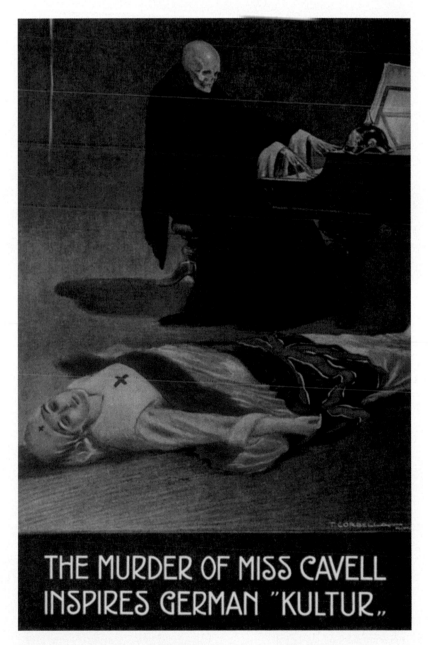

THE MURDER OF MISS CAVELL
INSPIRES GERMAN "KULTUR.„

Figure 5.43. **Tito Corbella (1885–1956). "The Murder of Miss Cavell Inspires German 'Kultur.'"**
England. 1915. *(See note.)*

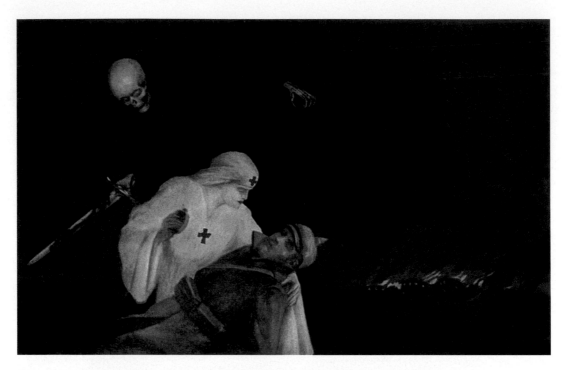

Figure 5.44. Tito Corbella (1885–1956). "'Kultur' threatens Miss Cavell nursing a wounded enemy."
England. 1915. *(See note.)*

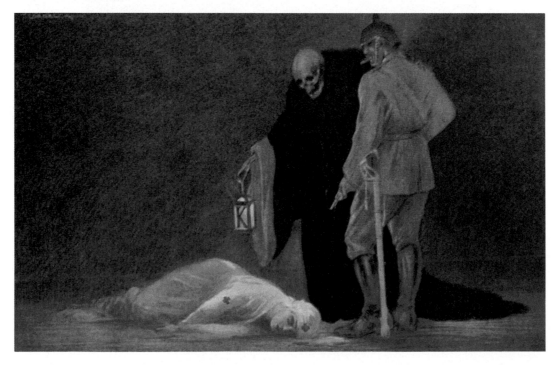

Figure 5.45. Tito Corbella (1885–1956). The Murder. *"Well done,"* *said "Kultur."*
England. 1915. *(See note.)*

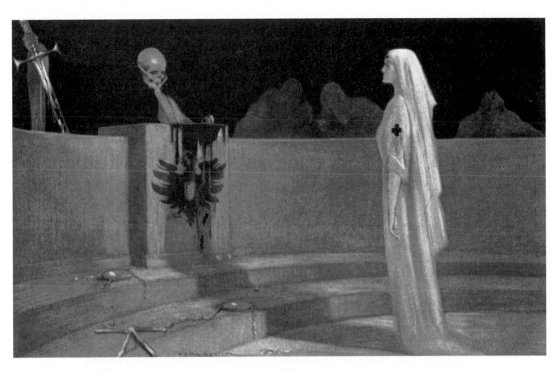

Figure 5.46. **Tito Corbella (1885–1956). "The parody of justice at the court of 'Kultur.'"**
England. 1915. *(See note.)*

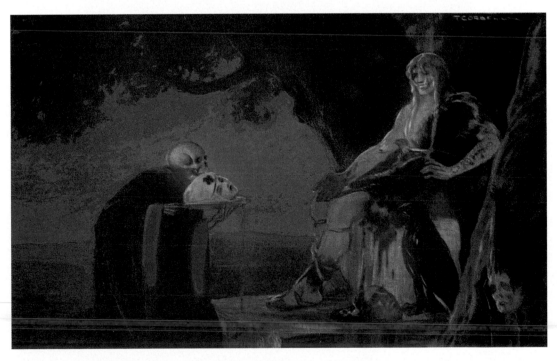

Figure 5.47. **Tito Corbella (1885–1956). "A welcome gift for Kaiser's birthday."**
England. 1915. *(See note.)*

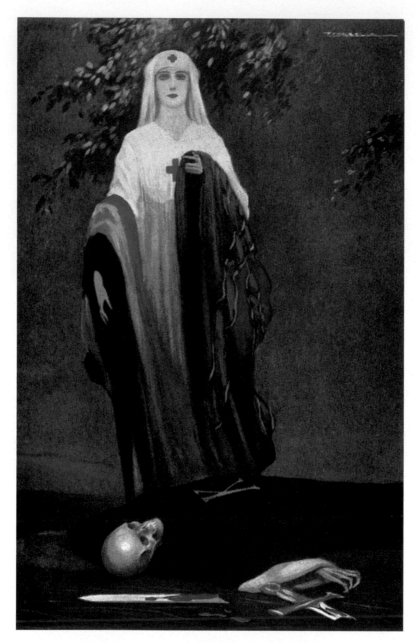

Figure 5.48. **Tito Corbella (1885–1956). "The victory of the victim."**
England. 1915. *(See note.)*

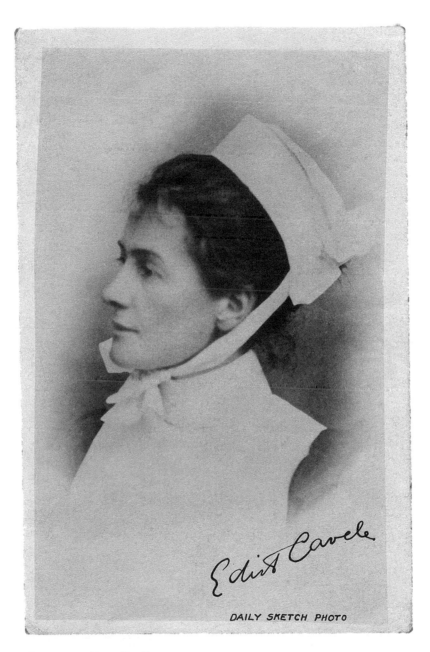

DAILY SKETCH PHOTO

Figure 5.49. Nurse Cavell.
England. 1915. *(See note.)*

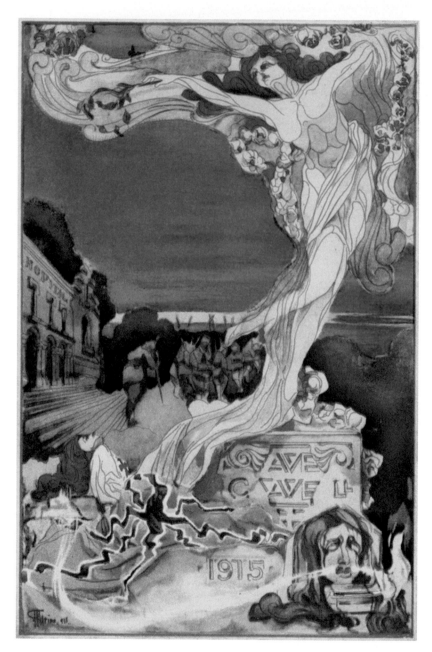

Figure 5.50. **"Ave Cavell."**
Italy. 1916.

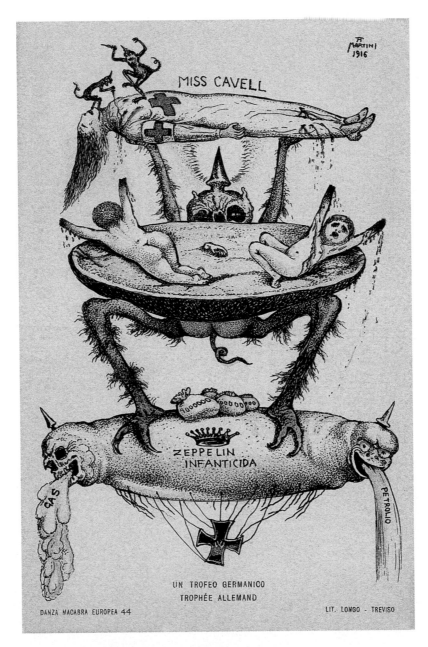

Figure 5.51. A. Martini. "German Trophy."
France. 1915. *(See note.)*

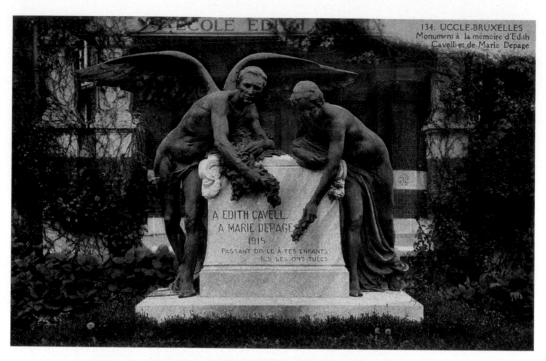

Figure 5.52. **Monument to the memory of Edith Cavell and Marie Depage.**
Belgium. 1920. *(See note.)*

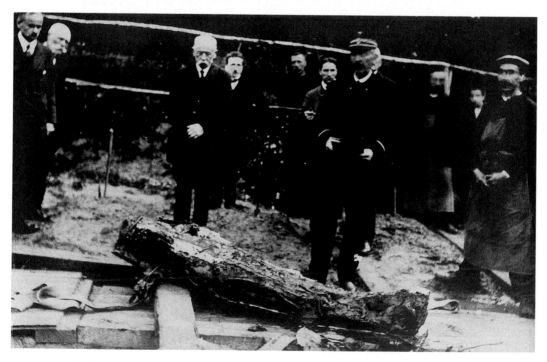

Figure 5.53. **"Miss Edith Cavell disinterment."**
England. 1919.

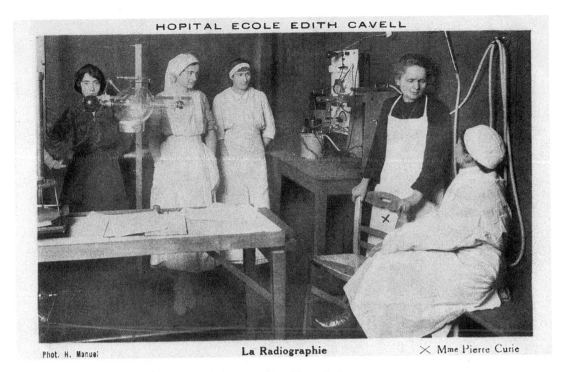

HOPITAL ECOLE EDITH CAVELL

Phot. H. Manuel   La Radiographie   ✕ Mme Pierre Curie

Figure 5.54.   Edith Cavell Hospital School. X-ray. Madame Pierre Curie.
France. 1918. *(See note.)*

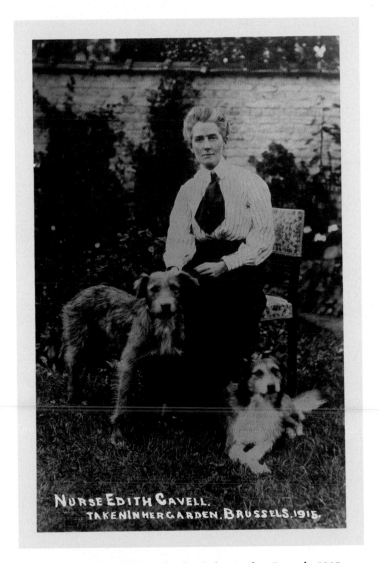

NURSE EDITH CAVELL. TAKEN IN HER GARDEN, BRUSSELS, 1915.

Figure 5.55.   Nurse Edith Cavell, taken in her garden, Brussels, 1915.
England. 1916. *(See note.)*

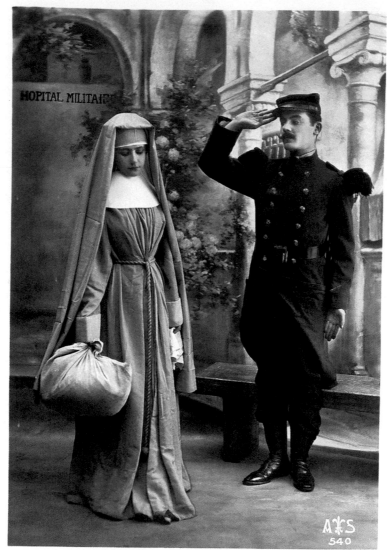

Ces anges des champs de bataille
O France, tu les as chassés !
Qui donc ira sous la mitraille
Un jour relever nos blessés ? –

Figure 5.56.
France. 1914. *(See note.)*

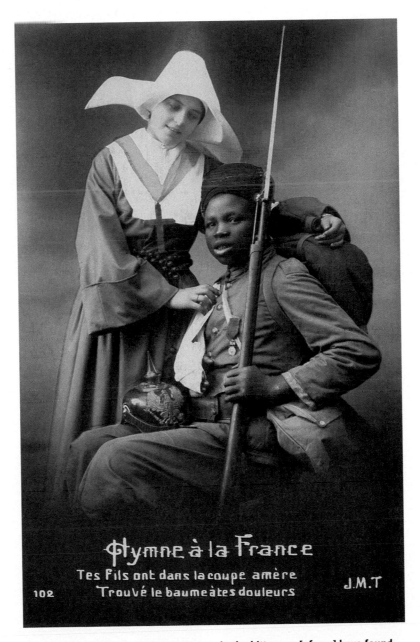

Figure 5.57.   **"Hymn to France. Your sons in the bitter cup [of war] have found balm in your sorrow."**
France. 1914. *(See note.)*

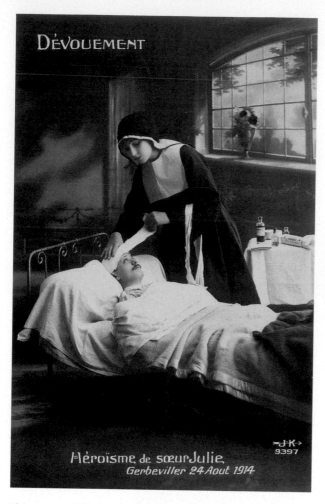

Figure 5.58. **The Heroism of Sister Julie, Gerbeviller, August 24, 1914. "Devotion."** France. 1914. *(See note.)*

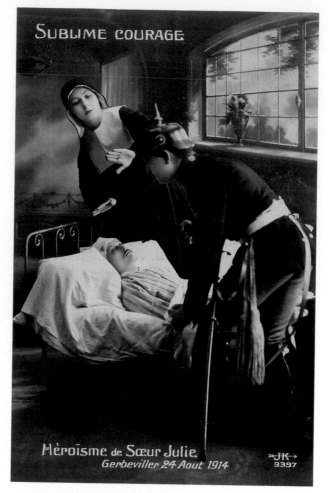

Figure 5.59. **"Sublime Courage."** France. 1914. *(See note.)*

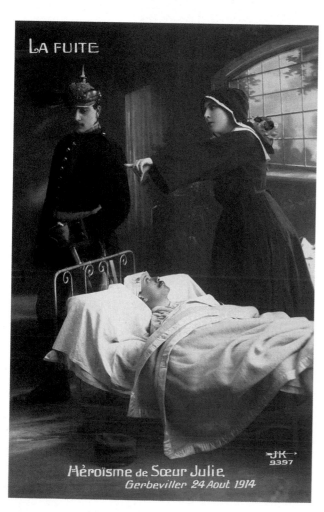

Figure 5.60. **"Admonishment."** France. 1914. *(See note.)*

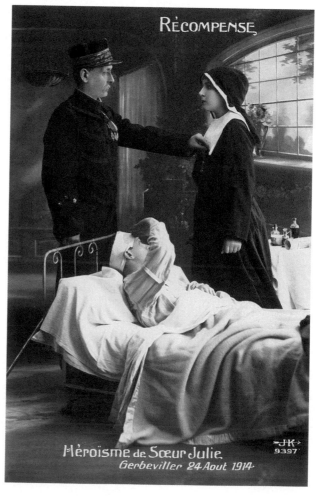

Figure 5.61. **"Reward."** France. 1914. *(See note.)*

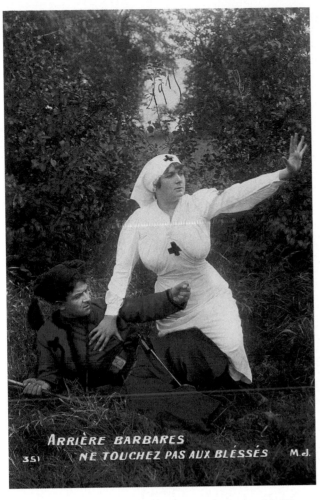

Figure 5.62. "Stop barbarians! Do not touch the wounded!" France. 1914.

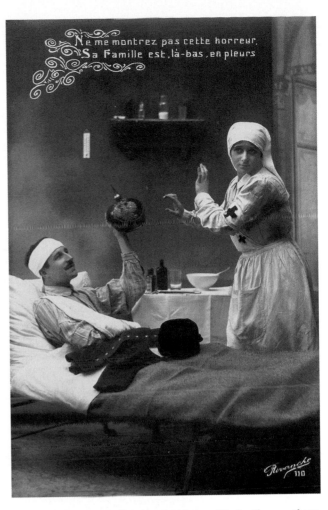

Figure 5.63. "Do not show me that horror. His family, over there, is in tears." France. c. 1915.

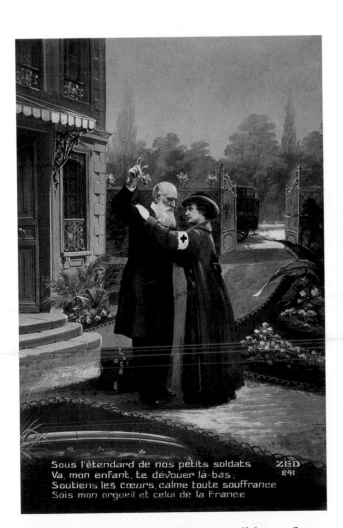

Figure 5.64. "Go, my child, and devote yourself there. . . ." France. 1914. *(See note.)*

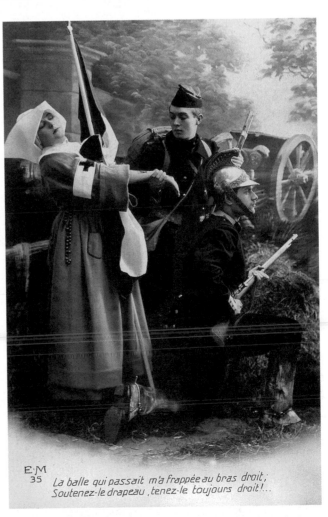

Figure 5.65. "The passing bullet has struck my right arm; Take the flag, always hold it high!" France. 1914.

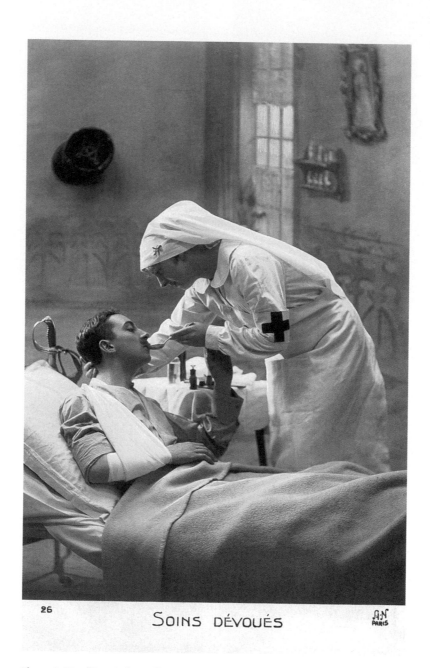

Figure 5.66. **"Devoted care."**
France. c. 1915. *(See note.)*

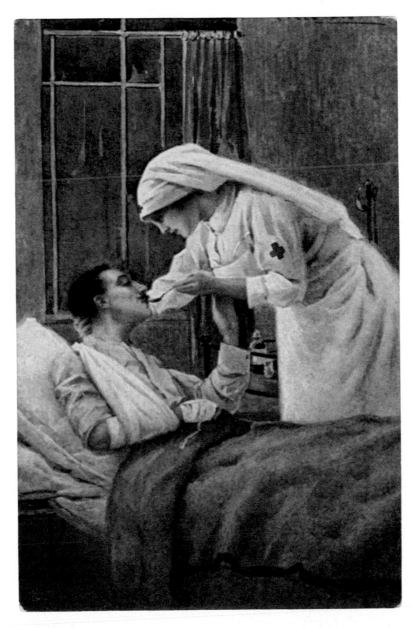

Figure 5.67.
Italy. c. 1915. *(See note.)*

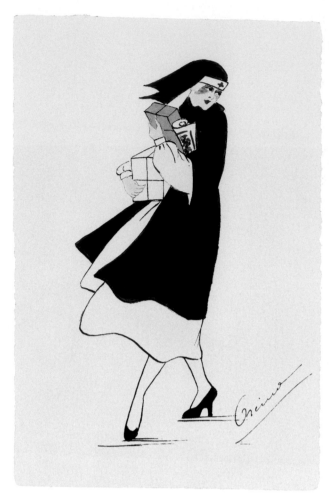

Figure 5.68. **Untitled.** Hand drawn.
France. 1917. *(See note.)*

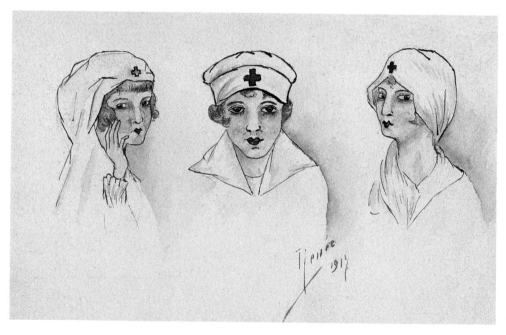

Figure 5.69. **Untitled.** Hand drawn.
France. 1917. *(See note.)*

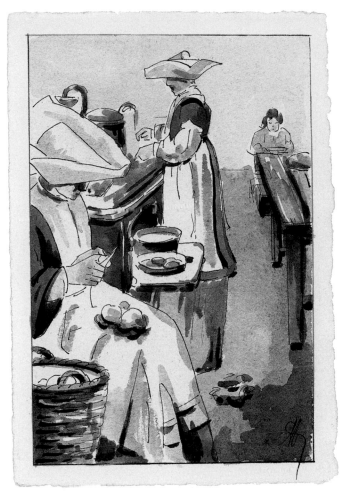

Figure 5.70. **Untitled.** Hand drawn.
France. 1917. *(See note.)*

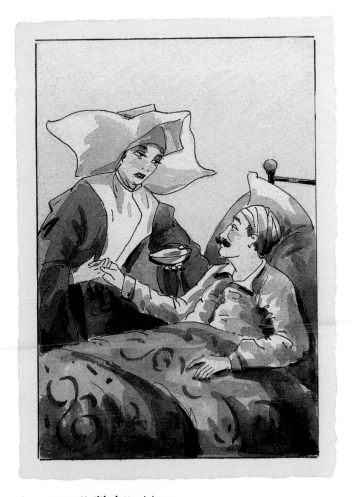

Figure 5.71. **Untitled.** Hand drawn.
France. 1917. *(See note.)*

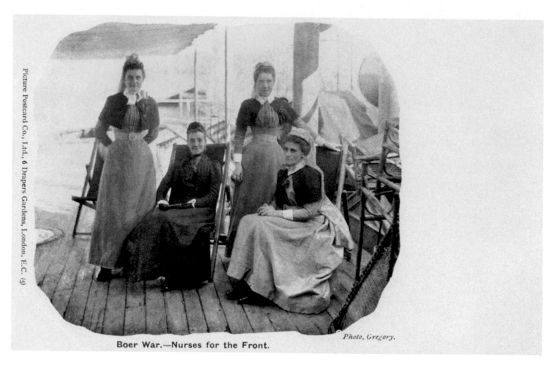

Figure 5.72. **Boer War. Nurses for the Front.**
England. 1900. *(See note.)*

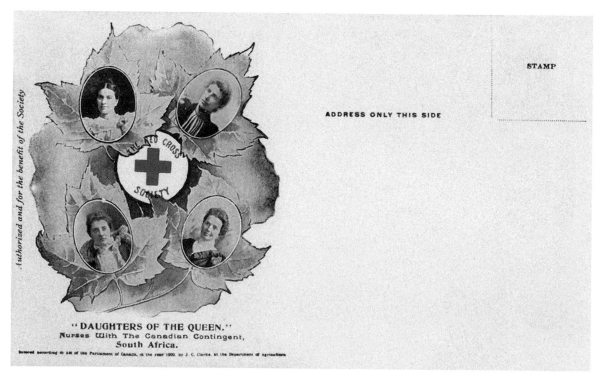

Figure 5.73. **Boer War. Nurses with the Canadian Contingent, South Africa.**
Canada. 1899. *(See note.)*

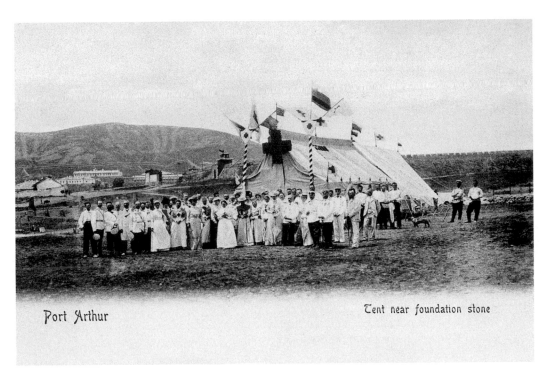

Port Arthur

Tent near foundation stone

Figure 5.74. **Russo-Japanese War.**
Port Arthur. 1904. *(See note.)*

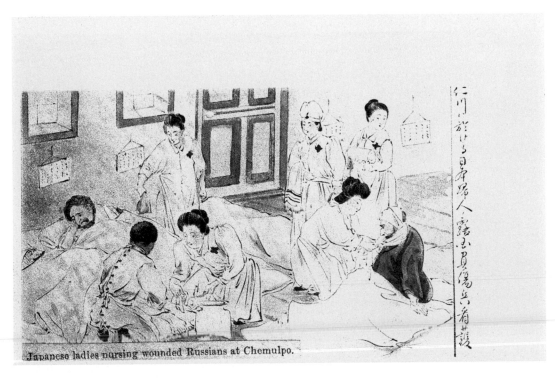

Japanese ladies nursing wounded Russians at Chemulpo.

Figure 5.75. **Russo-Japanese War. "Japanese ladies nursing wounded Russians at Chemulpo."**
Japan. 1904. *(See note.)*

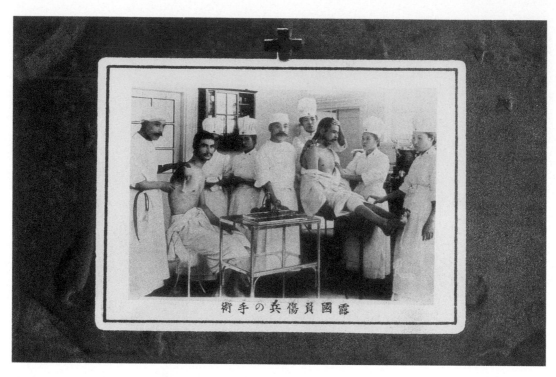

Figure 5.76. **Russo-Japanese War. "Performing surgery on wounded Russian soldiers."**
Japan. 1904. *(See note.)*

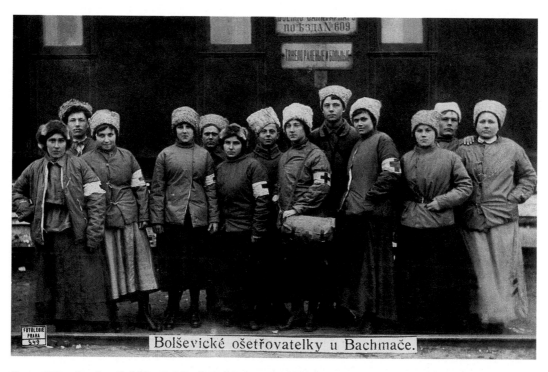

Bolševické ošetřovatelky u Bachmače.

Figure 5.77. **Russian Civil War. Bolshevik Red Cross nurses at Bachmac.**
Russia. c. 1918. *(See note.)*

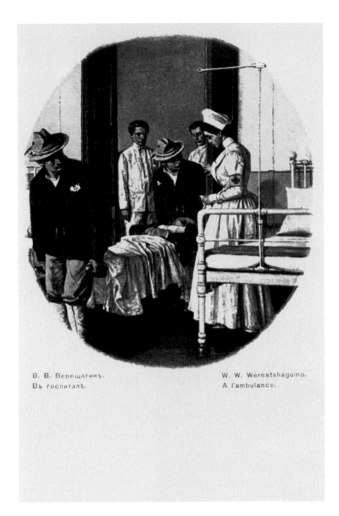

В. В. Верещагинъ.
Въ госпиталъ.

W. W. Wérestshaguino.
A l'ambulance.

Figure 5.78. Spanish-American War. V. Vereschagin (1812–1904). "At the hospital."
Russia. c. 1906. *(See note.)*

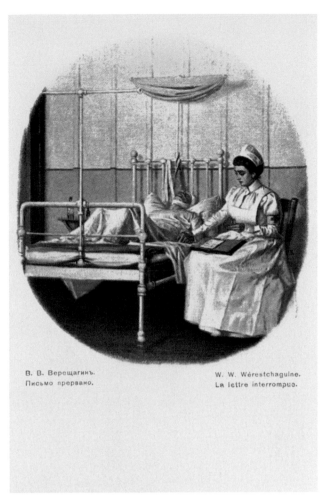

В. В. Верещагинъ.
Письмо прервано.

W. W. Wérestchaguine.
La lettre interrompue.

Figure 5.79. Spanish-American War. V. Vereschagin (1812–1904). "Letter to mother."
Russia. c. 1906. *(See note.)*

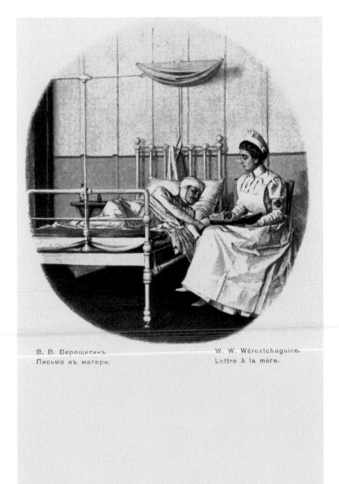

В. В. Верещагинъ.
Письмо къ матери.

W. W. Wérestchaguine.
Lettre à la mère.

Figure 5.80. Spanish-American War. V. Vereschagin (1812–1904). "The letter interrupted."
Russia. c. 1906. *(See note.)*

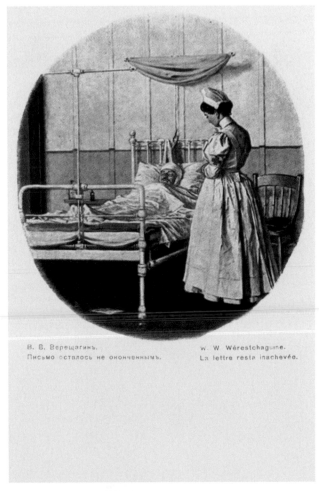

В. В. Верещагинъ.
Письмо осталось не оконченнымъ.

w. W Wérestchaguine.
La lettre resta inachevée.

Figure 5.81. Spanish-American War. V. Vereschagin (1812–1904). "The letter remains unfinished."
Russia. c. 1906. *(See note.)*

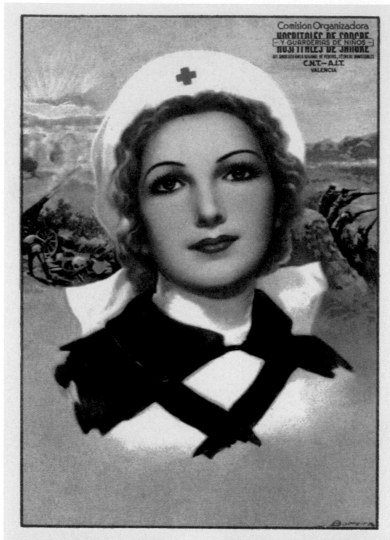

Figure 5.82. **Spanish Civil War. "Help the blood hospitals by subscribing and acquiring numbers for this popular raffle, stamps and postcards." Issued by the CNT-AIT in Valencia.**
Spain. 1936. *(See note.)*

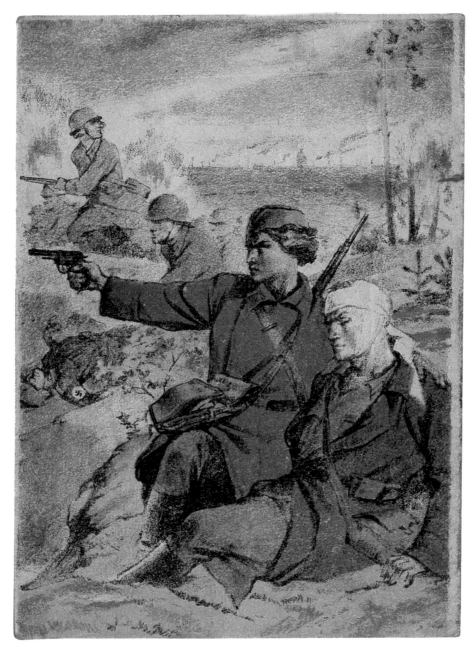

Figure 5.83. **World War II.**
Russia. c. 1944. *(See note.)*

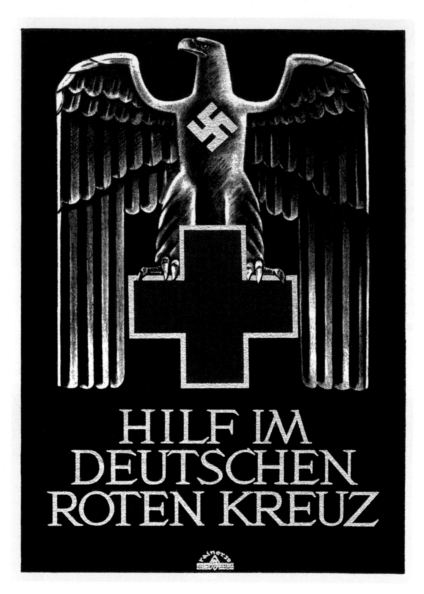

Figure 5.92. **"Help the German Red Cross."**
Germany. 1941. *(See note.)*

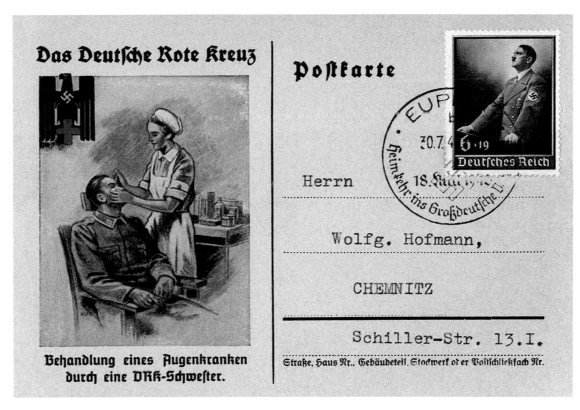

Figure 5.93. **"Treatment for an eye ailment from a Red Cross nurse."**
Germany. 1941. *(See note.)*

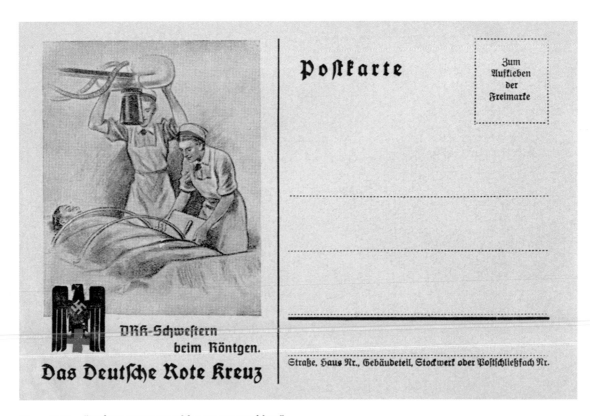

Figure 5.94. **"Red Cross nurses with an x-ray machine."**
Germany. 1941. *(See note.)*

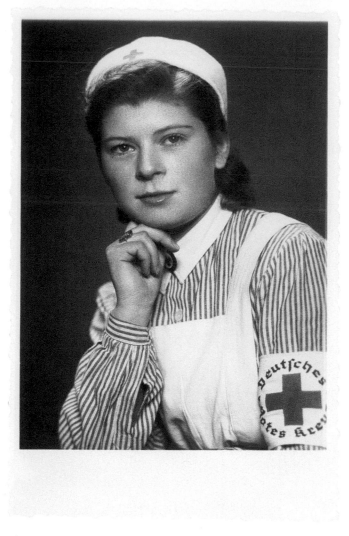

Figure 5.95.
Germany. 1941. *(See note.)*

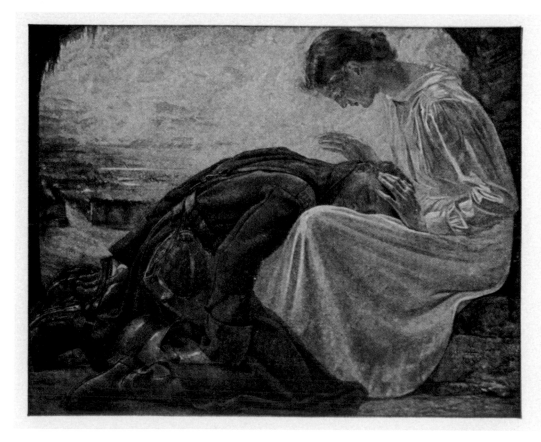

Figure 5.96.   **Hans Buhler. "Returning Home."**
House of German Art. Germany. 1942.

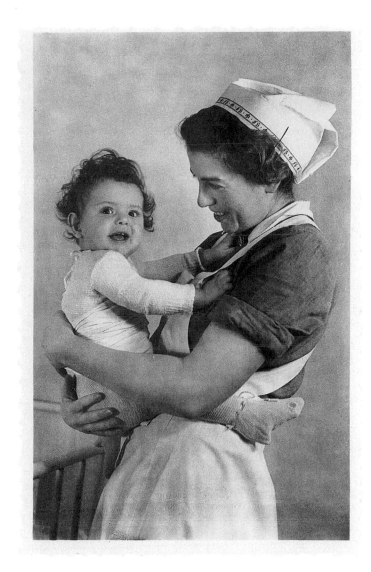

Figure 5.97.
Germany. c. 1940.

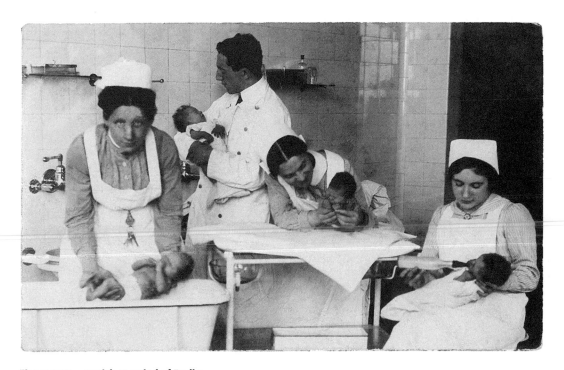

Figure 5.98. Jewish Hospital of Berlin.
Germany. c. 1914. *(See note.)*

5.1. The postcard reads, "Dear Aggie, I am sending you one of our new cards which has just been designed for Mrs. McGifferts' Dept. of the Red Cross to see how you like it. Am looking for a letter every day haven't heard from Fred lately, have you? Max." Postmarked Duluth, Minnesota, July 18, 1917.

5.2. **Robert Stephenson Smyth Baden-Powell** is best known as the founder of the **Boy Scouts,** officially begun in 1908. His sister Agnes (1858–1945) founded the Girl Guides in 1910.

Baden-Powell joined the army in 1876, served in India and Afghanistan, and won fame during the **Boer War** as the defender of Mafeking. Colonel Baden-Powell and a detachment of British troops were besieged there by the Boers from October 1899 until May 1900. The news of their relief aroused public hysteria in Britain, and a new word entered the vocabulary: participating in wild celebrations and public outpourings of joy became known as "mafficking."

Baden-Powell formed a Cadet Corps of boys aged 9 and older to deliver messages and supplies, help in the hospital, and act as lookouts. These Mafeking Cadets were given their own khaki uniforms and wide-brimmed hats, similar to the Boy Scout in the postcard, handing supplies to the soldier. They took themselves quite seriously, and made themselves useful. When not working, they would study and drill, and learn how to tie knots, make fires, and so on. Baden-Powell resolved to form a civilian corps of Scouts on similar lines as soon as the war was over.

5.3. **Harry Payne** (1858–1927) is one of the most celebrated illustrators of British military subjects, known for his accurate detailing of uniforms and equipment.

5.4. The nurse's cap: "**Moscow**." The box at the top: "Moscow Local Committee of the Russian Red Cross"; and at the bottom: "War wounded." The basket: "War wounded." This image represents the commitment of Moscow's aristocracy to the war effort. It was accurate at least in that the women of the royal family did become working nurses, and some voluntarily gave up all their wealth to do it. (See also Figs. 4.87 to 4.95.)

5.5. The card depicts Russian forces fighting either German or Austrian troops on the Eastern front.

5.7. The central figure is an infantry sergeant. The young man in the blue tunic is a senior private of hussars. **Hussars** were traditionally Hungarian light cavalry regiments dating from the 15th century, but by World War I several European countries, including England, Austria-Hungary, and Germany, had hussar regiments. The uniform on the postcard was worn from 1914 to 1915. By 1915, the regiments that remained had switched to less flamboyant, more practical apparel.

5.10. **Harrison Fisher** (1877–1934) was one of the most prolific of all American illustrators. His postcards of beautiful ladies are collected by more people than postcards of any other American artist (Mashburn, 1997).

This postcard is No. 11 of a 1920 French series of 47 postcards titled *Affiches de la Grande Guerre* (Posters of the Great War). The poster itself was produced in the United States in 1918, just before the end of the war, and copies are relatively easy to find. The postcard, on the other hand, is the most rare of all the known Fisher postcards (see Fig. 2.57).

5.11. **Clara Dutton Noyes** (1866–1936) graduated from Johns Hopkins School of Nursing and later became its head nurse. She was superintendent of nursing at St. Luke's Hospital in New Bedford, the Hospital for Women and Children in Boston, and Bellevue Hospital in New York City. When the United States entered the war in 1917, she became director of the **Red Cross Nursing Service.**

Noyes was responsible for the enrollment, organization, and assignment of nurses to duty. For nurses who are up to their ears in paperwork, consider what Noyes had to coordinate: "the publicity necessary to reach every nook and cranny of the country for qualified women [21,000 of them], the letters and telegrams necessary before assurance of loyalty and of the exact address and date for assignment could be turned over to the War Department, the speeding up of enlistments by advancing graduation dates, the subordination of the needs of private hospitals, physicians and wealthy chronic patients to the greater war need, the assembly of special units, and the distribution of clothing and equipment" (Pennock, 1940).

One of the Ms. Noyes' major problems was that most of the volunteers were completely unqualified. During the first 3 years of the war, nursing had been heavily promoted via postcards and other media as a romantic adventure. Young women in the United States were confident that they could carry out the "angel of mercy" role. World War I battlefields were not real to a population that had neither television nor other accurate graphic portrayals to show what was happening. It was impossible to visualize ten thousand men wounded in one battle, much less consider what it might be like to be in the midst of their suffering. Many thought that dispensing large quantities of morphine would be the extent of their duties (Kalisch and Kalisch, 1986).

On April 8, 1917, Clara Noyes wrote to **Adelaide Nutting** in desperation:

Surely we need your prayers. There are moments when I wonder whether we can stem the tide and control the hysterical desire on the part of thousands, literally thousands, to get into nursing or their hands upon it.

. . If I were not convinced before, I should be now that the most vital thing in the life of our profession is the protection of the word nurse. Everyone seems to have gone mad. I talk until I am hoarse, dictating letters to doctors and women who want to be Red Cross nurses in a few minutes, not knowing the meaning of the word nurse and what a Red Cross nurse is (Kalisch and Kalisch, 1986).

In 1918, just as the Allies were starting the greatest offensive in the Meuse-Argonne area, the influenza epidemic struck.

The following is excerpted from *1918: The Great Influenza Pandemic* (Emerson, 2002), © The Bostonian Society, used with permission, all rights reserved.

The Influenza Pandemic of 1918

Each winter, 20,000 Americans die of flu. In the pandemic years of 1957 and 1968 the numbers were closer to 50,000. The plague which hit in 1918 dwarfs every other epidemic of the 20th century. Deaths from the epidemic worldwide at a very conservative estimate, were twenty million. Some estimates of the death toll are as high as 100 million. India alone claimed 20 million. If a similar virus hit today, it is estimated that it would kill more people in a single year than heart disease, cancer, stokes, chronic pulmonary disease, AIDS and Alzheimer's disease combined. Strangely, we seem to have collective amnesia about this episode in our history.

Early cases of the flu had started in February, 1918 on the northern coast of Spain, and in March, at Fort Riley, Kansas, in an army camp. It traveled with the troops to Europe and made them, and the enemy, even more miserable in the muddy trenches of the Argonne. But late in summer, the virus mutated into something quite horrific. It left Brest, France, on a troop ship and arrived at the Commonwealth pier in Boston.

On August 27, sailors on board the receiving ship began reporting to sickbay. Within 3 days, 60 men were sick with the "Spanish Influenza." By the third day in September, the first civilian flu casualties were admitted to City Hospital.

The virus was astonishing. Victims went from robust health to complete prostration in a matter of hours. Fifty percent of cases developed full-blown secondary pneumonia. Fevers soared to 105 degrees and many people sickened and died within a single day. Physicians and nurses attending the patients fell ill. Within weeks of the flu's onset, Camp Devens in Massachusetts had 17,000 sick.

At the beginning of September, few had noticed that an epidemic was on. On September 3rd, four thousand soldiers marched through Boston in a "Win-the-War-for-Freedom Parade." A week later, 6-year-old Fenway Park filled with a wildly enthusiastic crowd as Babe Ruth led the Red Sox to their last World Series victory of the century. In Quincy Market the same day, three men dropped dead on the sidewalk.

The Boston press at the time saw little sign of alarm. The Boston Globe noted on September 13 that doctors had the Spanish flu "pretty well in hand." On September 26, the day the Allies began their great offensive in the Meuse-Argonne, 156 Bostonians died of the flu and an estimated 50,000 citizens statewide were morbidly ill. Between September 1918 and mid-March 1919, 6,225 Spanish flu deaths were recorded in Boston. More than half a million died in the United States as train lines carried the flu to every corner of the country.

Schools were soon requisitioned as emergency hospitals and soup kitchens and the newspapers of the time are full of reports of individual women doing historical work—and putting themselves at great risk.

Twenty five percent of all Americans got the flu. Philadelphia was hardest hit and the morgues there were so overwhelmed that corpses had to be put out on the sidewalk to be collected by horse-drawn carts. Unlike most flus, this strain hit healthy people in their prime the hardest, leaving an extraordinary number of orphans in their wake.

No vaccine was ever effective while the flu raged. There is no evidence that any precautions, from the distribution of masks by the Red Cross to closings of all businesses and pubic gatherings, had any preventive success. The flu simply ran its course.

Jane A. Delano (1862–1919) graduated from Bellevue Nursing School in 1886 and took her first post as superintendent of the Sandhills Hospital in Jacksonville, Florida during a yellow fever epidemic. She was subsequently a pioneering industrial nurse in the copper mines of Bizbee, Arizona, Superintendent of Nurses at the University Hospital in Philadelphia, in full charge of delinquent girls at Randall's Island and, finally, Superintendent of Nursing at Bellevue.

From 1909–1912 she held dual positions: chairman of a committee to build up a professional nursing service within the Red Cross, and superintendent of nurses in the **Army Nurse Corps.** In 1912 she resigned her army position to give her full time to the Red Cross. She is most recognized for her efforts in marshaling nurses for World War I.

"She had to gather 21,480 nurses for war work without jeopardizing the health of the civilian population. She had to plan for the teaching of home nursing to thousands of women. She had to place these trainees as aides in local hospitals and homes, knowing that she might be jeopardizing the professional standards of the profession. She had to extend the services of public health nursing. She had to adjust administrative difficulties resulting from the unforeseen relation which developed between military and non-military nursing forces in Europe, all the while being constantly and painfully notified through official communications (which never reached the public) of the appalling need for nurses. Above all, she had to endure the huge burden of the preservation of human life which rested on her shoulders" (Pennock, 1940).

Jane Delano died in France while on a tour to spur healthcare workers to do their utmost during the post-armistice period.

Much has been written about **Florence Nightingale.** Although she made many significant contributions to the nursing and social welfare professions, she is best known for her system of education, her book *Notes on Nursing,* and her actions during the Crimean War.

The **Crimean War** began as a quarrel between Russian Orthodox monks and French Catholics over who had precedence at the holy places in Jerusalem and Nazareth. At the time, the Turkish Ottoman Empire controlled Palestine, Egypt, and large areas of the Middle East. In 1850, Louis Napoleon III, Emperor of France, requested the restoration to French Catholics of the possession of the key to the Church of the Nativity in the old city of Jerusalem and the right to place a silver star on Christ's birthplace in Bethlehem. The French threatened military action if the Ottoman Empire did not agree, and the Russians threatened to occupy Moldavia and Wallachia (principalities in the Ottoman lands) if France acted (Rempel, 2002).

To back up the threat, the French sent a warship to Constantinople and a squadron of ships to the Bay of Tripoli. In response, Russia mobilized two army corps and sent an ambassador to Constantinople. Because Russian domination of Constantinople and the Dardanelles was a perennial nightmare of the British, the British decided it was worth a war to expand their interests in the area and sent their fleet to join with the French fleet.

In July 1893, the Russian army invaded Moldavia and Wallachia. The Anglo-French fleet entered the Dardanelles (the strait that separates Asia from Europe), and anchored in the Bosporus (where the Dardanelles widens into the Black Sea). Meanwhile, the Russians sailed down the Black Sea from the north, and engaged and defeated the Ottoman fleet. Turkey then turned to France and England, with whom she made a formal alliance. The Anglo-French fleet sailed into the Black Sea. Austria, seeking some advantage in the conflict, joined France and England, and along with the Turks demanded that Russia withdraw from Moldavia and Wallachia. Facing international pressure backed by military strength, Russia was forced to withdraw.

The conflict should have ended there, but the French and British decided that the great Russian naval base at Sevastopol was a direct threat to the future security of the region (ie, a threat to British and French expansion). In September 1854, the French and British, never having left the Black Sea, landed their armies on the Crimean peninsula. From their landing beaches, they marched southward to Sevastopol. The advance ended in trench warfare, bombardment, and siege. The winter of 1854–1855 brought great misery to the troops, particularly the British, as their commissary department was grossly incompetent. For months the men, clothed in rags, were cold, hungry, and short of everything. Finally, in early 1856, Sevastopol fell, and a treaty ending the war was signed. The only bright light in this tale of wartime misery and governmental negligence was the work of Florence Nightingale (Rempel, 2002).

When the war broke out in 1854, the French had the Sisters of Charity at the front, but the British government had not made provisions to care for British wounded. As usual, the expected casualties were grossly underestimated. Hastily, an old barracks at Scutari (the Greek name for the district of Istanbul now known as Üsküdar) was pressed into service as the main hospital. **The Barrack Hospital,** constructed 60 years earlier to house Turkish army troops, was made of stone, with wooden floors, and had room for 3000 beds in more than 4 miles of corridors.

It was built above a grid of latrine trenches, which traveled the width and breadth of the building and had no outlet. Fumes and particulate matter wafted up through the floors and settled on surfaces or hung in the air. There were lots of windows, but they were kept closed. Istanbul is cold in the winter; charcoal braziers, which would have given off a lot of smoke, supplied heat. The rotting wood floors retained spilled fluids. Kitchen utensils, mops and buckets, sheets, dressings, clean clothing, medical equipment, and even food and clean water were in short supply. Amputations were performed in front of other patients, and body parts were heaped in piles on the floor. Frostbite, scurvy, dysentery, cholera, gangrene, and sepsis were rampant. War wounds accounted for only one death in six.

Reports of these conditions, sent back to Britain, came to Miss Nightingale's attention. She immediately dispatched a letter to the British Secretary of War, volunteering her services. At the same time, unaware of her action, the Minister of War (a different official) proposed that she assume direction of all nursing operations at the front.

On October 21, 1854, Miss Nightingale set out for **Scutari,** accompanied by 38 nurses. Under Nightingale's supervision, and with less than enthusiastic cooperation from the military (whose leaders resented the presence of women in general and of women with authority in particular), efficient nursing departments were established at Scutari and later at Balaklava, near Sevastopol.

The British had no real ambulance corps active in the Crimea; the wounded were dumped onto ships that had not been cleaned after transporting horses and cavalry to the Crimea. It is estimated that the mortality rate of the passengers on the 2-day trip to Scutari was about 30%. Most who did arrive at the hospital were in terrible condition, and there was little that nursing care could have done for them. Mortality rates began to drop when the British finally improved the ambulance corps and got better transportation, and when Florence Nightingale and her nurses took responsibility for conditions in the Barrack Hospital (Bullough, 2002).

Within the first 6 months of her 20-month stay, the mortality rate dropped from 42% to a little over 2%. At its peak, the hospital held 2500 sick and wounded at one time. Therefore, prior to and shortly after Miss Nightingale's arrival, 1050 of them would have died. Six months later, due to both nursing intervention and the British Sanitary and Engineer Corps' cleaning out the latrine trenches, only 50 would have died. The thousands of saved lives finally changed the military's opinion of war nursing from negative to positive.

Florence Nightingale's "shift" was 18 to 20 hours per day. Three trips across the Black Sea, the harsh weather, lack of sleep, and being in the midst of thousands of suffering and dying men took their toll. Her constant letter-writing in the cold and damp, coordinating the procurement of supplies, patrolling the hospital and grounds, maintaining discipline among her nurses, and finally, contracting Crimean fever (brucellosis) all contributed to the post-traumatic stress disorder from which she subsequently suffered and which affected her for the rest of her life. She was not only the first modern war nurse and nurse commander, but its first documented psychological casualty (McDonald, 2000).

Since post-traumatic stress syndrome was not recognized in the 19th century, most researchers note simply that her debilitation was a result of the chronic effects of brucellosis and exhaustion. As with any popular but enigmatic figure, rumors arose (and continue to emerge) of everything from schizophrenia to syphilis to explain her withdrawal from public life (Howe, 2002).

At the close of the war in 1860, with a fund raised in tribute to her services, Nightingale founded the Nightingale School and Home for Nurses at Saint Thomas's Hospital in London. The opening of this school marked the beginning of professional education in nursing.

The Barrack Hospital building is still existence, put to its original use, now as the Selimiye Barracks of the Turkish First Army Group.

5.12. From 1917 through 1918, the Red Cross undertook a massive nationwide enlistment and support campaign. This is a mock field hospital tent, complete with patient and nurse inside, and "rescue dog" outside.

5.13 to 5.14. **Mons** was the first protracted battle of World War I involving British troops. It took place on August 23 along the Mons-Conde canal in Belgium, as British troops, under the command of Sir John French, attempted to hold the line against the advancing Germans. The Germans were numerically a much larger force; although they fought with great tenacity, the British were overwhelmed by the advancing German army and had to retreat.

In retrospect, the Battle of Mons became endowed with the very quality of greatness. "The deeds of every named regiment were chronicled down to the last hour and bullet of the fight until Mons came to shine mistily through a haze of such gallantry and glory as to make it seem a victory" (Tuchman, 1980, p. 292).

Shortly after the battle, a story appeared in the *London Evening News* which began the legend of the **Angel of Mons.** Apparently, at one stage, a German assault had considerably weakened the British lines, to the point where they expected that the line would be overwhelmed in the next wave. An angel clad all in white and mounted on a white horse appeared over the field of battle, was seen by both sides, and forbade the German troops to advance.

In fact, the *Evening News* story was an openly fictional romantic tale, written by Arthur Machen and printed on September 29, a month after Mons. In Machen's story, the ghosts of the English bowmen killed at Agincourt came to the assistance of their 20th-century countrymen by shooting arrows that killed Germans without leaving visible wounds. Within a week, Machen's fictional ghost bowmen had been transformed into angels, and what he had written as fiction was soon credited as fact. He was embarrassed and distressed at the confusion, but he was assured, especially by the clergy, that he was wrong: the angels were real and had appeared in the sky over Mons. Many reports confirming the vision were received from troops of both armies and in Britain it became unpatriotic and almost treasonable to doubt it (Fussell, 1975).

5.14. The model for the nurse in this painting was **Barribal's wife,** and the soldier is a modified self-portrait (see Fig. 2.28).

5.15 to 5.16. **Rosa Zenoch** (1898–1915), a 16-year-old girl from a small town near Innsbruck, Austria, served with one of the Austrian Kaiserjägers (Imperial Rifles) line infantry regiments as a nurse's aide. On August 18, 1914, the regiment joined the Austrian Fourth Army opposing the Russians along the Ukrainian border.

On the morning of September 7, the Austrian forces were attacked from all sides by Russian forces in **Rawaruska** (a town about 10 miles south of the Ukrainian border) and suffered heavy losses. Throughout the battle, Rosa remained on the field, bringing water to the troops and binding their wounds. She herself was wounded. After the battle, while recuperating in an Austrian hospital, she was decorated with the Honor Decoration of the Red Cross, visible in the photograph.

On the May 23, 1915 Italy declared war on the Habsburg Empire. By the beginning of June, Italian troops were attempting to invade Austria through the Dolomites, a section of the Alps bordering Italy and the Austrian province of Tyrol. The Austrian defense consisted of troops trained especially for mountain warfare, backed up by *Standschützen. Standschützen* (standing guard) were a home guard formed by boys under 18 and men over 45 years of age. Rosa Zenoch was among them. She was killed in a battle at Sella, one of the passes through the mountains.

5.17. *Boche* is French slang for the Germans, derived from *alboche,* which was a combination of two words—*allemand* (German) and *caboche* (pate, head). *Jerry,* another nickname for a German or Germans collectively, used first by the British and later by the Americans, was an old colloquialism for chamber pot. It referred to the shape of an upturned German helmet.

This is the only postcard I have seen that depicts a sinister, evil nurse. Figure 3.80 is anti-Red Cross, but the nurse is not particularly sinister. Although military medics on both sides in both World Wars carried sidearms and exchanged fire, in clear violation of Red Cross regulations, there is no evidence that nurses did. There is also no evidence that the German Red Cross behaved less honorably in the field than their Allied counterparts.

5.19. This postcard is a **propaganda** effort. Although nurses may have been casualties during the battle, there is no evidence that this event took place as described. Podvolochisk, now in the Ukraine, was on the Austrian side of the Zbruch River, separating Austria from Russia.

5.20. The following article is adapted from Spartacus Educational of Great Britain, © 2002 Spartacus Educational, used with permission. All rights reserved.

The French Army were the first to employ **gas as a weapon** when, in the first month of the war, they fired tear-gas grenades at the Germans. The German Army first used chlorine gas cylinders in April 1915 against the French Army at Ypres. French soldiers reported seeing yellow-green clouds drifting slowly toward the Allied trenches. They also noticed its distinctive smell, which was like a mixture of pineapple and pepper. At first the French officers assumed that the German infantry were advancing behind a smoke screen and orders were given to prepare for an armed attack. When the gas arrived at the Allied front-trenches, soldiers began to complain about pains in the chest and a burning sensation in their throats.

Most soldiers now realized they were being gassed and ran from the scene. An hour after the attack had started, there was a 4-mile gap in the Allied line. Concerned about what the chlorine gas would do to them, the German soldiers hesitated to move forward in large numbers. This delay enabled Canadian and British troops to retake the position.

After the first German **chlorine gas** attacks, Allied troops were supplied with masks of cotton pads that had been soaked in urine. It was found that the ammonia in the pad neutralized the chlorine. These pads were held over the face until the soldiers could escape from the poisonous fumes. Other soldiers preferred to use handkerchiefs, a sock, or a flannel body-belt, dampened with a solution of bicarbonate of soda, and tied across the mouth and nose until the gas passed over. Soldiers found it difficult to fight like this, and attempts were made to develop a better means of protecting men against gas attacks. By July 1915, soldiers were given efficient gas masks and anti-asphyxiation respirators.

One disadvantage of gas was the unpredictability of the weather. (When the British Army launched a gas attack on September 25, 1915, the wind blew it back into the faces of the advancing troops.) This problem was solved in 1916, when gas shells were produced for use with heavy artillery. This increased the army's range of attack and helped to protect their own troops when weather conditions were not ideal.

Chlorine gas destroyed the respiratory organs of its victims, which led to a slow death by asphyxiation. There was no method of successfully treating chlorine gas poisoning.

However, a disadvantage of chlorine gas was that it made the victim cough and therefore limited his intake of the poison. Both sides found that **phosgene** was a more effective poison: only a small amount was needed to make it impossible for the soldier to keep fighting. It also killed its victim within 48 hours. Advancing armies also used a mixture of chlorine and phosgene called "white star."

Mustard gas (Yperite) was first used by the German Army in September 1917. The most lethal of all the poisonous chemicals used during the war, it was almost odorless and took 12 hours to take effect. Yperite was so powerful that only small amounts had to be added to high-explosive shells to be effective. Once in the soil, mustard gas remained active for several weeks. Mustard agents rapidly penetrated clothing and skin, so only a full protective suit (mask with charcoal filters, over-garments, gloves, and boots) afforded protection.

The skin of victims of mustard gas became blistered, the eyes became very sore, and vomiting occurred. Mustard gas attacked the bronchial tubes, stripping off the mucous membrane. This was extremely painful; most soldiers writhed so much, in spite of administrations of morphine, that they had to be strapped to their beds. It usually took 4 or 5 weeks to die of mustard gas poisoning.

It has been estimated that the Germans used 68,000 tons of gas against Allied soldiers. The French and British used 61,000 tons against the Germans. An estimated 91,198 soldiers died as a result of poison gas attacks and another 1.2 million were hospitalized. The Russian Army, with 56,000 deaths, suffered more than any other armed force. (See Fig. 5.24.)

5.21. The Armenian Genocide.

"Who, after all, speaks today of the annihilation of the Armenians?" (Adolf Hitler, less than 25 years after the Armenian Genocide, while persuading his associates that the West would tolerate the extermination of the Jews.)

The following is excerpted from *Genocide Research,* © 2001 The Armenian National Institute, used with permission, all rights reserved.

The Armenian Genocide was planned and administered by the Turkish government against the entire Armenian population of the Ottoman Empire. On the eve of World War I, there were an estimated two million Armenians living in the Ottoman Empire. Between 1915 and 1923 one and a half million of them perished, hundreds of thousands butchered outright. The others were forcibly removed from Armenia and Anatolia to Syria, where the vast majority were sent into the desert to die of thirst and hunger. Women and children were abducted and horribly abused. The entire wealth of the Armenian people was expropriated.

Tens of thousands of the Armenians living along the periphery of the Ottoman Empire fled to the Russian border to lead a precarious existence as refugees. In 1918, however, the Turkish regime took the war into the Caucasus, where approximately 1,800,000 Armenians lived under Russian dominion. Ottoman forces advancing through East Armenia and Azerbaijan engaged in systematic massacres.

The Turks also made use of a newly created clandestine organization, called simply the **Special Organization.** Consisting of irregular troops and released convicts, the Special Organization formed "butcher battalions," whose primary function was the carrying out of the mass slaughter of the deported Armenians. The head of the Special Organization was a medical doctor, Behaeddin Shakir.

After only a little more than a year of calm at the end of the war, the atrocities were renewed between 1920 and 1923, and the remaining Armenians were subjected to further massacres and expulsions, adding tens of thousands of more victims. By 1923, the entire landmass of Asia Minor and historic West Armenia had been expunged of its Armenian population. The destruction of the Armenian communities in this part of the world was total.

There were many witnesses to the Armenian Genocide. Foremost among them were U.S. diplomatic representatives and American missionaries. They were the first to send news to the outside world about the unfolding genocide. Some of their reports made headline news in the American and Western media. The international community condemned the Armenian Genocide. In May 1915, Great Britain, France, and Russia advised the Young Turk leaders that they would be held personally responsible for this crime against humanity. There was a strong public outcry in the United States against the mistreatment of the Armenians. Relief efforts were mounted to save "the starving Armenians." The American, British, and German governments sponsored the preparation of reports on the atrocities and numerous accounts were published.

On the other hand, despite the moral outrage of the international community, no strong actions were taken against the Ottoman Empire either to sanction its brutal policies or to salvage the Armenian people from the grip of extermination. Moreover, no steps were taken to require the postwar Turkish governments to make restitution to the Armenian people for their immense material and human losses.

Countries such as France, Argentina, Greece, and Russia have officially recognized the Armenian Genocide. However, as a matter of policy, the present-day Republic of Turkey adamantly denies that a genocide was committed, dismissing the evidence as mere allegation.

Days of Tragedy in Armenia (Riggs, 1997) is one of the most detailed local accounts of the Genocide written in English. The book reproduces a manuscript prepared in 1918 by **the Reverend Henry Riggs,** an American missionary present from 1915 to 1917 in Harpoot, Turkey, where the massacre took place on a large scale. The manuscript was originally submitted to the U.S. government commission investigating various aspects of World War I, including the destruction of the Armenian communities. The postcard depicts the hospital where Riggs was stationed during the Genocide.

The Annie Tracy Riggs Memorial Hospital. Although the writing on the back of this postcard locates it in Harpoot, the hospital was actually located in Mezireh, a suburb 3 miles from the city. The hospital is named after Annie Tracy Riggs, a teacher and nurse, and wife of the Reverend Henry H. Riggs (1875–1943). Henry Riggs was a third-generation American Protestant missionary in the Ottoman Empire, and President of Euphrates College in Harpoot.

The college was started in 1878 by the American Board of Commissioners for Foreign Mis-

sions to send American missionaries to the Middle East. It was originally named Armenian College, but in 1888 it was forced to change its name because of pressure from city officials. Its official teaching language was Armenian, with basic English provided for comprehension of textbooks written in English. The staff consisted of approximately 20 Armenians under the supervision of 3 or 4 American teachers. The American missionaries formed the governing body and did all the administrative tasks. The college was involved in two specific areas, education and health. Approximately half of the students were trained to be teachers; the other half were trained to be nurses and medical researchers. The nurses trained at the Annie Tracy Riggs hospital after its completion in 1910. The total number of students in the college averaged about 550 per year, with a peak of 998 in 1898.

Henry Riggs married Annie C. Tracy in July 1904 in Athens, Pennsylvania. She traveled with him to Harpoot, where she taught as a nurse instructor at the college, but she became ill and died in July 1905. When the missionary hospital was completed in 1910, it was named in her memory.

When the war broke out in Europe in August 1914, the Turks found themselves more or less manipulated into siding with Germany, mostly due to their interest in preventing Russian expansion into Turkey. A conscription order went out to the Turks in the cities and villages to report to encampment sites, Harpoot being one of the largest. Thousands simply ignored the order, but thousands more gathered and waited to be mustered into the army. Harpoot rapidly filled with uneducated countrymen who, upon arrival, found nothing organized for them. Some stayed in private houses and public buildings. More of them camped in small groups in the streets and pitched tents or simply slept in the open. They made bonfires and scrounged for food. Hundreds simply wandered off. Since there were no sanitary facilities, the thousands who remained left feces and urine on the open ground. Eventually, some of the conscripts were issued uniforms and equipment, but there were no plans for debarkation.

The Commandant of Turkish troops in Harpoot notified the head of the hospital, **Dr. Atkins,** that the facility was to be requisitioned for military purposes. The hospital was thrown open for the soldiers, who were treated there by military surgeons. This arrangement lasted for 3 months, after which the Constantinople chapter of the American Red Cross authorized Dr. Atkins to admit one hundred soldiers and care for them at the expense of the Red Cross. The hospital was once more in the hands of American management. This arrangement lasted for 15 months, and at any time during that period "upwards of one hundred of the miserable wreckage of the Turkish military inefficiency were given the best of care that the hospital could provide" (Riggs, 1997).

Dr. Atkins remained the director of the hospital and **Mrs. Atkins** (in picture) acted as matron. Miss Campbell of Jamaica and New York was in charge of nursing until her departure in 1915. She was replaced by **Miss Maria Jacobsen** (in picture) of Denmark, a trained nurse who was also engaged in district and general relief work. Miss Jacobsen, although attached to the American Red Cross, was actually supported by the Danish Foreign Missionary Board.

In 1915, a typhus epidemic swept the city and the hospital, and every one of the hospital staff contracted the disease. Most recovered, but among the fatalities were Dr. Atkins and Henry Riggs' small daughter.

Harpoot was not spared the genocide. The College was closed in 1915 by the local Turkish government due to its involvement in the Armenian cause. The Armenian nurses (in picture) simply failed to show up for work one day and were never seen again. The hospital was finally closed in May 1917 and its remaining staff ordered out of Harpoot. For 2 years, Reverend Riggs was witness to the ensuing atrocities; using the facilities of the hospital and the resources of the Red Cross, he did his best, to assist the Armenians. Little could be done.

5.27 to 5.41. King George Military Hospital

A single photographer took all the postcards in Figures 5.27 through 5.41 in 1915. He penciled the details (staff names, room numbers, and so on) in a distinctive handwriting on the back, and numbered the cards, but he never signed his name. Virtually everything was photographed: the building itself, everyone inside it, every room, and even individual pieces of equipment. He took at least 380 photographs and made them all into postcards. All those that appear here were obtained by Mr. Chris Butler, in London, who also wrote the essay on the hospital specially for this book.

The introductory essay (© 2002 by Chris Butler, used with permission, all rights reserved.) is followed by notes on the individual postcards.

The declaration of war on Germany by Britain on August 4, 1914 was greeted with an outpouring of patriotic fervor and optimism. A general view was that the war would be over by Christmas. The initial contribution of the British army to the fight in the form of the British Expeditionary Force (BEF) was small: 100,000 men, at most. Few could have imagined the scale of the slaughter to come, and the mobilization and direction of society that would be needed before the struggle was over. Men and munitions en masse would be flung at each other, casualties pitiful and blood spilled in torrents, not so much in the end for abiding victory, but for armistice. Two decades later the main contenders would return to finish the match.

The BEF may have been tiny in relation to the German and French armies, but it soon played a vital role in plugging a gap in the Allied line, in checking the German advance at the Mons-Condé canal (as early as August 23), and in blunting the thrust of the German Schlieffen Plan to sweep around the French armies via Belgium. When the German advance was blocked, the opposing armies began repeatedly to try to hook around each other to the extent that the battle line eventually stretched 460 miles from Switzerland to the North Sea. The British withstood—just—the first big German attempt to rupture the line in the Battle of First Ypres later in 1914. As the line settled and the men entrenched, the war of attrition began.

By the end of 1918, more than 5,700,000 men had been through the British army; attrition demanded men to be fed into its maw. Attrition meant that coping with the casualties had to be turned into a mechanized industrial process. Before the war, there were but 2000 occupied beds in military hospitals. In 1914, 70,815 sick and wounded men were treated in British hospitals; in 1915, 337,457; in 1916, 553,633; in 1917, 692,794; and in 1918, 681,783. This enormous demand for bed space was met by requisitioning government buildings, schools, and offices.

Cornwall House was built between 1912 and 1915 for His Majesty's Stationery Office (HMSO) to warehouse Government official publications. It was revolutionary in its construction. Of fireproof iron and concrete construction, it had six large load-bearing floors covering 80,000 square feet, with 10 capacious, electrically powered main elevators. It was centrally heated by a boiler housed in the basement. It had kitchens fitted with steam and "other cooking arrangements." Its loading platforms were in a side street, under cover and at the right height to receive from ambulances. All these features made it highly suitable for converting into a hospital. Besides, it was a stone's throw away from the railhead at Waterloo, the station serving the South Coast, and receiving so many of the wounded soldiers from the front. So, on May 25, 1915, Cornwall House opened as the King George Military Hospital, partly supported by the British Red Cross and Order of St. John.

Thousands of injured were shipped and entrained to Waterloo, then trundled through the private tunnel between the station and this new hospital—hiding men's mutilations from the public eye. What met the men was a large, busy, effective community that gave them care, the best—and often pioneering—medical care, and good up-to-date facilities. They even had a one and a half acre roof garden laid out by a Royal Academician with revolving summerhouses to catch the sun.

The *Times* reported in May 1915 under the heading, "New Ideals of Healing": "In these, during hot summer days, sick men will be able to enjoy the advantage of a relatively high altitude without incurring discomfort from the wind . . . Wounded soldiers weary of foreign campaigning, see the beloved city and win comfort and cheer from the spectacle . . . [A] wealth of originality and organization . . . have gone to make up the completed scheme. Beneath lies one of the most gigantic hospital constructions in the world, an institution in which some 2,000 men and women will live, which will accommodate upwards of 1,600 patients, every floor of which will be as large as the Middlesex Hospital, for which the very floorcloth will extend to 9½ acres, and which will have as many separate departments as there are specialised branches of medicine. The complexity and sheer size of the undertaking, indeed, produce a sense of bewilderment . . . The common rooms where the men will be able to sit and talk or read are privately funded by generous donors; every patient is to have a special electric light over his bed capable of being turned off and on independently, a ward locker, and a neat folding chair. He will have the services of a sister and two doctors resident in the wards at his command night and day; and hosts of willing helpers will minister in various ways to his requirements . . . The wards here are very large and roomy and splendidly lighted."

The hospital contained 63 wards varying in size from 3 beds to more than 65. Someone calculated that the beds laid end to end would stretch for 3 miles. The ground floor was dedicated to medical cases. The floors above had two operating theaters each, one for septic and one for aseptic cases. In the operating theaters, corners were rounded to prevent dust and bacteria accumulating; stone with the "smoothness of glass" was used to allow for "scrupulous cleanliness." Lighting was arranged so that no shadows would be cast. Operations could take place under X-ray, and there was a "magnificent" X-ray department in the basement. Much emphasis was placed on dental work; the Battle of the Marne had demonstrated the need for work on damaged teeth and jaws.

From 1915 to 1919, the King George treated 71,002 patients in all. The results of some of the surgical operations are carefully recorded in two volumes of professionally taken photographs housed in the Imperial War Museum (IWM) library. They record the progress of successive plastic surgery interventions with breathtaking acuity. Dr. Albert Norman, Human Scientific Photographer, took the photographs. Such is the clarity and power of these photographs that I suspect that it is the same Dr. Norman who took the fine photographs upon which the King George V postcard suite was based.

What was life like for the nurses and orderlies? We can guess it was rushed and busy, and no doubt exhausting at times: the hospital cared for an average of 2356 patients a month in 1917. Life was a community life, very much centered within the building. The ground floor had barracks for 200 orderlies; nurses and officers resided in the semi-detached block facing Waterloo Road. Sometimes RAMC staff would escape the building briefly for a quick snack at the YMCA hut in Waterloo Road. Staff could sleep in the nearby Union Jack Club with their visiting wives and families and still get back to duty in good time.

We can guess it must have been satisfying to assist in the mending of men. There were losses, to be sure, but the death rate was not that high, only 1039 in total, about 1.5% of the total number of cases.

We know there were enjoyments. The hospital had its own "cinematograph," its own choir and orchestra, and its own concert hall. Celebrities of the day, such as Ivor Novello and Clara Butt, entertained the men in a series of concerts. The Lord Mayor's Band came every Wednesday. Lectures were often given by "men of note" and illustrated with "lantern pictures." Lady Wynne arranged "Joy Rides" for the men in private cars or by "omnibus." Royalty visited several times. The King and Queen gave up their Christmas afternoon to visit in 1915. The King and Queen of Romania visited in 1919.

What emerges from the records and the postcards is a strong sense of the full involvement of the whole of society in this institution, as indeed the whole of society was mobilized on the "Home Front." Aristocracy was very much in evidence: for instance, Adeline, Duchess of Bedford had furnished the chapel in the basement. The Marchioness of Ripon initiated the Compassionate Fund and worked 7 hours a day running the Gift Stores. (See Fig. 5.38.) Gifts flooded in for the men from all walks of life. Each bed in the hospital had been endowed: by farmers, foreigners, industrial hands, some even by children in primary school. Ladies came in to teach the men embroidery in the afternoons. Middle class and upper class girls volunteered as VADs. Coming from privileged backgrounds, it must have been an eye-opening experience for them to see men's suffering at its worst, but sharing perhaps some of the dogged cheerfulness of so many working class young men.

We know it was a moving, seminal experience because some of the men and women who worked here felt the need to record life in the round in the hospital. The postcards, more of which are housed in the IWM and the Wellcome Library, are the best and fullest example of this. The IWM even has pieces of the brown linoleum and scraps of chintz curtain from the nurses' common room: such was the motivation of some to let succeeding generations have a real feel of what it was like to be there. We hear it, too, in the poignant poetry written on the "death" of the hospital on June 15, 1919, written by V. C. Hassan, Sgt. RAMC. In his verse he refers obliquely to a bombing raid by German Gothas nearby:

"I took them in for all were kings
And nestled then beneath my wings.
Their wounds I healed with tender care.
In me they looked for all repair.
And, when the Huns were overhead
I hid them from their dread."

One must conclude at least some of the staff were sad to leave.

After the hospital closed, the building was used mainly by humdrum HMSO but it still had its moments. It was hit by a flying bomb in World War II. There are rumors that some outpost of the secret services may have been based here, and that "The Man Who Never Was"—the exhumed corpse that was used to mislead the Germans over the invasion of Sicily—began his journey to the sea from a fridge in Cornwall House. The Office of the Government Chemist had a floor there for some time. There are stories of winos drinking from the drainpipes as spirits in floors above were being tested for their alcoholic proof, and of students chasing marijuana plants around the streets nearby after the plants had blown off the roof where the Government Chemist was growing them for research. By the 1990s the building was looking very down at heel. It is a tribute to its original solid construction that it was not demolished. It has been refurbished, and is now back full of eager life, occupied by Kings College, University of London. Cornwall House has been converted into halls of residence with 557 rooms for students. There is a gym, and a lecture theater, but the strains of Ivor Novello have long faded away.

5.31. Lady Constance Gladys, Countess de Grey, later **Marchioness of Ripon** (?–1917), wife of the Earl de Grey (later Marquess of Ripon), was a philanthropist who devoted much of her time and energy to the hospitals in Britain. She envisioned and planned a facility to care for those who were permanently disabled in the war. Though she did not live to see it completed, the Queen Alexandra Hospital Home was founded in 1919. John Singer Sargent painted her in 1914. The obscuration of her birth date was probably deliberate: a society beauty hiding her age.

5.33. The kitchens were capable of cooking for more than 2000 people. The kitchen staff was engaged and salaried by the Joint War Committee. Food was distributed to the dining rooms on different floors in closed trolleys. The RAMC man on the left is an Honorary Lieutenant and Quartermaster; the one on the right is a Company Sergeant Major.

5.35. **Sir Launcelot Edward Barrington-Ward** (1884–1953) was Surgeon to George VI. Apparently the doctor led a colorful life and was a known public figure in London. The character of Sir Lancelot Spratt, in the 1954 movie **Doctor in the House** from the novel of the same name by Richard Gordon, was based on Dr. Barrington-Ward (North of Scotland Institute, 2002).

5.37. The white pillar at the head of the table is an **eye magnet** (for removing ferrous bodies from the eye). The box on the wall with the two glass doors is a faradic/galvanic unit, which could be used for pulsed stimulation, cautery, or as a power supply for lights (eg, in endoscopes). The cylindrical machine in the lower left is a **Ruhmkorff coil,** a high-voltage transformer often used to power X-ray tubes. On the table is an X-ray collimator (the object on the far left showing the cross-hair lens and cloak) and directly in front of it, a pair of headphones. The purpose of the headphones is not known, but they could be part of an electronic stethoscope, in use from the 1890s. A regular stethoscope pickup led to a carbon microphone, which would amplify the sound and transmit it to the headphones.

The scientific and professional equipment was under the supervision of **Sir Frederick Treves** (1853–1923). Treves was a famous pioneer in abdominal surgery. In 1902 he performed an appendicectomy (not an appendectomy—he drained an abscess, but did not remove the appendix) on King Edward VII. Today he is mostly remembered as the physician to John Merrick, the Elephant Man. It was Treves who first had the idea of making the Stationery Office over to be a hospital. He presented the idea to the Joint War Committee.

5.39. These kettles were steam heated and were used to make soups, stews, and other such dishes.

5.40. The **refuse destructor** or incinerator came into widespread use around 1880. It reduced burnable waste at the expense of the air, into which it poured thick smoke and noxious odors.

5.41. The roof was used as a promenade. There were 20 swiveling summerhouses in which the soldiers would sit on pleasant days and swivel to follow the sun. Because the building was centrally heated (as opposed to coal fires) the roof could be flat, without a multitude of chimneys. The "accident" was a distraught soldier leaping over the roof barrier to his death.

5.42 to **5.55.** Notes on the individual postcards follow the essay on Edith Cavell.

Edith Cavell is the 20th century's most famous nurse. She was Matron of a Red Cross hospital and nursing school in German-occupied Belgium during World War I. In that position, she assisted in the escape across the border of more than 200 Allied soldiers. The plot was discovered and a trial was held.

On October 12, 1915, Miss Cavell was executed by firing squad. A massive propaganda campaign was launched following the execution. Her death did more to stoke the fires of hatred against the Germans than any other incident in the war.

Edith Louise Cavell (1865–1915) was born in Swardeston, England, and grew up there. She had a great respect and love of nature, and she seems always to have surrounded herself with plants and animals. She became an accomplished artist. She had a flair for French, which she had learned easily and quickly; after several jobs as a governess, in 1890 she was recommended for a post in Brussels. In 1895 she returned to Swardeston to nurse her father through an illness; this inspired her to take up nursing.

At about this time, **Antoine Depage,** a Belgian surgeon, had grown frustrated with the religious orders that controlled Belgian nursing. He wanted to shift to a nondenominational system with professionally trained personnel, as developed by Florence Nightingale in England. He proposed to start a nurses' training school at his Berkendael Institute, which was a combination hospital and nursing home. To implement it, he sought a matron who had administrative experience, teaching capabilities, an understanding of the Belgian people, and fluency in French, and who had been trained in the manner of Florence Nightingale. Edith Cavell qualified on all counts. She opened the **Berkendael Institute Training School** on October 1, 1907 (Unger, 1997). By 1911, she was training nurses for 3 hospitals, 24 schools, and 13 kindergartens in Belgium.

Upon the outbreak of the war, the nursing home was taken over by German authorities and turned into a Red Cross hospital for the care of German wounded. Despite being offered the chance to return to Britain, Miss Cavell decided to remain with her nurses and was permitted to remain as Matron of the Institute.

In November 1914, two stranded British soldiers found their way to the training school. After an overnight stay, they were whisked away by the Belgian underground to neutral territory in Holland. In the 8 months that followed, an organized underground lifeline was established, masterminded by **Prince and Princess De Croy,** at a chateau in Mons, with the help of Brussels architect **Philippe Baucq.** The group combed the fields around Mons for fugitive troops, whom they then hid, provided with food, money, and civilian clothes, and relocated. More than 200 French, English and Belgian soldiers were guided over the Dutch border.

As part of that apparatus, Cavell provided a refuge in the nursing home and cared for the men until they could continue their escape. She saw to it that each man had 25 francs for his journey. If he lacked identification papers, she supplied them. If he needed guides, she found them, and she often led the soldiers through the streets of Brussels to the meeting place with those guides (Unger, 1997).

The Institute came under suspicion by the German authorities. As evidence against her mounted, colleagues urged Edith to escape while she could, but she refused. She arranged for 60 of her nurses to return to Britain, but Cavell remained at the Institute.

On July 31, 1915, the Germans seized Philippe Baucq, and on August 5 they arrested Edith Cavell. She was brought to trial on October 7. She was arraigned, with 35 other persons, on the charge of having facilitated the escape of enemy subjects from Belgium into neutral territory. This was, naturally, an offense against German military law, but it was not a capital offense. However, the prosecution further asserted, and was prepared to prove, on Miss Cavell's own confession, that she had provided English and French soldiers with funds and with guides to enable them to get across the frontier and so back to their own countries. It was also said that she had admitted to having received letters (in fact, she had received only one) from repatriated soldiers, thanking her for enabling them to "fight another day." If that were so, she was guilty of attempts to conduct soldiers back to the enemy fronts; for that, under the German military code, the penalty was death.

There were many opportunities for Ms. Cavell to speak words that might have resulted in either her release or a lesser punishment, but she chose not to speak them.

The court found her guilty and sentenced her to death. Edith Cavell was executed by an 8-man firing squad, firing from a distance of six paces at the Tir Nationale (National Rifle Range), just outside Brussels, at dawn on October 12, 1915.

Stories were told that the men fired wide of Edith, that she fainted, that she was finally dispatched by a German officer with a pistol. Reliable witnesses report nothing of this. It seems the executions were carried out without incident, with the exception that one of the firing squad did refuse to take part in the execution. A Private Rammler is said to have thrown down his rifle when ordered to fire at Nurse Cavell, and was shot on the spot by a German officer for refusing to obey orders.

Permission was given for the English chaplain, Stirling Graham, to visit Nurse Cavell the night before her execution. She is quoted as saying, "I have no fear or shrinking; I have seen death so often that it is not strange or fearful to me. I thank God for this 10 weeks' quiet before the end. Life has always been hurried and full of difficulty. This time of rest has been a great mercy. They have all been very kind to me here. But his I would say, standing as I do now in view

of God and eternity: I realize that patriotism is not enough. I must have no hatred or bitterness towards anyone." (See also Note 5.42.)

The rest of the world had no such compunction. **Britain's most extensive propaganda effort of the war** was launched around Nurse Cavell. In the month following her execution and attendant publicity, enlistment in the army went from 71,000 men the previous month to 113,000 (Judson, 1941).

After the war, Cavell's remains were disinterred (see Fig. 5.53) and brought to Westminster Abbey for the first part of a burial service on May 15, 1919, attended by His Majesty, King George V. A special train then brought her to Thorpe Station, Norwich. A great procession followed her to Norwich Cathedral, where she was laid to rest, just a few miles from her native Swardeston.

5.42. The words at the top of the postcard, "I am happy to die for my country," although they appear on numerous items commemorating Cavell's death, were never spoken by her. The quote is a misinterpretation of her actual words, "I have seen death so often that it is not strange or fearful to me," spoken to her chaplain the night before the execution.

5.43 to **5.48.** **Tito Corbella,** an Italian artist, studied at the Academia di Belle Arti in Venice. He became famous for his postcards of women and engaged couples, which he began designing at the beginning of World War I and continued to produce until the 1920s. There are over 300 known designs.

Kultur is the term the Germans used for what they felt was their superior civilization, which they wished to see propagated over the European continent. In fact, they felt it was their obligation to do so lest humanity lose its chance to evolve. Here, of course, Kultur is seen as death. Note that in Figure 5.47 the Kaiser is shown dressed as a Teutonic mythical figure associated with Wagner's *Der Ring des Nibelungen* (*Ring of the Nibelung*). The Kaiser's birthday was on January 27, 1859, and since Cavell was killed on October 12, the caption is a propaganda embellishment.

5.49. This is an autographed picture taken circa 1909, which was reproduced in the *London Daily Sketch* a few days after Cavell's execution. It was also made into a postcard, which was distributed for the duration of the war. The reverse of this one states: "November 6, 1915. Here is a postcard for your collection. I got it today at an exhibition of needle work that the Daily Sketch has got up."

5.51. **Alberto Martini** was a painter, engraver, lithographer, illustrator, and graphic designer. In 1898 he located in Munich and did work for the art magazine *Jugend*. Between 1905 and 1908 he did a series of drawings inspired by the works of Edgar Allan Poe, and between 1908 and 1915 he did works based Shakespeare, Mallarmé, and Rimbaud.

Between 1915 and 1916 he produced 54 designs in five series of postcards titled **"La Danse Macabre Europeenne."** This postcard is number

44, from the fifth series. Martini is one of the few artists who accurately interpreted the war for what it was: grotesque, bloody, and obscene.

5.52. The monument is in front of the Edith Cavell Nursing School, which is affiliated with the Edith Cavell Hospital in Brussels. The inscription reads, "To Edith Cavell. To Marie Depage. Passing, say to your children, 'They have killed them.' " Marie Depage was the wife of Dr. Antoine Depage, the Belgian surgeon who founded the Berkendael Institute. She was a friend of Miss Cavell who perished in the sinking of the *Lusitania* by a German U-boat off the coast of Ireland, May 7, 1915.

5.54. The Nursing School of the Hospital Edith Cavell in Paris in Paris is part of Miss Cavell's legacy, dedicated to her and named in her honor.

Marie Sklodowska Curie (1867–1934) was born in Poland. At age 24, she went to Paris to study physics and mathematics. There she married physicist Pierre Curie and began research on her doctoral thesis. Choosing radioactivity as a thesis topic, Madame Curie examined several substances and found that thorium and its compounds behaved the same way as uranium. So exciting were her initial findings that Pierre gave up his own work to join her. Marie's marriage to Pierre gave her access to scientific resources usually barred to women.

In 1897, the Curies were credited with the discovery of two radioactive substances, **radium and polonium,** for which they received the Nobel Prize in 1903. After Pierre's death in 1906, Marie went on to become the first woman professor at the Sorbonne. In 1910 she succeeded in isolating pure radium metal. She was the recipient of a second Nobel Prize in 1911, in chemistry.

During the First World War, Marie Curie found that radiologic services for military hospitals in France were lacking. She established field X-ray stations, and donated to the army 20 X-ray-equipped cars, called *petites curies* (little curies). She drove her own radiologic car to the front, where she and daughter Irene, then 17, trained personnel and assisted in radiographing the wounded. Irene had studied nursing, and was able to direct an X-ray facility on her own. The French Health Service, on Marie's advice, added a department of radiology to the **Nurses' School of the Edith Cavell Hospital.** From 1916 to 1918, Marie and Irene Curie trained 150 nurse X-ray technicians in the theory and practice of electricity, X-rays, and anatomy (Penn State University, 2001).

Since very little was known about the immediate or cumulative biological effects of **radiation,** these early X-ray units were used with little or no shielding. However, within a few months after Roentgen's discovery, erythema and severe burns had already been observed. Early radiologists suffered severe local radiation damage, especially to the hands, and later developed skin cancer and leukemia. Becquerel, who had discovered radioactivity, experienced radiation burns from carrying radium samples in his pockets. Marie Curie and her daughter both died of leukemia. Pierre Curie developed leukemia as well; however, he died as a result of a carriage accident.

From the reverse of 5.54:

Mrs. Grantly Ross
30 Williams Street
Bradford, Mass.
Etats-Unis
Nurse and company. Jan. 28, '18.
Dear Florence and Folks,

I have moved again, Living in Latin Quarter and studying x-ray under Madame Curie—the woman who discovered radium. Of course it's a wonderful chance, but awfully hard course, all in French—Photography, Anatomy, Physics, Electricity and actual x-ray manipulations. The electricity is the worst—work is easy but the theory & problems are hard, & trying to recite about condensers, accumulators, magnetic fields & poles, etc. in French is dreadful. I've often wished I could get hold of Harry or Jake to ask questions. We have to learn to repair our machines too.
Love, Polly

5.55. Although the caption states 1915, the photo was taken about 3 years earlier. Cavell's dogs, who went with her everywhere, were Don, on the left, and Jack.

5.56 to 5.66 are examples of **French real photo studio postcards,** each hand-tinted individually on the print. The French were the undisputed masters of this genre, producing innumerable varieties in great quantities. Sometimes wings or smoke and such were painted in to create fantasy effects. The larger postcard companies employed dozens of people to brush the watercolor paint onto the postcards. Sometimes, for glow-in-the-dark effects, radium paint was used, and the painters later went blind.

Before the war, France based its strategy on **élan and patriotism.** The military and political leaders were entirely convinced that the army with the greatest will and spirit would prevail, no matter what the odds. In other words, if the spirit were high enough, a cavalry charge with saber-wielding men could overwhelm a superior force of entrenched machine-gunners. The French implemented this strategy. Every time the French were defeated, the leaders would say the cause was poor resolve on the part of the troops.

In any case, during the early years of war there was rampant propaganda to build up élan. These postcards were produced to that effect. The professional models were often posed as if in a still shot from a silent movie, where gesture and facial expression are exaggerated to convey emotion in the absence of words. About half of the photographers knew how to position their models and props at least reasonably well; the other half seemed to be completely inept, but the cards were patriotic; so, good or simply awful, they sold.

5.56. The verse reads, "Those angels of battlefield, Oh France, you have dismissed them! Who, then, will go under the machine guns one day to pick up our wounded?" It refers to the fact that the military authorities, despite lessons learned in the Crimean War, felt that religious nursing orders should not be allowed to serve in military field hospitals, since it would offend everybody's sensibilities. Fortunately, the orders knew better and the nurses remained available.

The soldier is wearing the **red pants** that made the men such excellent targets. When this was pointed out at a parliamentary hearing, M. Etienne, a former war minister, spoke for France. "Eliminate the red trousers?" he cried. "Never! *Le pantalon rouge c'est la France!*" (Tuchman, 1980). In May 1915, light blue uniforms were issued, which hid the men relatively well in smoke. The nicknames for the soldiers changed from *les pantalons rouges* (red-pants) to *les horizons bleus* (sky-blues).

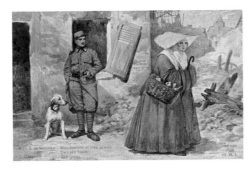

**S. Solomko. Sky-blue and heavenly-blue.
Lapina Gallery.**
France. 1916.

5.57. The verses on this sort of postcard were often generic and could be applied to any number of scenarios. The soldier is a member of the forces of French-occupied Algeria. Those men distinguished themselves well in the war, and were held in high esteem, even though they were kept segregated from the regular French troops. They were usually under command of a French officer. They were among the troops who were first exposed to poison gas, at **Ypres.** The German **Pickelhaube** (spiked helmet) on French artwork was a symbol of German defeat. The men took them from dead Germans as souvenirs. The helmets were made of leather and offered little protection.

5.58 to 5.59. On August 24, 1914, the Germans, who had occupied **Gerbéviller** for 4 days, withdrew, but not before atrocities had been committed against civilians. During their brief occupation and subsequent retreat, the Germans set fire to every house that had not already been damaged by their earlier bombardment (Gilbert, 1994, p. 52). It is possible that the scene depicted in the postcards actually took place, but it is more likely that it was simply invented for propaganda purposes.

5.64. The translation is "Away, my child, to devote yourself under the banner of our young soldiers. Lift their spirits and calm all suffering for my pride and that of France!" In French, it rhymes in singsong anapestic tetrameter. "Tum, ta ta tum, ta ta tum, ta ta tum," typical of the verse associated with this type of postcard.

5.66 to 5.67. An Italian artist obtained a copy of the French postcard shown in Figure 5-66 and drew his own interpretation of it. The Italian and French nursing uniforms were similar, so few modifications were required.

5.68 to 5.71. These postcards are one-of-a-kind originals, hand drawn by soldiers recovering in hospitals.

5.70 to 5.71. From a series of 14 cards by the same artist.

5.72 to 5.73. **The Boer War**

In 1899 the British Empire was at its zenith in power and prestige, but the High Commissioner of Cape Colony in South Africa, **Alfred Milner,** wanted to create and rule over a Cape-to-Cairo confederation of British colonies to dominate the African continent. British expansionists lobbied strongly for Milner's plans, and the order was finally given to undertake the annexation of what they defined as unlawful Boer Republics (Emuang, 1999). As usual, overconfident generals and politicians predicted the war would be "over by Christmas." However, as disaster piled on disaster, military careers were destroyed, and 22,000 British men were laid to rest in "some corner of a foreign field that is for ever England."

The Boers, who were Dutch settlers, had no more claim to the land than the British, other than having displaced the native people earlier and more extensively than the British had. Nevertheless, having settled the land, they were going to defend it. On October 11, 1899, the Boers took the offensive and invaded Natal and Cape Province. They quickly surrounded three towns: **Ladysmith, Mafeking** (see also Note 5.2), and **Kimberly.** This forced the British to abandon their original offensive plans in order to lift the sieges. After achieving overwhelming superiority in the field with the arrival of the British main forces, the British lifted the sieges and captured the cities in May and June 1900. With this, Britain considered the war over.

The truth about the siege may have been different from the heroic action depicted by the British press. It has been alleged that the white garrison survived in reasonable comfort as the result of appropriating the rations of the blacks, who were faced either with starvation or with running the gauntlet of the Boers by escaping from the town (Scouting Resources, 2001).

The second phase of the conflict began as Boer commando units, the **"bitter-enders,"** escaped into the vast bush country and continued to wage unconventional guerrilla warfare by blowing up trains and ambushing British troops and garrisons. The British Army, unable to defeat the Boers using conventional tactics, adopted many of the Boer methods, and the war degenerated into a devastating and cruel struggle between British might and Boer nationalist desperation (Ice, 1995).

The British crisscrossed the countryside with blockhouses to flush the Boers into the open. They burned farms and confiscated foodstuffs to prevent them falling into Boer hands. They herded Boer women and children to concentration camps as "collaborators." Due mostly to British neglect, 25,000 Boer civilians (mainly women and children) and 14,000 natives died in these infamous camps. The last of the Boer commandos, left without food, clothing, ammunition, or hope, surrendered in May 1902, and the war ended with the Boers reluctantly signing the Treaty of Vereeniging (Ice, 1995).

5.73. The nurses pictured clockwise from upper left are **Elisabeth Russell, Georgina Pope, Minnie Affleck,** and **Sarah Forbes.**

During the Boer War the **Canadian Nursing Service** was organized as part of the Army Medical Corps. Canadian nurses were granted the rank, pay, and allowance of Lieutenant in the Army. On October 30, 1899, one thousand men of The Royal Canadian Regiment of Infantry left for South Africa on the troopship *Sardinian* and arrived at Cape Town on November 29. Accompanying them were the first Canadian nurses to be sent to South Africa.

For 5 months after their arrival, the nurses, with Georgina Fane Pope (1862–1938) as senior, served at British hospitals just north of Cape Town. Then in May 1900, Miss Pope and another nurse proceeded north to Kroonstadt where they took charge of the military hospital and, despite shortages in food and medical supplies, successfully cared for 230 sufferers of enteric fever. Pope returned to South Africa a second time, in 1902 (Canadian War Museum, 2000).

In 1906, Miss Pope began work as a member of the permanent Canadian Army Medical Corps at the Garrison Hospital in Halifax. Two years later, she attained the position of matron, the first in the history of the Canadian Army Medical Corps. She went overseas in 1917, but was invalided back to Canada at the end of 1918 (Canadian War Museum, 2000).

Elisabeth Russell worked with the Canadian troops in the relief of Mafeking. She went on to become matron of The Duchess of Connaught Red Cross Hospital, in World War I (see Fig. 4.85).

5.74 to 5.76. The Russo-Japanese War

Japan had fought a very successful war against the crumbling Chinese Empire in 1894–1895 and had imposed a severe treaty, demanding from China a heavy war indemnity: the island of Formosa, and **Port Arthur** together with the Liaotung Peninsula on which it stood. The European powers, while having no objection to the indemnity, did feel that Japan should not gain Port Arthur, for they had their own ambitions in that part of the world. Japan was obliged to relinquish Port Arthur. Two years later, Moscow forced the Chinese into leasing Port Arthur to Russia. For Russia, this meant the acquisition of an ice-free naval base in the Far East to supplement Vladivostok. For Japan it was a case of adding insult to injury (Madison, 2002).

Meanwhile, Japan was heavily engaged in Korea. Russia also had interest in Korea, and although at first Russians and Japanese managed to coexist peacefully, tensions on both sides soon led to hostilities. Negotiations between the two nations began in 1901 but made little headway. During the negotiations, Russia did not expect the Japanese to go to war. The Japanese had other plans. They knew they could not win a long war fought over a vast expanse, but they could win a short, localized war. The Russo-Japanese War began on February 8, 1904, when the Japanese launched a surprise attack on Russian naval vessels at Port Arthur.

Despite all the attention it has received from historians, the attack on Port Arthur was just a covering operation for the real target of Japan's opening move of the war, the **invasion of Korea** on February 9, at Chemulpo (Inchon). The Japanese advance detachment entered the harbor at Chemulpo and commenced the debarkation at once. The soldiers streamed ashore while Togo's declaratory assault was being delivered at Port Arthur. The Russian ships, moored in the harbor, ignored them. By the next morning the transports had discharged their passengers and withdrawn from the harbor. The Japanese next delivered an ultimatum to the Russian commander to vacate the harbor by noon. The Russians ran and were caught by Japanese ships blocking the harbor. The Japanese prevailed. The surviving Russians were able to return to the anchorage where they scuttled their damaged ships, and their wounded were brought ashore to be treated by the Japanese.

5.77. The Russian Civil War.

After the abdication of the Tsar, Russia was governed by a Provisional Government, under **Kerensky** (see also Fig. 2.15). On November 7, 1917, the government was placed in the hands of the Soviet Council of People's Commissars with **Vladimir Lenin** as its elected chairman. Other members included Leon Trotsky, Alexei Rykov, Anatoli Lunacharsky, and Joseph Stalin, all leading Bolsheviks. By December, central Russia and Siberia were under the control of Lenin's government (Spartacus, 2000).

Opposed to Lenin's Bolsheviks, known as the **Reds,** were a group of disparate factions, socially and politically lacking in unity and coordination. They were known collectively as the **White Movement.** The White Movement's strongest forces initially were a Volunteer Army organized by General Lavr Kornilov, numbering 3000 men. In May 1918, the Czechoslovak Corp, wishing to go to the French front to fight for an independent Czechoslovakia, quarreled with Soviet authorities. They then seized the Trans-Siberian Railroad, aided the Whites, and cleared the Reds from most of Siberia.

The Bolsheviks, on the other hand, were unified under **Trotsky,** who became War Commissar in 1918. Bolshevik forces became a regular army, with conscription and severe discipline imposed by former imperial officers. The Red Army had more than 500,000 soldiers in its ranks, including more than 40,000 officers who had served under Nicholas II. This was an unpopular decision with many Bolsheviks, who feared that given the opportunity, the tsar's former officers would betray their own troops. Trotsky's method of overcoming this problem was to impose a strict system of punishment for those judged to be disloyal. To get Red soldiers to obey their officers, Trotsky appointed political commissars whose families were often held hostage to ensure the officers' loyalty (Spartacus, 2000).

The Bolsheviks gradually reasserted military and political control. In 1920, Red forces restored the rule of Ukrainian communists wholly subservient to Moscow, thus ending the abortive Ukrainian struggle for independence (see Note 3.76). The civil strife between Reds and Whites laid the foundations of the autocratic Soviet system. The Bolshevik Party was hardened and militarized, systematic terror began, extreme economic policies were adopted, and implacable hostility developed toward the West (Rempel, 1998).

5.78 to 5.81. The Spanish American War.

Figure 5.78 depicts a soldier being brought into the U.S. General Hospital in Key West, Florida. The other figures show a nurse writing a letter for the soldier to his mother: while the nurse is writing, the soldier quietly dies. The images are from a series of oils titled *Spanish American War*, painted in 1901 by the Russian artist V. Vereschagin (1812–1904). The postcards were issued in 1906 by **the Society of St. Eugenia,** the publishing house of the Community of the Sisters of Mercy of St. Eugenia, a nursing order in Russia. The Society, which began in 1898, went on to become one of the major postcard publishers in Russia. The proceeds from the sale of the postcards were used to support the order itself and the St. Petersburg chapter of the International Red Cross.

On February 15, 1898, the United States Battleship *Maine* moored in Havana Harbor exploded, killing 266 crewmen. By April 22, America was at war with Spain. By July, 20% of the U.S. forces participating in the war were suffering from typhoid fever and **yellow fever.**

At that time, it was not known whether yellow fever was contagious, or what, if anything, conferred immunity. It was suspected, but not known, that mosquitoes might be the only source. In a desire to help spare present and future yellow fever patients, **Clara Maass,** a 25-year-old nurse from New Jersey who was stationed in Havana, volunteered to be bitten by a carrier mosquito, knowing she would probably become infected. She was bitten on the hand; when the subsequent attack of yellow fever was not considered sufficiently immunizing, she was bitten several more times. She perished from these infections, and added her life to those given for the sake of the sick, (Kalisch and Kalisch, 1985).

On August 12, 1898, the Spaniards signed an armistice. By that time, the U.S. army was so debilitated with disease that an immediate evacuation was ordered to prevent the entire force from perishing. On August 14, when the men began debarking at the 5000 acres selected for them on **Montauk Point,** four fifths of them were ill and 10,000 required hospitalization (Kalisch and Kalisch, 1985). As was often the pattern, there was no facility ready for them. The hospitals were half-completed, so the men were forced to sleep for days on the ground in tents, without bedding, and on short rations. The nurses attended them there. During the calendar years 1898–1899, the army suffered 968 battle casualties and 5438 deaths from disease (Kalisch and Kalisch, 1985).

Following the war, most of the women serving with the army were summarily dismissed, in accordance with the military's well-established anti-women rationalizations: impossible to preserve discipline, negative effect on the corpsmen, nurses too coddling, and so on. In response to that came the U.S. Army Nurse Corps, established on February 2, 1901 (see also Note 3.42), with Dita H. Kinney as its first superintendent. The Navy Nurse Corps was established in 1908 (Kalisch and Kalisch, 1985).

5.82. The Spanish Civil War (1936–1939)

was a military revolt against the new Republican government of Spain. The Republicans had assumed control in 1931 after a public vote to rid the country of monarchy and King Alfonso III. The Republicans were comprised of socialists, communists, and anarchists all in disagreement with each other ideologically. As a result they never formed a fully cohesive army. In opposition to them were the Nationalists, under **Franco,** with troops he brought from Morocco, moving up from the south in a broad coordinated wave. The Nationalists received support from fascist Italy and Nazi Germany. The Republicans received aid from the Soviet Union, as well as from International Brigades, composed of volunteers from Europe and the United States.

Many artists and intellectuals took up arms in the Spanish Civil War. Among the most notable artistic responses to the war were the novels *Man's Hope* by André Malraux, *Homage to Catalonia* by George Orwell, *The Adventures of a Young Man* by John Dos Passos, and *For Whom the Bell Tolls* by Ernest Hemingway, as well as Pablo Picasso's painting *Guernica* and Robert Capa's photograph *Loyalist Soldier, Spain* (Spartacus, 2002).

The **postcard** in Figure 5.82 was issued by the *Confederación Nacional de Trabajo—Asociación Internacional de los Trabajadores* (National Labor Confederation—International Association of Labor), a trade union founded in 1910, whose members believed in the revolutionary overthrow of capitalism. Being fervently anti-Franco, the CNT played an active part in the Revolution. Today, the CIT-AIT is the largest union organization in Spain (Spartacus, 2002).

The logo on the card states, "Blood Hospitals And Day Care Centers. Organizing Committee of the Single Regional Union of Industrial Experts and Technicians." Blood hospitals treated people involved in accidents or fighting, or who, for some other reason, had bleeding wounds. Diseases were treated elsewhere.

5.83. **World War II.** As in World War I, Russian and German medics often exchanged fire in violation of the Geneva Convention prohibiting the use of firearms by anyone displaying the logo of the Red Cross. The woman in the picture is probably a medic rather than a nurse. In Russian forces, women served in both capacities in the field, but the medics were more likely to be armed.

5.86. The full cancel reads "Tetschen a.d. E (Tetschen on the Elbe), Day of Liberation, October 3, 1938." Tetschen is a small city, now called Decin, on the river Elbe, in the Czech Republic. The Day of Liberation refers to the **German annexation of Czechoslovakia's Sudetenland** under the Munich Agreement. Although the Agreement was signed on September 29, the Day of Liberation was designated as October 3, the date of Hitler's speech in the "liberated" territory.

In the summer of 1938, Hitler had voiced support for the demands of the German population of the Sudetenland, in Czechoslovakia, for annexation of the region into Germany. Britain's Prime Minister, **Neville Chamberlain,** believed that Germany had been badly treated by the Allies after the First World War, that the German government had genuine grievances, and that these needed to be addressed. He also thought that by agreeing to the demands being made, he could avoid a European war.

European leaders met in a conference at Munich on September 29. Eduard Daladier represented France, Neville Chamberlain represented England, Benito Mussolini represented Italy, and Adolf Hitler represented Germany. Representatives of Czechoslovakia and the Soviet Union were not invited. The ministers submitted to Hitler's demands very quickly: the conference was over the next day. Afterwards Chamberlain boasted that "Peace in our time" had been achieved. By October 10, the Sudetenland was fully annexed into Germany. Germany's annexation of the Sudetenland, with its military industries, gold reserves, communications system, coal mines, and anti-German defense lines, simply made it that much easier for Hitler to wage war. In March 1939, the German Army seized the rest of Czechoslovakia, breaking the treaty. The Munich Agreement became one of the most infamous treaties of the century, a symbol of failed appeasement, and Chamberlain was ever after associated with his part in it.

5.88 to **5.89.** Both cards are issued by the Ersatzkommando Flandern der Waffen-SS, (Flemish Reserve Unit of the Armed Protection Force), Belgium.

The Germans occupying Belgium were not without supporters, and aimed their recruitment propaganda at those individuals. The Belgian lion is shown in the background of 5.88 and on the arm patch of the nurse. The soldier in 5.89 is Jules Geurts, first Flemish winner of the Iron Cross. **DRK** stands for Deutsche Rotes Kreutz (German Red Cross).

The **SS runes** were derived from the Sigrune, which is part of the Norse alphabet. They were adopted by Julius Schreck (1891–1936). In April 1925, Hitler ordered Schreck, who was his chauffeur, to form a new headquarters guard that initially consisted of only 8 men. A week later, it was christened Schutzstaffel (Protection Force).

The **SS** was at the heart of the German political and social revolution and later attempts to control all aspects of German life. It was a complex political and military organization consisting of three separate and distinct branches, all related but unique in their functions and goals. The Allgemeine-SS (General SS) was the main branch, and assumed the political and administrative role. The SS-Totenkopfverbande (SS Deaths Head Organization) presided over the concentration camps. The Waffen-SS, formed in 1940, is often mistaken for the SS itself, but although a part of the larger structure, the Waffen-SS was a front-line fighting organization, which included more than 500,000 members by the end of the war. At the head of the entire organization was **Heinrich Himmler,** Reichsfuhrer SS, head of the Gestapo and the Waffen SS, Minister of the Interior from 1943 to 1945. When Himmler took over the SS in 1929, it had 280 members. By the time the Nazi Party gained power in 1933, Himmler's SS had grown to a strength of 52,000.

Himmler was the principal organizer of the rounding up and the mass murders of all the "undesirables," including Jews, Gypsies, and others not of Aryan blood. By 1933 he had set up the first concentration camp in Dachau; in the next few years, with Hitler's encouragement,

Himmler established other camps and extended the range of persons who qualified for internment. Himmler's wife, **Margarete Himmler,** was a nurse during World War I.

5.92. **The swastika** has had a long history as a symbol of luck and happiness and as a protection against evil spirits. It has been found in ancient Rome, in excavations in Grecian cities, on Buddhist statues, and on Chinese coins from 300 BC. It appears in the art of the Ashanti of Africa, the Tlingit of Alaska, the Cuna in Panama, and the Navajo and the Hopi in the United States. It is a very prominent symbol in Hinduism and a heraldic form of the Christian cross.

It was first used in Germany by the German Freikorps. After the First World War, former senior officers in the German Army began raising private armies called Freikorps, whose purpose was to defend the German borders against the possibility of Russian invasion. Later they were used against attempts at revolution in Germany. The Freikorps were dissolved in 1921.

By the summer of 1920, the swastika was in use in Germany as the symbol of the **Nazi party.** Nazi is short for Nazional-socialistische Deutsche Arbeiterpartei (NSDAP) or National Socialist German Workers' Party. Most historians agree that it was Hitler himself who chose the swastika as the official symbol of his Third Reich, but there are many theories about who or what influenced him into making that decision. After its adoption by the Nazis, few other symbols in the history of mankind have become so widely associated with evil.

The chief propagandist of the Nazi party was **Joseph Goebbels** (1897–1945). He joined the NSDAP in 1924. Initially he was one of Hitler's opponents, but he became an ardent admirer after 1926. Goebbels became party provincial chief of Berlin-Brandenburg in 1926, Reich propaganda director of the NSDAP in 1929, and Reich propaganda minister in 1933. Goebbels controlled the German movie industry and the ideological orientation of the press. Thousands of independent propagandists and hundreds of advertising firms operated under his auspices and he issued monthly rules, specifications, and guidelines for the works to be created. Under his direction, Germany became completely saturated with propaganda in every form. No media were overlooked, which explains why propaganda postcards were employed in Germany during the war when they were all but abandoned for that purpose in other countries. In 1944, Goebbels was appointed general deputy for the "total war" effort, becoming, in effect, Hitler's sub-dictator. Goebbels took his own life, and that of his wife and 6 children, on May 1, 1945.

5.93 to **5.94.** From a series of 10 postcards issued by the German Red Cross in 1941.

5.98. When the Nazis began their racial purification and extermination programs, the *Jüdischen Krankenhaus Berlin* (**Jewish Hospital in Berlin**) was converted to a Gestapo headquarters and deportation center. After the war it was restored to its original function, and is still in operation today.

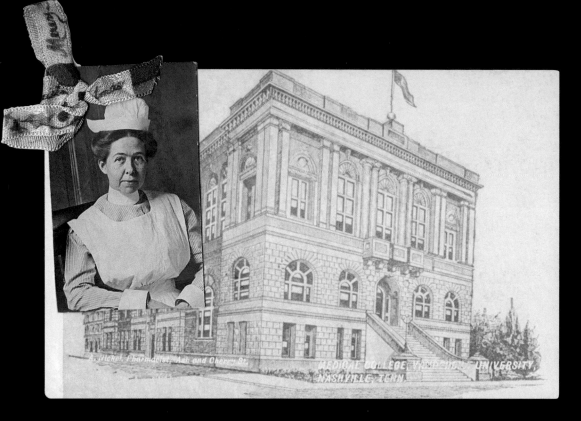

Figure 6.1. **"Who I am and where I stay."** *(See note.)*

An American Photo Postcard Album

*R*ural free delivery, inexpensive paper-film cameras, and the introduction of the postcard made it possible for anyone to create and send a picture, easily, reliably, and cheaply. Before those necessary components came together in 1907, most people had no clear image of where their distant friends and family lived, what their homes looked like, or even what they looked like. As a result, when photo postcards became possible, everything was photographed. This is not hyperbole: the subject matter on postcards is so diverse you can hardly dream up a subject that you can't find photographed. No one and nothing was overlooked. There are pictures of every item imaginable, natural, handcrafted, or manufactured. Every relative and neighbor, every street, every building in town inside and out, the shed out back, the rock behind the shed . . . all were photographed. Naturally, events of note were documented too: celebrations, disasters, haircuts, dinner, the sale of the cow, or a visit to the store. Although postcards were produced in every mechanized country in the world, only in America were there so many real photos that captured the day-to-day lives of the people.

Eventually, the postcards found their way into the postcard collectibles community. A medium-size postcard show, of which there are hundreds each year around the world, can have several million postcards for sale in one room. At any given time, there are tens of thousands more being offered on Internet auction sites. A good number of the amateur photographic ones are out of focus, poorly composed, and of unidentified people and places. However, if you are willing to mine this vast repository, you can discover many postcard gems that perfectly capture the spirit of the golden times. And, no matter how many years you have been collecting, no matter how many postcards you have seen, you will always find something you haven't seen on a postcard before.

The postcards in this chapter, with one exception, were produced between 1907 and 1917.

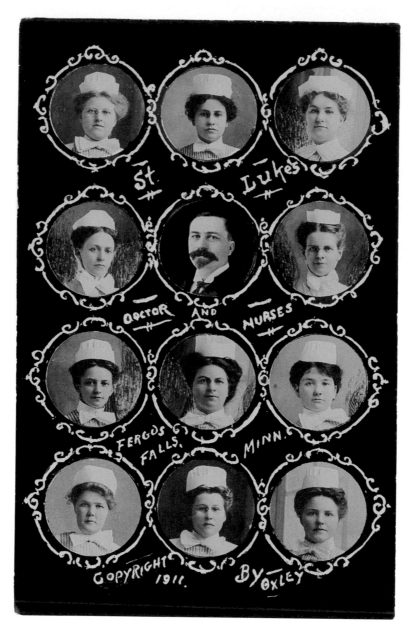

Figure 6.2. **St. Luke's Doctor and Nurses.**
Fergus Falls, Minnesota. 1911.

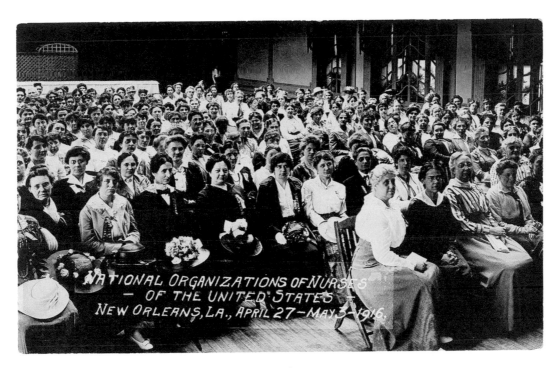

Figure 6.3. **National Organization of Nurses of the United States.**
New Orleans, Louisiana. 1916.

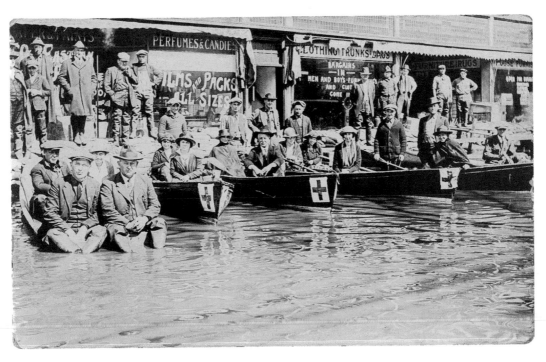

Figure 6.4. **Mississippi River flood.**
St. Louis, Missouri. c. 1912.

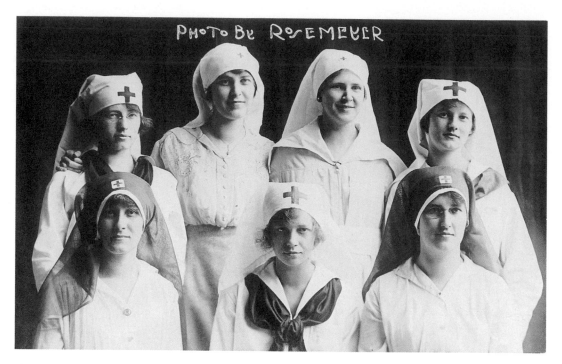

Figure 6.5. **Nurses and Camp Fire Girl.**
c. 1915.

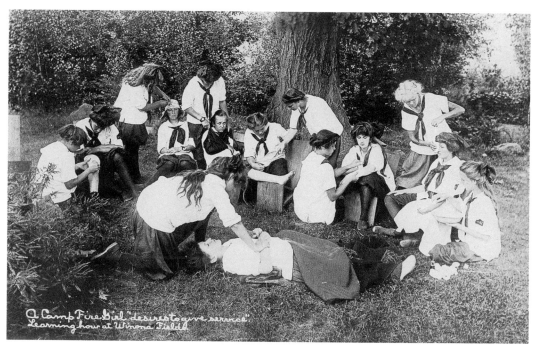

Figure 6.6. **A Camp Fire Girl "desires to give service."**
c. 1915. *(See note.)*

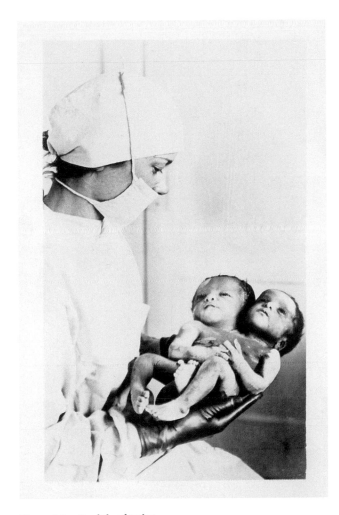

Figure 6.7. Conjoined twins.
c. 1940.

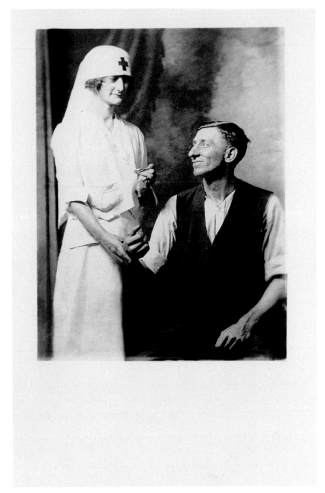

Figure 6.8. Fraternal twins.
c. 1910.

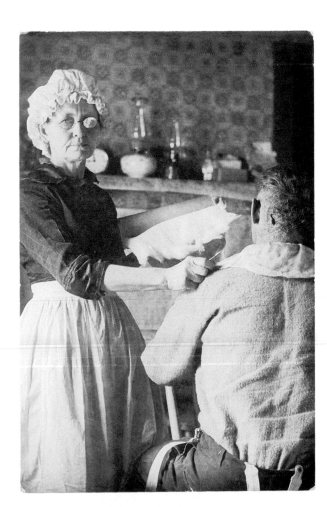

Figure 6.9. Unidentified community nurse.
c. 1914.

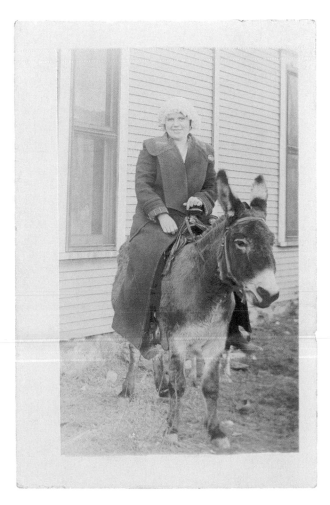

Figure 6.10. "John's nurse."
Oklahoma City. 1914.

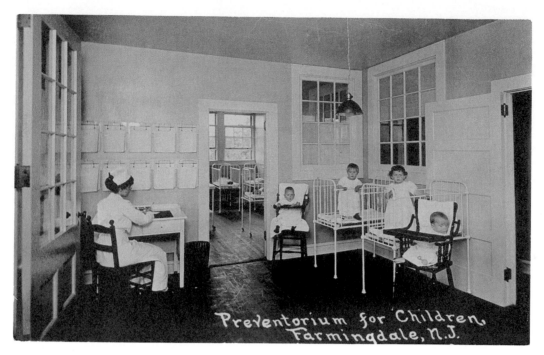

Figure 6.11.   Preventorium for Children.
Farmingdale, New Jersey. c. 1910.

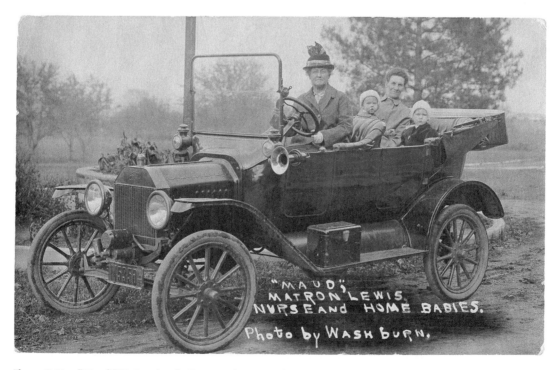

Figure 6.12.   "Maud," Matron Lewis, Nurse and Home Babies.
Iowa. 1915. (Maud is the car.)

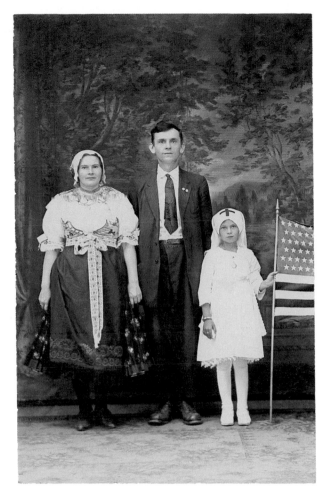

Figure 6.13. Immigrant photo.
c. 1914. *(See note.)*

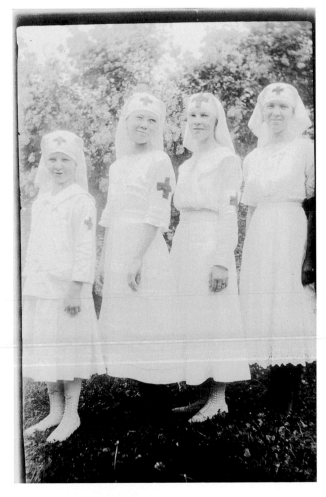

Figure 6.14. Unidentified.
c. 1917.

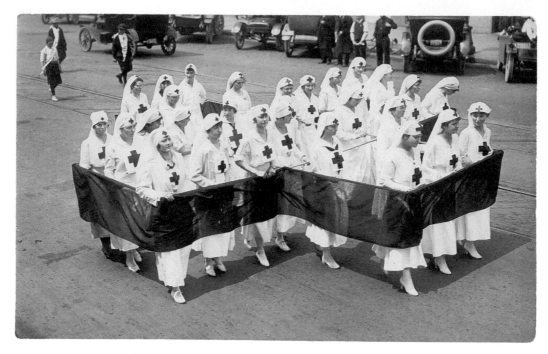

Figure 6.15. **Unidentified.**
c. 1917.

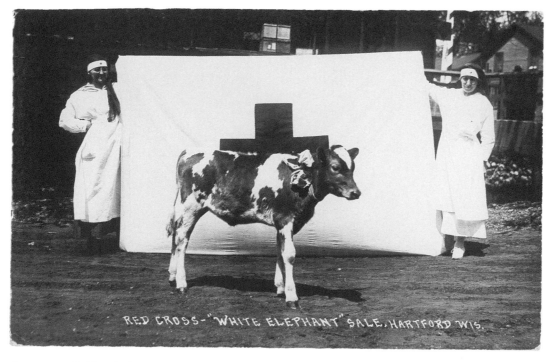

Figure 6.16. **"White elephant" sale.**
Hartford, Wisconsin. c. 1917.

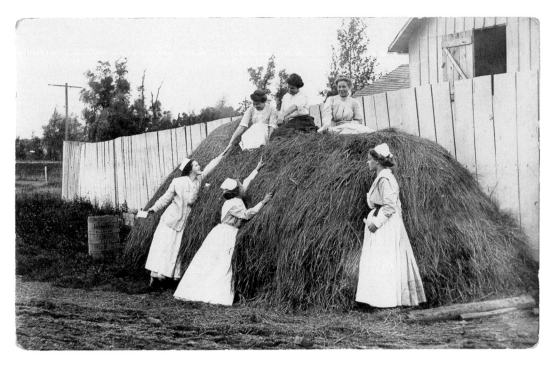

Figure 6.17.
Madison, Wisconsin. c. 1910.

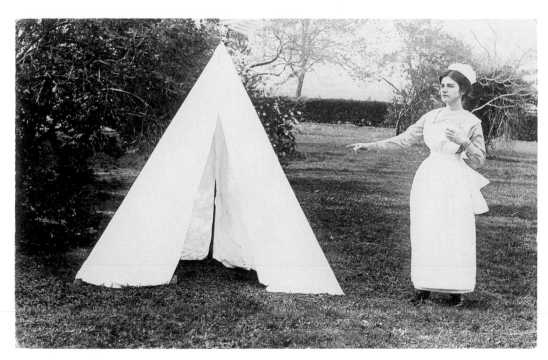

Figure 6.18.   **Unidentified.**
c. 1910.

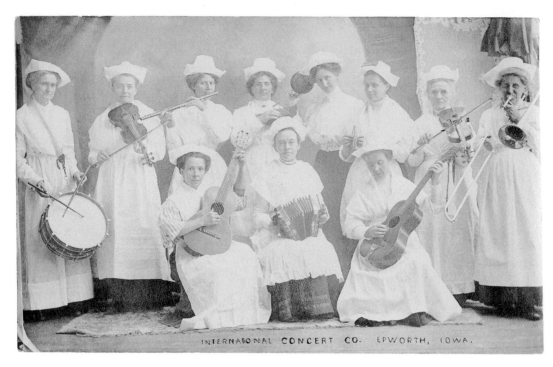

Figure 6.19.   **International Concert Company Nurse Band.**
Epworth, Iowa. c. 1910.

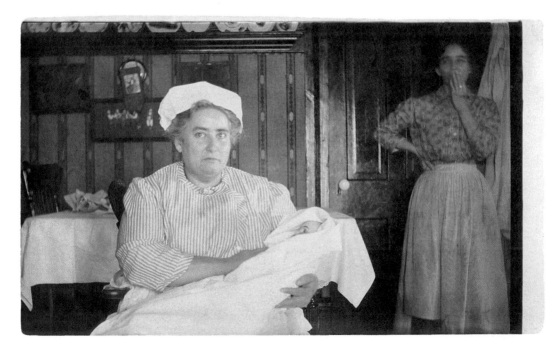

Figure 6.20.   **From reverse: "Mable did not think she was going to show but haint it good torne apron and all the baby is Vera's doll."**
c. 1910.

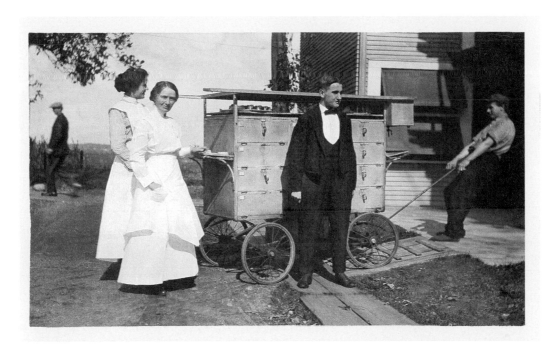

Figure 6.21.   **Hospital food cart.**
c. 1910.

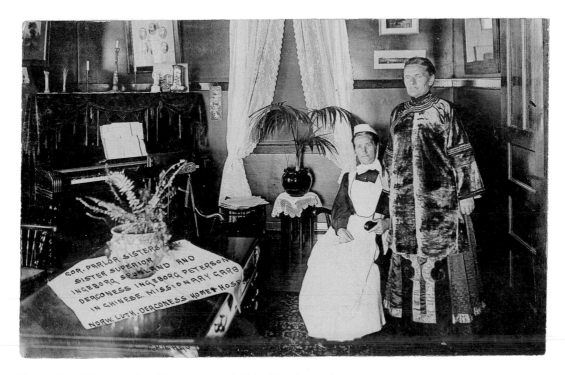

Figure 6.22.   **"Corner parlor sisters apartment. Sister Superior Ingeborg Sponland and Deaconess Ingeborg Peterson in Chinese missionary garb. Norwegian Lutheran Deaconess Home and Hospital."**
Chicago, Illinois. 1909. *(See note.)*

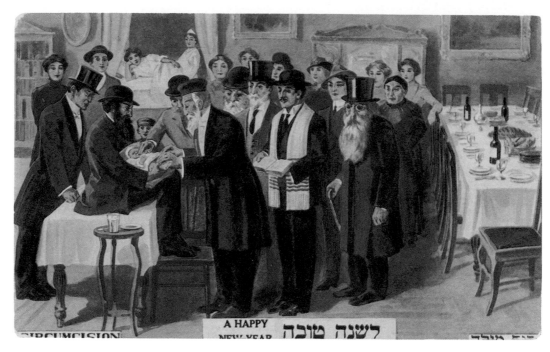

Figure 6.23.   Circumcision. A Happy New Year.
1917. *(See note.)*

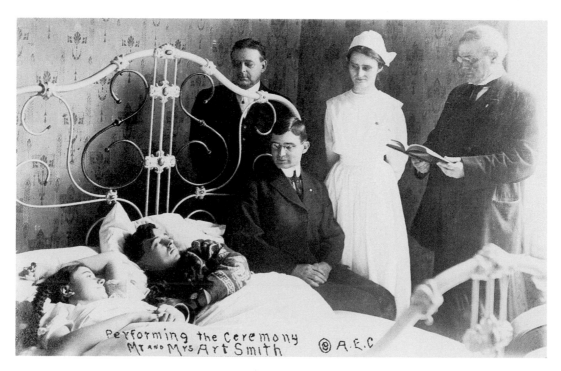

Figure 6.24.   Performing the Ceremony. Mr. and Mrs. Art Smith.
Art Smith was an aviation pioneer. His marriage was performed after a crash during the
first elopement by airplane.
Hillsdale, Michigan. 1912. *(See note.)*

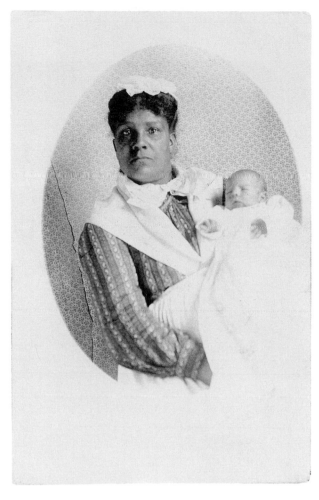

Figure 6.25. Unidentified.
c. 1910. *(See note.)*

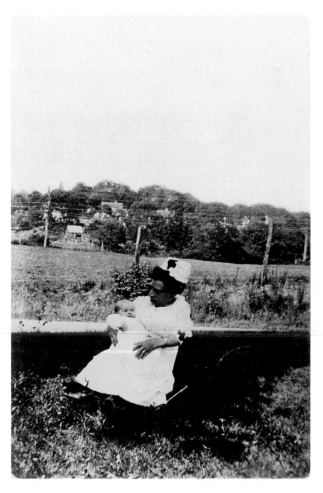

Figure 6.26. Unidentified.
c. 1910. *(See note.)*

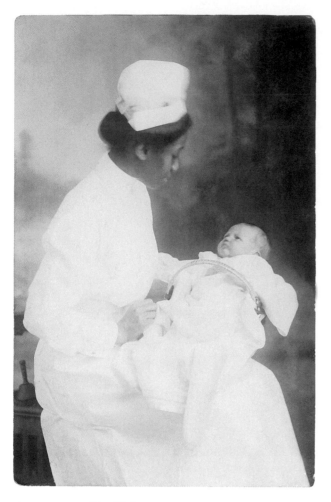

Figure 6.27. **Unidentified.**
Oblong, Illinois. c. 1910. *(See note.)*

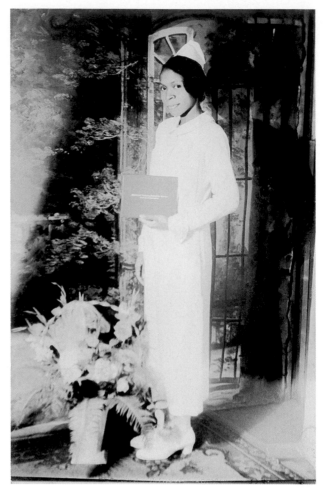

Figure 6.28. **Unidentified nurse with diploma.**
c. 1935. *(See note.)*

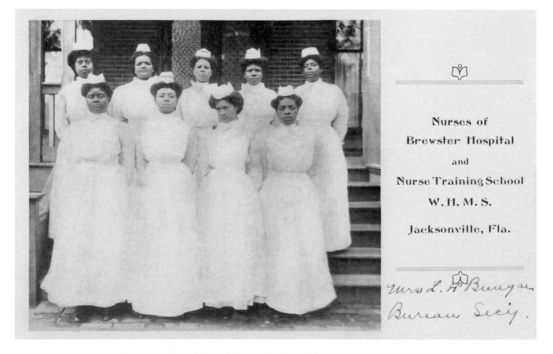

Figure 6.29. **Nurses of Brewster Hospital and Nurse Training School.**
Jacksonville, Florida. c. 1908. *(See note.)*

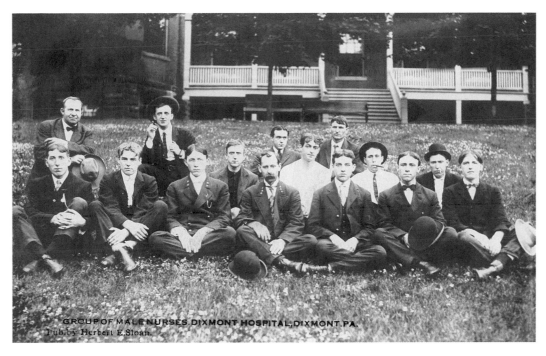

Figure 6.30. **Group of male nurses.**
Dixmont Hospital, Dixmont, Pennsylvania. c. 1910. *(See note.)*

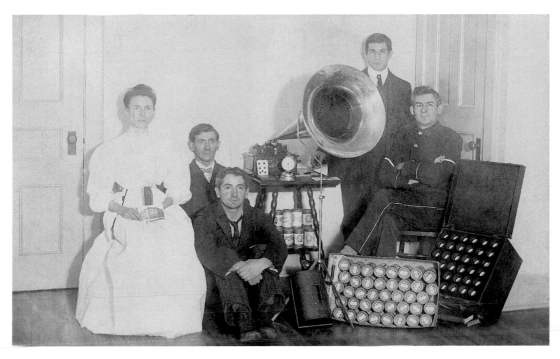

Figure 6.31. **Sonyea, New York.**
The nurse is the man on the far right.
1907. *(See note.)*

6.24. **Art Smith** (1890–1926), from Fort Wayne, Indiana, was an aviation pioneer who built and flew his own plane for the first time at age 20. He became internationally famous as an exhibition flyer, became one of the first airmail pilots to fly at night, and had many crashes and brushes with death. He died in a crash while on one of his night mail flights.

In 1912, after courting his childhood sweetheart, Aimee Cour, Smith asked Cour to elope. In October 1912, after one last exhibition before a crowd of enthusiastic Fort Wayne fans, they flew together in Smith's plane toward Hillsdale, Michigan, about 70 miles from Fort Wayne. As he leaned against the controls to swing the machine in the direction of a smooth landing field near Hillsdale, he discovered his ailerons would not respond. Smith brought the machine down in a farmer's field. The wheels sank into the soft sand, and the airplane flipped over, throwing both pilot and passenger. They later woke up in a Hillsdale hotel that served as a makeshift hospital.

When Smith came to, he asked for a preacher right away, and they were married with Smith lying on the bed beside Cour. The nurse and doctor, already present at the bedside, acted as witnesses. Aimee had sustained a broken arm and was in considerable pain throughout the ceremony, but had readily agreed to it. Newspapers all over the country played up the story as the first elopement by airplane. The next flying season, Smith toured the country with his wife at his side.

6.25. to **6.35.** Notes on individual postcards follow. The two most prominent **minority groups** in nursing in the United States are African Americans and men (of course, there is overlap, since African American men are in both groups). Each of these groups currently represents approximately 5% to 7% of the nursing workforce.

The definition of "minority" must be a functional definition. Everyone belongs to at least one minority group, if only based on surname. Zwerdlings in nursing, for example, are in the minority when compared to all nurses. However, the Zwerdlings historically have not been denied educational and placement opportunities, nor have they been treated any differently from the

"majority" of nurses. Moreover, the number of Zwerdlings is so small compared to all nurses that they have no representation as a group. Functionally, then, Zwerdlings are not a true minority.

Which groups, then, constitute the true minorities in nursing today? One organization that represents minority nurses declares "African-American, Hispanic, Asian, Native American and Filipinos comprise roughly 10% of the overall nursing population" (Minority Nurse, 2002). However, this definition does not include men as a separate minority, nor does it mention, for example, nurses with physical handicaps, nurses with European citizenship working in the United States, Islamic nurses, homosexual nurses, and so on, all of which can be considered minorities in nursing.

As a functional definition, then, we might say that a minority in U.S. nursing is any group that has been or is treated in a different manner than the group of white, fully able-bodied, American-born, heterosexual, English-speaking, Christian women who constitute the majority. Differences in workplace treatment and professional opportunities were more evident during the postcard era than now, reflecting the bias at the time against minorities in general. Fortunately, the country appears to be moving toward the understanding that competency and willingness to act responsibly are better measures of worth than racial origin, religious affiliation, gender, or sexual orientation. The history and contribution of minority groups in nursing is rich and detailed, and I refer you to *The Advance of American Nursing* (Kalisch and Kalisch, 1995) for an excellent examination of the subject.

6.25. This African American's occupation derived from a background of slavery and deprivation. She was a **mammy,** after the women slaves of the same name who, in the United States, were put in change of their owner's children, with duties similar to the British nanny. The mammy was every bit as qualified as her British counterpart. During the days of Jim Crow (a period of oppression, prejudice, and unequal treatment lasting from the end of the Civil War through the 1960s) she was still referred to as a mammy, even though she was a paid servant.

6.26. I can only imagine the obstacles this person had to go through to become a Red Cross nurse. She faced a double prejudice: she was black and she was a little person. There is nothing in this photograph to indicate she was part of an act (as might be expected for midgets at the time, showmanship being one of the few opportunities open to them). Therefore, the photograph must be taken at face value: this woman was a Red Cross nurse caring for an infant.

6.29. **Brewster Hospital** was built in 1885 as the Boylan-Haven Private School for African American Girls. **Hattie Emerson** started a nurse training program in the 1890s and became its first superintendent. By 1901, the school was deeded to the Women's Home Society of the Methodist Church and re-chartered as Brewster Hospital, the first for African Americans in Jacksonville. Its charter was unchallenged until the 1964 Civil Rights Act opened larger, more modern hospitals to African Americans. Underfunded, and thus less able to compete, in 1966 Old Brewster closed (Soul of America, 2002).

6.31. From the reverse: "Dear Jack, The people in the picture are: one behind me—Mr. Bixby. One behind the horn, Mr. Keith (runs phonograph). One in uniform, Mr. Brewster, our nurse. Lady, his wife. Picture taken in our room. Merry Christmas, Jor." If you look closely, you can see that the nurse's wife is holding a postcard showing the building.

The postmark is Sonyea, NY. December 23, 1907. Although Sonyea is a town near Rochester, in the Finger Lakes region of western New York, the initials originally stood for "State of New York Epileptic Association." The institution, in what is now the town of Sonyea, developed around a Shaker community. The grounds are now used as a site for two state prisons: Groveland and Livingston correctional facilities.

6.34. This is a photomontage. The two men are actually the same person. The seated version is draped in his missionary robes, which were intended to resemble native clothing as much as possible, with an American flag over one shoulder.

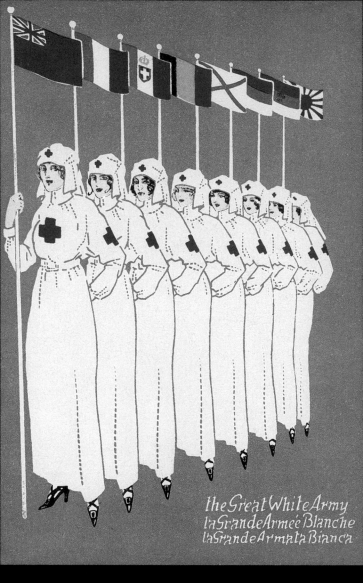

The Great White Army
la Grande Armée Blanche
la Grande Armata Bianca

Figure 7.1. "The Great White Army."
Italy. 1916.

Parade of Nations

*H*ow many countries produced postcards of nurses? There is no way to tell for sure because, unlike with stamps, there were never comprehensive postcard catalogs listing all the issues. Making an educated guess, I would venture that postcards of one kind or another were produced showing scenes or subjects of 200 countries, including colonies and occupied territories. (That is not the same as saying 200 countries produced postcards. Industrialized nations produced postcards showing scenes of less developed countries that lacked the technology to produce their own postcards.) Not all countries represented on postcards pictured nurses on the cards. Of the ones that did, over 70 are represented in this chapter or elsewhere in the book. Are there more nurse postcards from other countries waiting to be found? The answer is "almost certainly." Is there one in your attic?

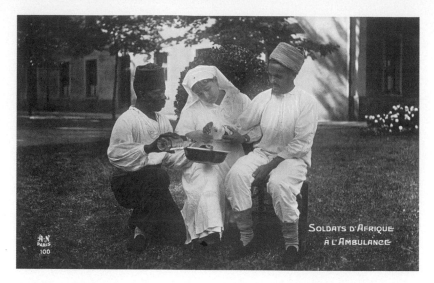

Figure 7.2. **Algeria.**
c. 1914.

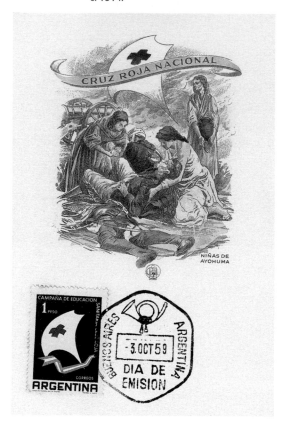

Figure 7.3. **Argentina.**
1959.

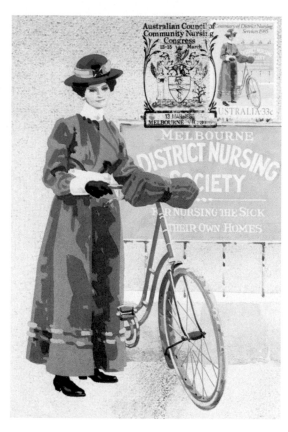

Figure 7.4. **Australia.**
1995. *(See note.)*

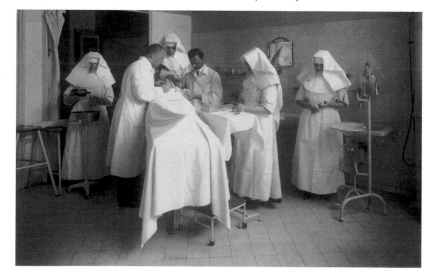

Figure 7.5. **Austria.**
c. 1910.

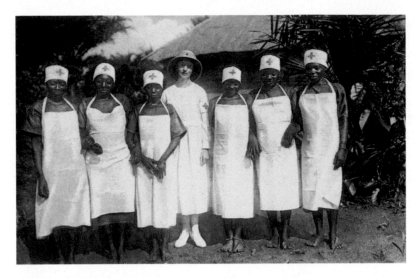

Figure 7.6. **Congo Free State.**
c. 1908. *(See note.)*

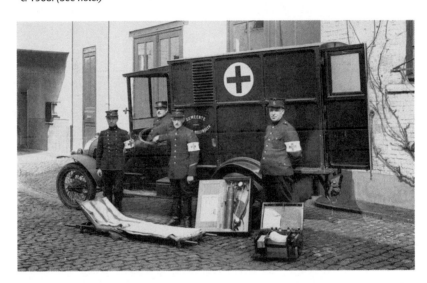

Figure 7.7. **Belgium.**
c. 1910.

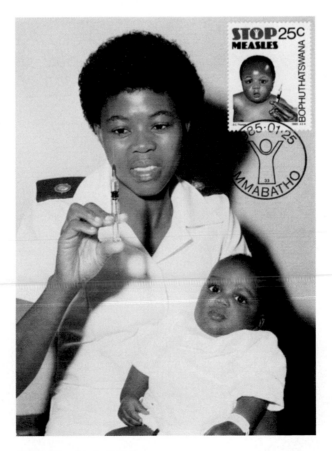

Figure 7.8. **Bophuthatswana.**
1985. *(See note.)*

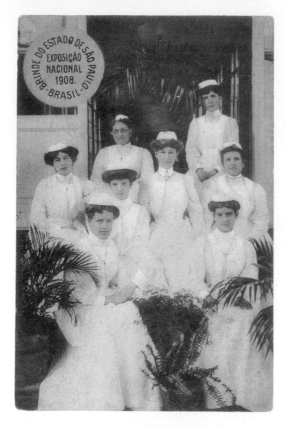

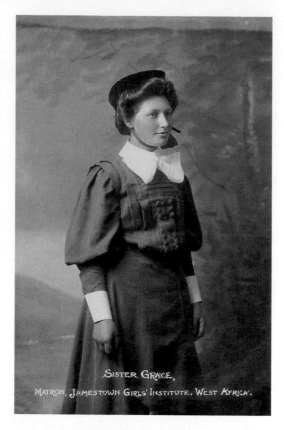

Figure 7.9.   **Brazil. Sao Paulo Isolation Hospital nurses.**
National Exposition of Brazil. 1908.

Figure 7.10.   **British West Africa. Sister Grace, Matron.**
Jamestown Girls Institute. c. 1908.

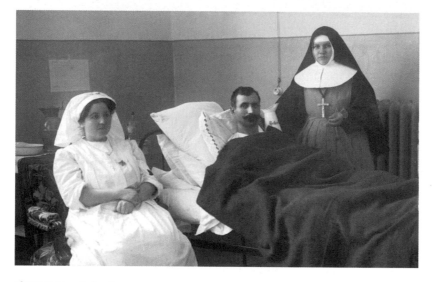

Figure 7.11.   **Bulgaria.**
c. 1914.

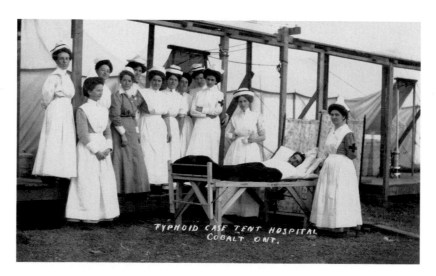

Figure 7.12.   **Canada.**
Typhoid case tent hospital, Cobalt, Ontario. c. 1910.

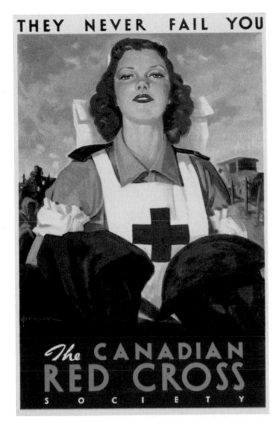

Figure 7.13. **Canada.**
Nursing Auxiliary Canadian Red Cross Corps. c. 1914.

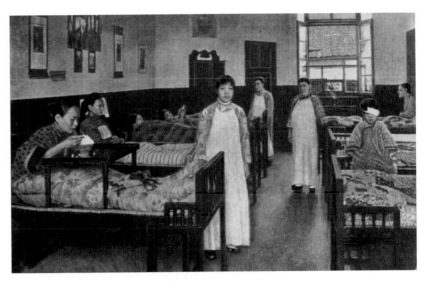

Figure 7.14. **China.**
c. 1908.

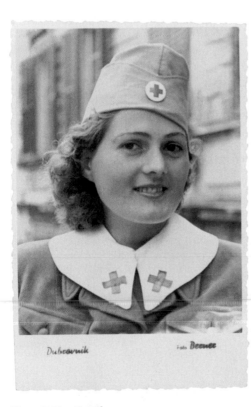

Figure 7.15. **Croatia.**
c. 1960.

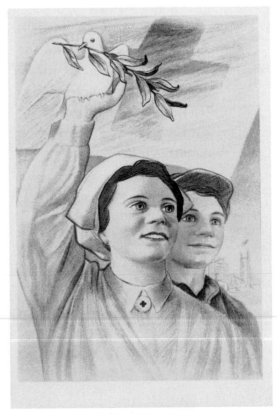

Figure 7.16. **Czechoslovakia.**
1951.

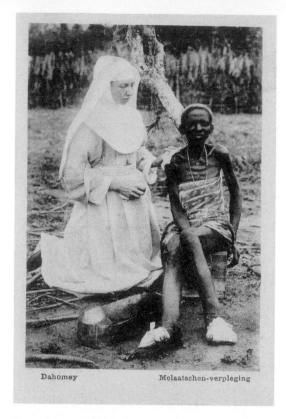

Dahomey   Melaatschen-verpleging

Figure 7.17.   Dahomey.
c. 1910.

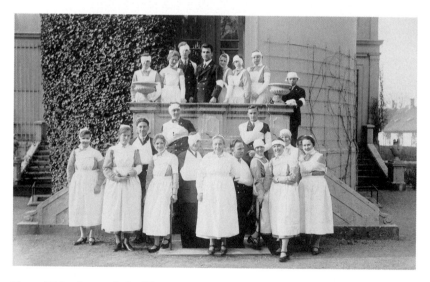

Figure 7.18.   Denmark. Staff has practiced bandaging skills on each other.
c. 1910.

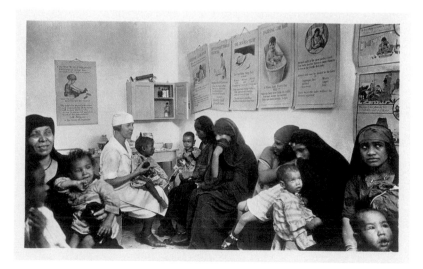

Figure 7.19.   Egypt. American Mission Child Welfare Clinic.
c. 1920.

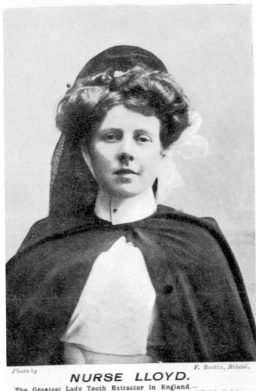

Photo by   F. Bastin, Bristol.

NURSE LLOYD.

The Greatest Lady Tooth Extractor in England.—
Vide Press and Public Opinion.

Figure 7.20.   England. Nurse Lloyd, The Greatest Lady Tooth Extractor in England.
c. 1910.

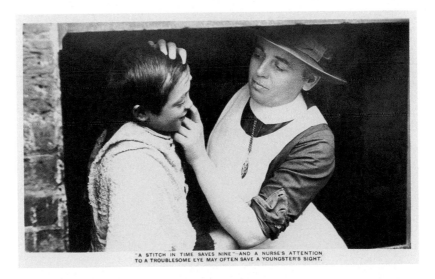

"A STITCH IN TIME SAVES NINE"—AND A NURSE'S ATTENTION
TO A TROUBLESOME EYE MAY OFTEN SAVE A YOUNGSTER'S SIGHT.

Figure 7.21.   England. National Memorial to Queen Alexandra.
1927. *(See Note 4.79.)*

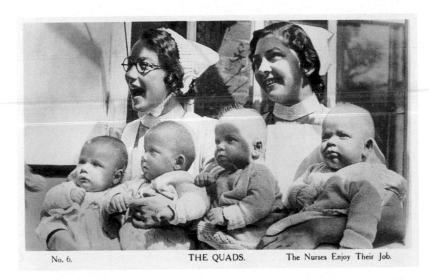

No. 6.   THE QUADS.   The Nurses Enjoy Their Job.

Figure 7.22.   England. The Quads.
1935. *(See note.)*

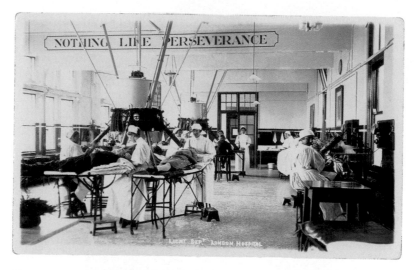

Figure 7.23. England. London Hospital. The patients are being treated with Finsen's therapy for tuberculosis of the skin.
c. 1914. *(See note.)*

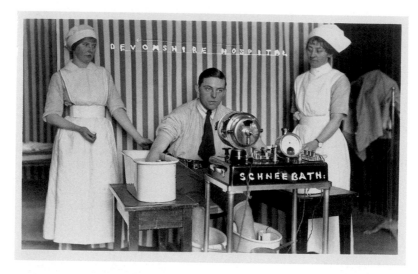

Figure 7.24. England. Schnee bath.
c. 1915. *(See note.)*

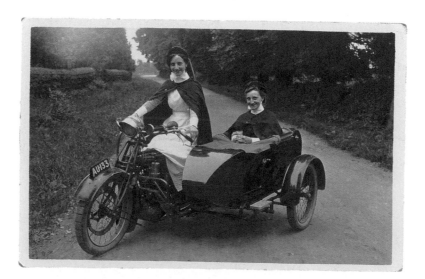

Figure 7.25. England. District nurses.
c. 1915.

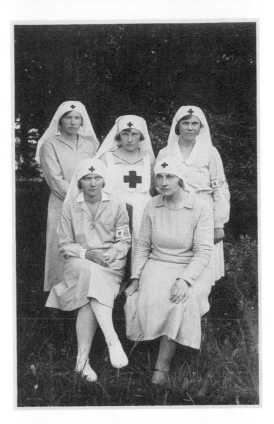

Figure 7.26. **Estonia.**
c. 1914.

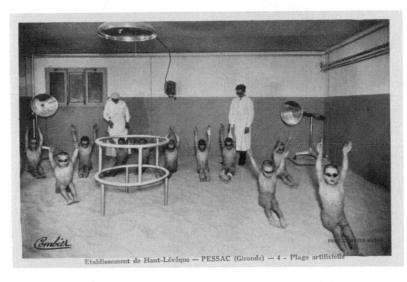

Figure 7.27. **France. Artificial seashore.**
(Note sand on floor.) c. 1910.

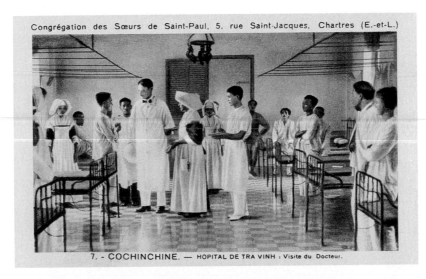

Figure 7.28. **French Indochina. Sisters of St. Paul in Tra Vinh.**
c. 1910. *(See note.)*

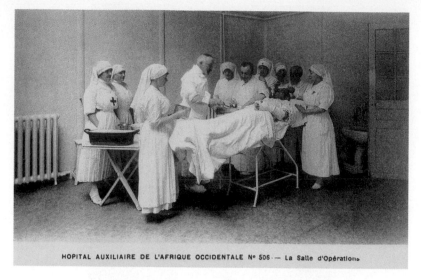

HOPITAL AUXILIAIRE DE L'AFRIQUE OCCIDENTALE N° 506 — La Salle d'Opération

Figure 7.29.   French West Africa.
c. 1910.

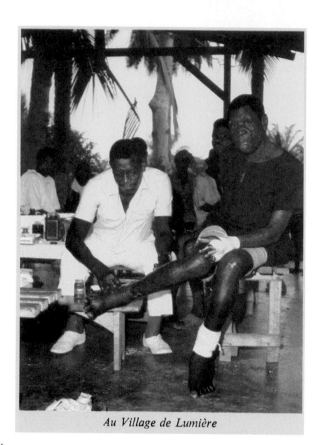

Au Village de Lumière

Figure 7.30.   Gabon. "At the Village of Light."
c. 1970.

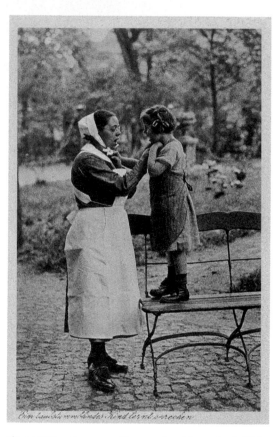

Figure 7.31.   Germany. "A nurse teaching a deaf child to speak."
c. 1908.

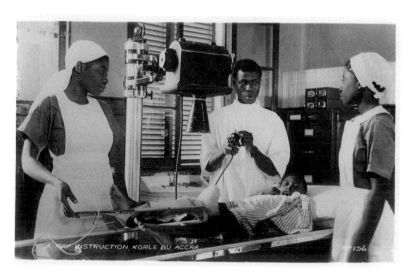

Figure 7.32.   Ghana. "X-ray instruction in Accra."
c. 1970.

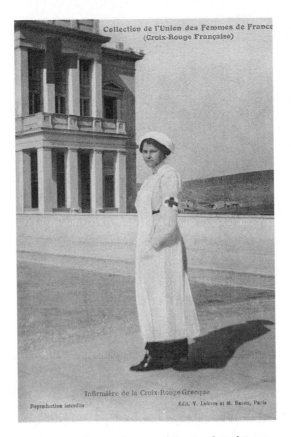

Figure 7.33. **Greece. A nurse of the Greek Red Cross.**
c. 1915.

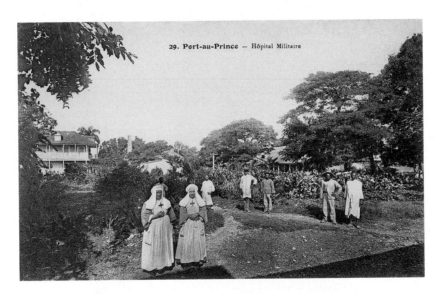

Figure 7.34. **Haiti.**
c. 1910.

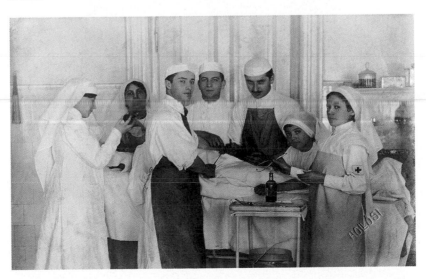

Figure 7.35. **Hungary.**
c. 1910.

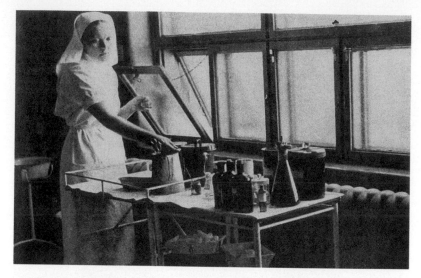

Figure 7.36.   Iceland.
c. 1925.

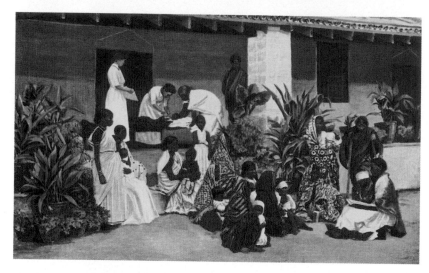

Figure 7.37.   India.
c. 1910.

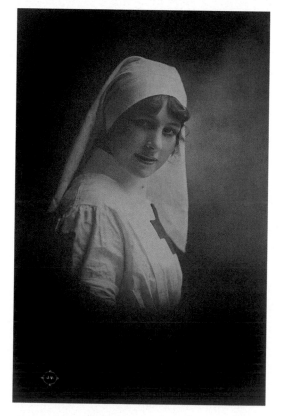

Figure 7.38.   Ireland.
1920.

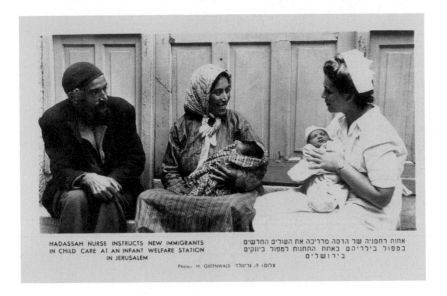

HADASSAH NURSE INSTRUCTS NEW IMMIGRANTS IN CHILD CARE AT AN INFANT WELFARE STATION IN JERUSALEM

אחות רחמניה של הדסה מדריכה את העולים החדשים בטפול בילדיהם באחת התחנות לטפול ביונקים בירושלים

Photo: H. GREENWALD   צלום: ה. גרינולד

Figure 7.39.   Israel.
c. 1950.

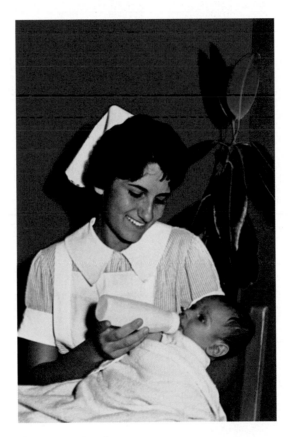

Figure 7.40.   Israel.
c. 1995.

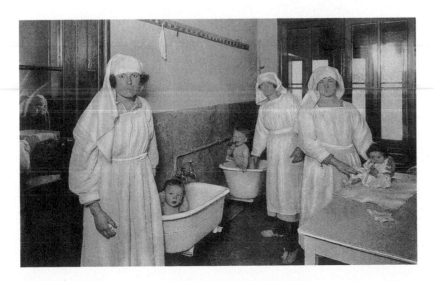

Figure 7.41.   Italy.
c. 1920.

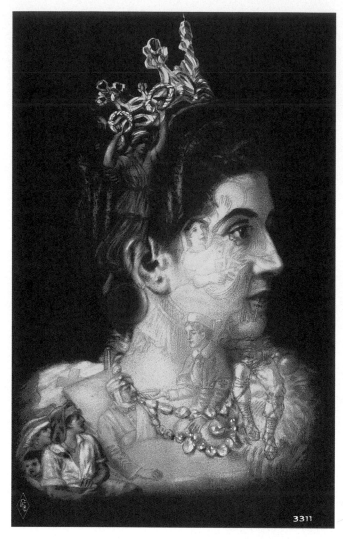

Figure 7.42. Italy. Can you find the four nurses?
c. 1910. *(See note.)*

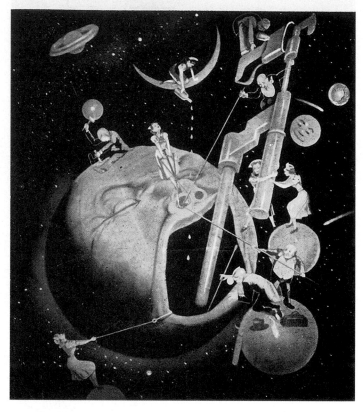

Figure 7.43. Japan.
c. 1950. *(See note.)*

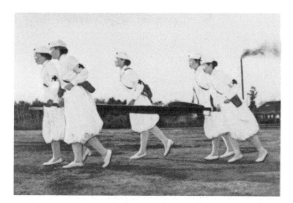

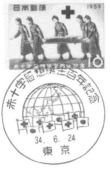

Figure 7.44. Japan.
1959. *(See note.)*

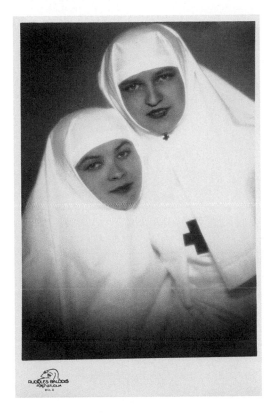

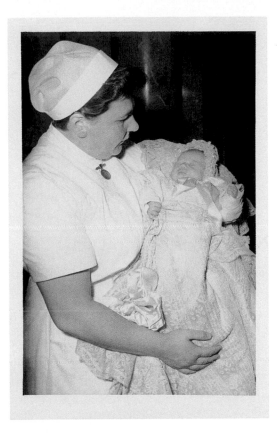

Figure 7.45. **Latvia.**
c. 1915.

Figure 7.46. **Luxembourg.**
1929.

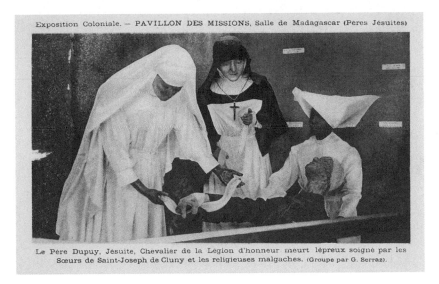

Exposition Coloniale. — PAVILLON DES MISSIONS, Salle de Madagascar (Pères Jésuites)

Le Père Dupuy, Jésuite, Chevalier de la Légion d'honneur meurt lépreux soigné par les Sœurs de Saint-Joseph de Cluny et les religieuses malgaches. (Groupe par G. Serraz).

Figure 7.47. **Madagascar. Father Dupuy.**
This is a tableau in an exhibition. c. 1931. *(See note.)*

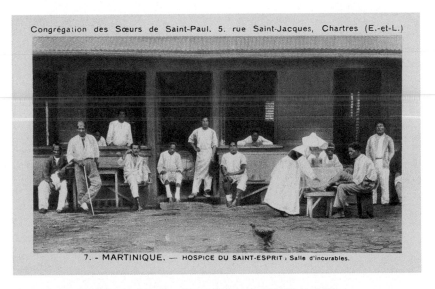

Congrégation des Sœurs de Saint-Paul. 5. rue Saint-Jacques, Chartres (E.-et-L.)

7. - MARTINIQUE. — HOSPICE DU SAINT-ESPRIT : Salle d'incurables.

Figure 7.48. **Martinique. Hospice of Saint-Esprit: ward of incurables.**
c. 1920.

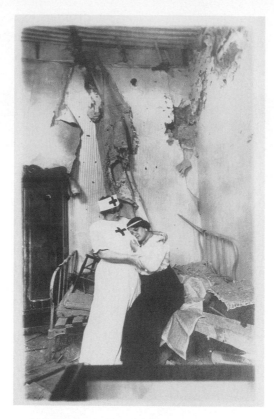

Figure 7.49. Mexico. Vera Cruz.
Mexican Revolution. 1914. *(See Note 3.16.)*

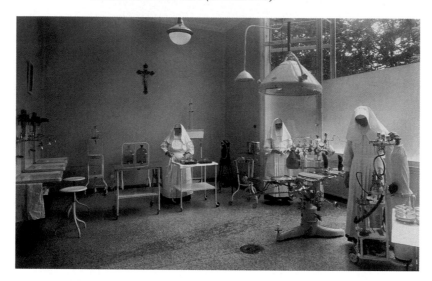

Figure 7.50. Netherlands.
1940.

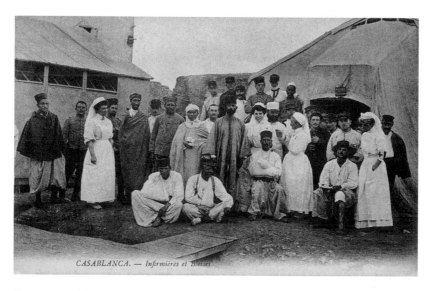

Figure 7.51. Morocco.
c. 1915.

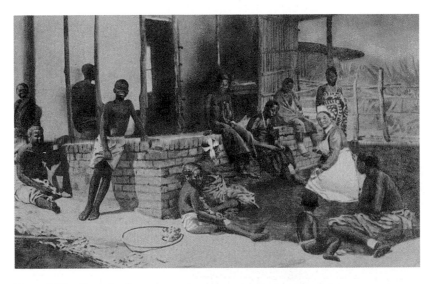

Figure 7.52.   Nyasaland.
c. 1910.

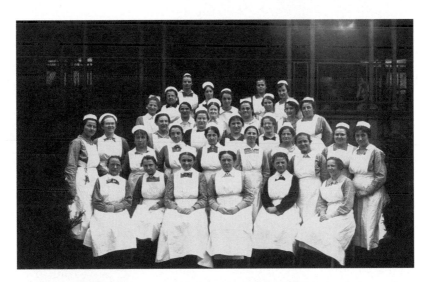

Figure 7.53.   Palestine. Sister Selma Mayer at the Shaare Zedek Hospital.
c. 1925. *(See note.)*

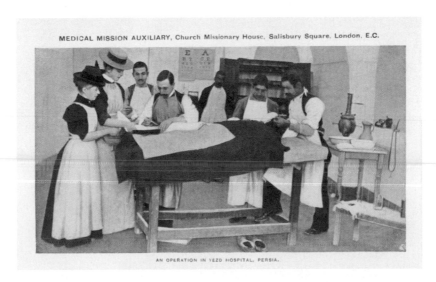

Figure 7.54.   Persia.
c. 1910.

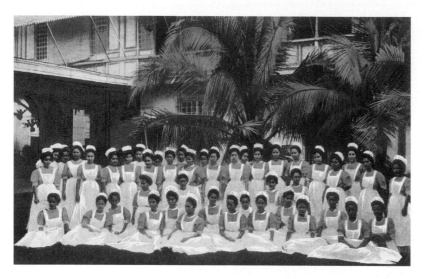

Figure 7.55.　Philippines.
c. 1920.

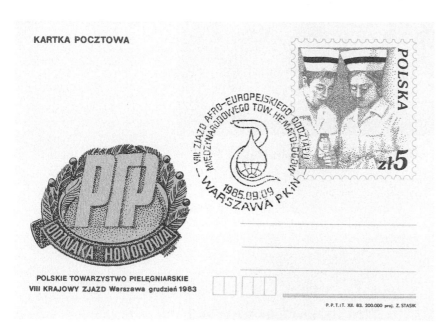

Figure 7.56.　Poland. Polish Nursing Association Badge of Honor.
1985. *(See note.)*

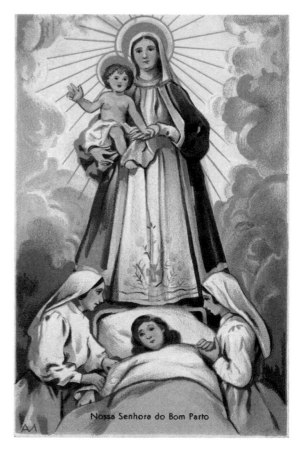

Nossa Senhora do Bom Parto

Figure 7.57.　Portugal. "Our Lady of Good Childbirth."
c. 1920.

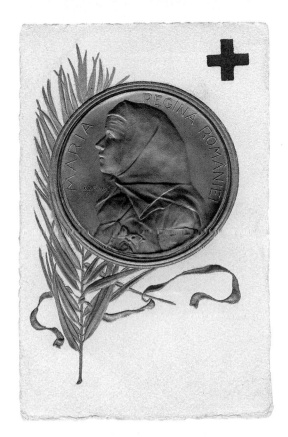

Figure 7.58. **Romania. Queen Maria of Romania.**
c. 1915 (See Fig. 4.98.)

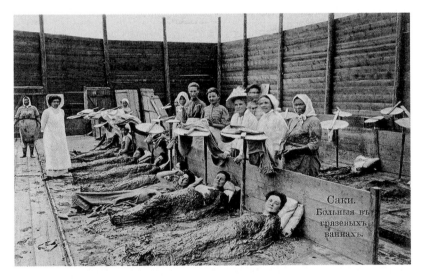

Figure 7.59. **Russia. Mudbath.**
c. 1920.

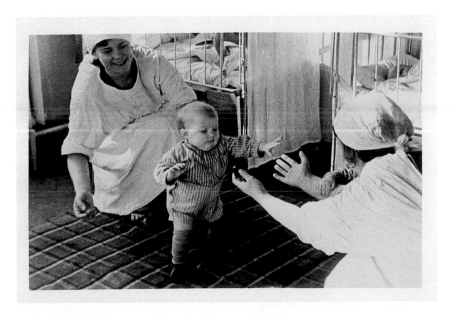

Figure 7.60. **Russia.**
c. 1940.

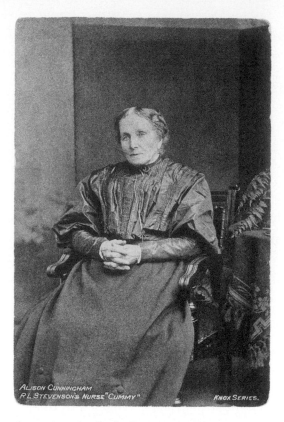

Figure 7.61.   Scotland. Alison Cunningham, Robert Louis Stevenson's nurse.
c. 1920. *(See note.)*

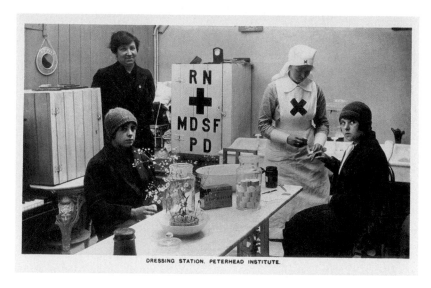

Figure 7.62.   Scotland. Dressing station.
Peterhead Institute. c. 1920. *(See note.)*

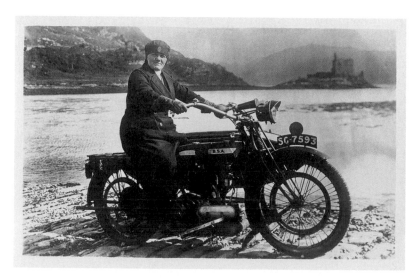

Figure 7.63.   Scotland. District nurse.
c. 1915.

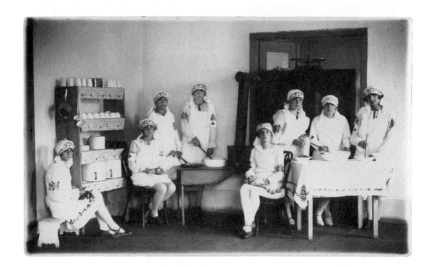

Figure 7.64. **Slovenia.**
1929.

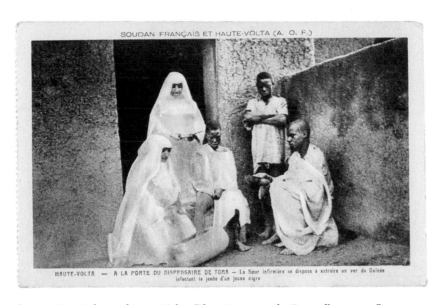

Figure 7.65. **Sudan and Upper Volta. "The entrance to the Toma dispensary."**
c. 1910.

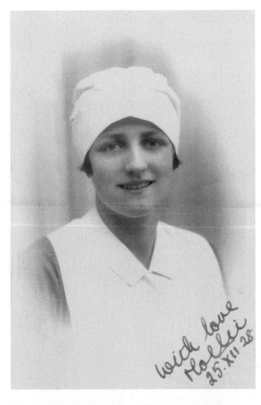

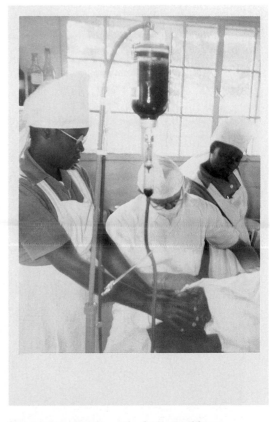

Figure 7.66. **South Africa. Nurse Molley Fellows.**
1928. *(See note.)*

Figure 7.67. **Southern Rhodesia. Washburn Memorial Hospital.**
c. 1985.

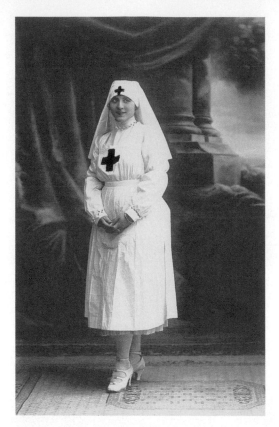

Figure 7.68. Spain.
c. 1910.

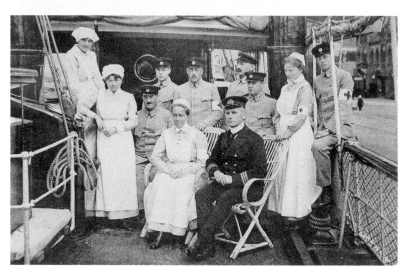

Figure 7.69. Sweden. Seated are Head Nurse Thomasine Andersson and Dr. C. G. Bostrom.
c. 1915.

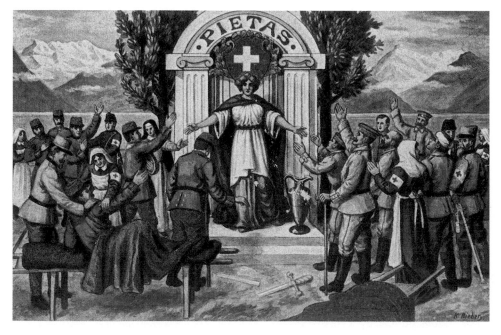

Figure 7.70. Switzerland. "Pity."
c. 1916.

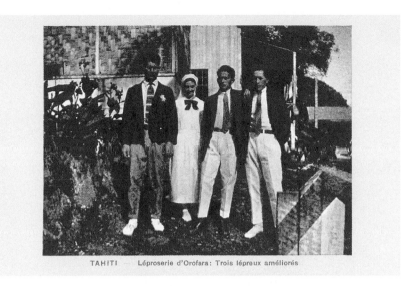

TAHITI — Léproserie d'Orofara : Trois lépreux améliorés

Figure 7.71. **Tahiti. Orofara Leper Colony. "Three improved lepers."**
c. 1930.

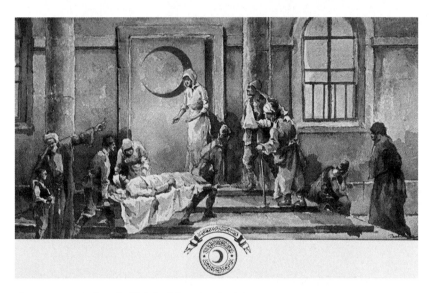

Figure 7.72. **Turkey. Turkish Red Crescent Society.**
c. 1915.

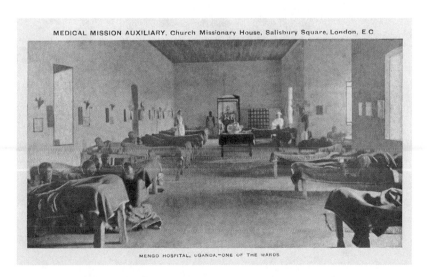

MEDICAL MISSION AUXILIARY, Church Missionary House, Salisbury Square, London, E.C.

MENGO HOSPITAL, UGANDA.—ONE OF THE WARDS.

Figure 7.73. **Uganda. Mengo Hospital.**
1911.

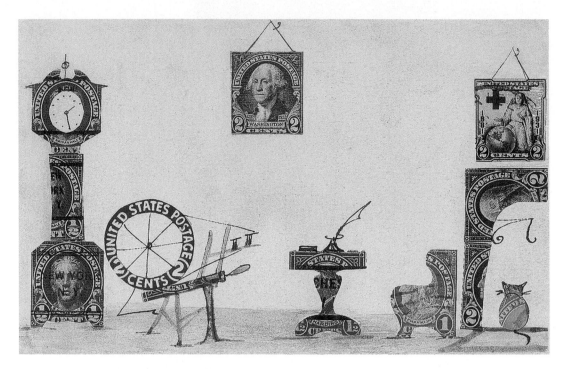

Figure 7.74. **United States.**
1932. *(See note.)*

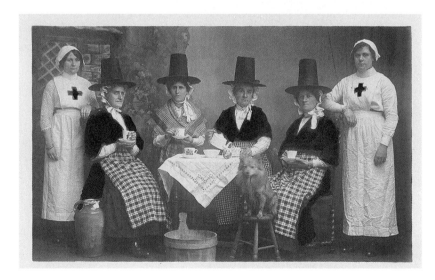

Figure 7.75. **Wales.**
c. 1915. *(See note.)*

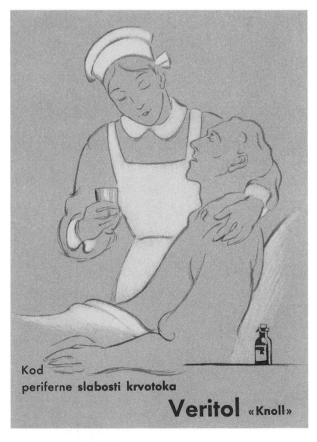

Figure 7.76. **Yugoslavia. "For peripheral circulation problems, use Veritol."**
1938.

7.4. From reverse: "On 17 February, 1885 a meeting was held . . . to discuss the need for an organised system of nursing care for the sick poor in their own homes. Home nursing services were subsequently formed in other states of **Australia** and a national co-ordinating body was set up in 1969. Stamp designed by Wendy Tamblyn. Art Work by courtesy of Australia Post."

7.6. For almost the entire period of the **Congo Free State** (1885–1908), the peoples of present-day Congo were subjected to a staggering sequence of wars, repression, and regimentation. Reduced to its essentials, Belgian paternalism meant that basic political rights could be withheld indefinitely from Africans as long as their material and spiritual needs were properly met (Congo, 2000). The country is now the Democratic Republic of The Congo, formerly Zaire.

7.8. **Bophuthatswana,** now part of the Republic of South Africa, comprised seven separate areas, one along the Botswana border, the remainder landlocked enclaves. The capital is Mmbatho.

7.22. From reverse: "Nurse Williams, left, and Nurse Murrant, right enjoying a joke with the photographer while Michael, Ann, Ernest and Paul, these much photographed babies, wonder what it's all about." **The Miles Quadruplets** (3 boys and a girl), born in England on November 28, 1935, were the first British quads to survive infancy.

7.23. Niels Ryberg Finsen (1860–1904) was the founder of modern phototherapy. As a student at the University of Copenhagen, he became interested in the effects of light on living organisms. In 1893 he discovered that lengthy exposure of smallpox sufferers to red light prevented the formation of the characteristic pockmarks.

Aware of the bacteria-destroying effects of sunlight, he developed a carbon arc ultraviolet treatment for **lupus vulgaris,** a form of skin tuberculosis. He first reported these cases in 1896, in his famous paper "The Treatment of Lupus by Concentrated Ultraviolet Light." Finsen's Medical Light Institute (now the Finsen Institute) was founded in Copenhagen in 1896. His work led to the use of **ultraviolet sterilization** techniques in bacteriological research. In 1903, Finsen received the Nobel Prize for Physiology or Medicine for the application of light in the treatment of skin diseases. Sequeira, a noted English dermatologist, introduced Finsen's techniques into England in 1900.

7.24. The back of this postcard has a penciled message that reads, "This is the electrical treatment I will be having this week only I shall have to undress and have a pad on my hip. Look how they watch your face to see if they are giving you too much. No running away from it like dad did." The therapy is hydrogalvanic diathermy, used for muscle rehabilitation and stimulation, called the **Schnee bath** after its inventor Paul Schnee, a German physician. (See Fig. 2.102.)

7.28. **French Indochina** comprised the current countries of Vietnam, Laos, and Cambodia.

7.42. This type of picture is called a **metamorphic,** because it changes in appearance depending how you look at it. The most famous metamorphic is called "Vanity," and shows either a skull or a woman looking into a mirror, depending on how you look at it. The main figure is of **Queen Elena of Italy** (see Fig. 4.114). In addition to her, there are three other nurses (Queen Elena herself was a nurse), a child, an adult patient, a soldier playing bagpipes, a tambourine player, a lute player, and a woman holding two wreaths. Can you find them all? The true metamorphic element is Queen Elena's eye, which is also the head of the lute player.

7.43. This is a fine example of a fantasy postcard. The clinic was in Tokyo and obviously catered to an English-speaking clientele.

7.44. "**Birth of the Red Cross.** To commemorate the Centenary of the inception of the Red Cross, a special stamp was issued on June 24, 1959. The illustration below shows the nurses's activities which are also shown in the design of the stamp." This is another example of a maximum card, where the stamp, image, and cancel are all related.

7.47. "**Father Dupuy,** A Jesuit, Recipient of the French Legion of Honor, dead from leprosy, attended by the Sisters of St. Joseph of Cluny and the Madagascan nuns." This is a wax tableau in the **Madagascar** Room in the Pavilion of Missions at the French Colonial Exposition, held at Vincennes, France, in 1931.

7.53. **Shaare Zedek** ("Gates of Righteousness"), the most modern hospital in the Middle East, opened in 1902 to serve the sick and needy of Jerusalem. The original building contained 20 beds. Today, the 500-bed Medical Center is located on a 14-acre site opposite Mt. Herzl in Jerusalem. The 1,300,000-square-foot complex consists of 10 linked buildings including inpatient facilities, comprehensive therapeutic and diagnostic services, outpatient clinics, teaching facilities for medical students, and a research center. The School of Nursing currently has 450 students (Shaare Zedek, 2002).

Schwester Selma Mayer (1884–1984) worked at Saloman Heine Hospital in Hamburg from 1906 to 1916. In 1916, during World War I, she left for Palestine to become head nurse at Shaare Zedek. She was the first nurse in Palestine with a nursing diploma. In 1936, she founded the Shaare Zedek School of Nursing. She remained head nurse of the hospital and the nursing school until her retirement in 1964 at age 80. Even when she was no longer able to work full time, she visited the patients every day to offer a kind word, a smile, and some good advice. In December 1975, *Time* magazine referred to her as "something of an angel" and later as a "Living Saint." She passed away in 1984, 2 days before her 100th birthday (Shaare Zedek, 2002).

7.56. The design (cachet) reads, "**Polish Nursing Association** Badge of Honor. Polish Nursing Association, 7th Countrywide Congress,

Warsaw, December, 1983." The cancel reads, "7th Congress of Afro-European Division of the International Society of Hematologists, 9 September, 1985. Warsaw PKiN (Palace of Culture and Science)."

7.61. **Robert Louis Stevenson** (1850–1894) suffered from tuberculosis as a child. He spent much of his time in bed during his early years. His nurse, whom he called "Cummy," fed his imagination with stories from the Bible and Scottish history that later became a source of inspiration for his own writing. His book, *A Child's Garden of Verses,* published in 1885, was dedicated to her.

> To **Alison Cunningham** From Her Boy
> For the long nights you lay awake
> And watched for my unworthy sake:
> For your most comfortable hand
> That led me through the uneven land:
> For all the story-books you read:
> For all the pains you comforted:
> For all you pitied, all you bore,
> In sad and happy days of yore:—
> My second Mother, my first Wife,
> The angel of my infant life—
> From the sick child, now well and old,
> Take, nurse, the little book you hold!
> And grant it, Heaven, that all who read
> May find as dear a nurse at need,
> And every child who lists my rhyme,
> In the bright, fireside, nursery clime,
> May hear it in as kind a voice
> As made my childish days rejoice!

7.62. **Scotland** has **St. Andrew's Ambulance Association,** whose members wear the diagonal Cross of St. Andrew on their uniform. Here, the nurse is on duty at a **Royal National Mission to Deep Sea Fishermen** dressing station (O'Neill, 1990).

7.66. From a newspaper clipping of unknown origin, which depicts the nurse in the postcard: "**Nurse Molley Fellows** of Grey's Hospital, Maritzburg, who has won no fewer than three gold and one silver medal during 1931. They comprise the Kenneth B. Gloag medal, awarded for the best nurse in practice and theory in the examinations open to the whole country held last April; the gold medal awarded by the Natal Provincial Administration for the best nurse in Natal taking the same examination; the silver medal for midwifery awarded by the Natal Provincial Administration in connection with the examination held in October and the gold medal awarded to the best practical nurse in the final examinations at Grey's Hospital by Dr. Odin-Taylor. Miss Fellows is staying on at Grey's Hospital as a nurse."

7.74. This postcard is a handmade collage, constructed from various portions of canceled US stamps and detailed with pen and ink and colored pencil. The nurse is on the 1931 2¢ commemorative, designed by Lawrence Wilbur, used for a picture above the fireplace. (See Fig. 3.32.)

7.75. The people around the table are dressed in the **Welsh national costume.** The postcard is hand-tinted.

Acknowledgments

*E*ach evening on my way home from my shift at the emergency room, I pass a gas station sign on which, each month, the owner posts a different inspirational message. Most of them more or less drift through me when I see them, but one night the new message said, "A dream is a goal with no energy behind it." That one hit a mental target dead center and stuck. It was the spark for what you hold in your hands, a dream with energy behind it.

In fact, most of the energy was not mine. If I had to balance my contribution against the sum of everyone else's, mine would come up short. I decided to keep a list of the people who helped. I did not count the folks who simply gave me a needed fact or pointed me to a reference because I could see right from the start that there would be hundreds of them, too many to list. So I kept a shorter list, of everyone who made a significant difference in the quality of the work. That list, a testimony to people's generosity, is here:

Frank Allard	George Miller
Jeff Behary	John and Sandy Millns
Patricia Casey	Susan Nicholson
Gordie Chamberlain	Daniel Pepper
Janet Christrup	Jane Pepper
Debra Cox	Don Preziosi
Allison Cusick	JD Rabbit
Nigel Edwards	Josephine Sapp
Stacey Farley	William F. Settle
Louis J. Forgione	Martin Shapiro
Tom Gibbons	Sally Pierce Silverman
Debra Gust	Sumner Silverman
Chris Hand	Ed Stephen
William Helfand	Ellen Stuter
Clyde F. Herreid	Damon Torsten
Dawn Johnson	Christopher Wagner
Ted Kole	Dennis Weidner
Judy McCann	Charlotte Zeepvat
Country Joe McDonald	Susan Zodin
Kathleen McFadden	Fritzi Zwerdling
Alison Wampler Mead	Harold Zwerdling
Don Mead	

There are, however, a few individuals without whose commitment this book would never have existed, and I would like to thank them individually.

Kay Stanton, a friend who saw the possibilities before I did, and supported me from the very beginning. The Zwerdling Nursing Archives, from which the postcards for this book were selected, should really be named the Stanton-Zwerdling Archives.

Nancy Tryon, who generously donated many days of research and her unparalleled expertise on European royalty, and who contributed images and information I would never have found on my own.

Paul Miriam, who not only translated all the European languages on the postcards, but who also did the bulk of the research on the East European countries.

Patrick Gariepy, an expert on military uniforms and aspects of World War I, who patiently answered question after question.

Yoshiko Yamamura, who translated the Japanese and helped me with matters Japanese.

Chris Butler, who wrote an essay especially for this book, and who informed me on United Kingdom history, customs, and politics.

Sabrina Abhyankar and Kim Boriskin, who proofread and copy edited each clumsy draft and who gradually taught me something about punctuation and style.

Brett MacNaughton and Carolyn O'Brien, the art and design team at Lippincott, who took my inexpert layouts and transformed them into a book more beautiful than I thought possible.

Megan Klim, the project coordinator who kept it rolling over all sorts of uneven terrain.

Steve Edson, who scanned and corrected the images to bring out the very best in each and every one.

With a surname of Zwerdling, one becomes used to being last on any alphabetized list. As a result, when I was younger, I considered being last the position of honor, and in some ways that still holds true. Therefore, since we're speaking of making real a dream, I decided that the person most responsible for it should be mentioned last. Without question that person is Alan Sorkowitz. Alan was the book's editor and primary advocate during every phase of its development, from original idea until finished product. He is my mentor and friend, and since there are no words sufficient to express my appreciation for his contributions, I shall simply say, "Thank you," and leave the rest unsaid, and understood.

Michael Zwerdling, R.N.
Post Office Box 917
Burtonsville, MD 20866
www.nursepostcard.com
zna@nursepostcard.com

Chicago, Rock Island, and Pacific Railroad Company. *Encyclopedia Britannica* [online]. Available at: http://members.eb.com/bol/topic?eu=24359&sctn=1. Accessed February 27, 2002.

Chilvers I, ed. *The Concise Oxford Dictionary of Art and Artists.* 2nd ed. Oxford: Oxford University Press; 1996.

Christopher Gregg Parnall, MD. ViaHealth [online]. Available at: http://www.viahealth.org/archives/parnallbio.html. Accessed May 15, 2002.

Connecticut State Employees' Campaign for Charitable Giving [online]. Available at: http://www.state.ct.us/csec/directory/ctunitedways/westcentral.htm. Accessed February 21, 2002.

Cook County Hospital [online]. 1999. Available at: http://www.cchil.org/Cch/cook.htm. Accessed March 18, 2002.

Cope D, Cope P. *Postcards from the Nursery: The Illustrations of Children's Books and Postcards 1900–1950.* London: New Cavendish; 2000.

Cox J. *Bizarre lives: Louis Wain* [online]. 2001. Available at: http://www.bizarremag.com/lives/wain.html. Accessed May 31, 2002.

Crimean War. *Encyclopedia Britannica* [online]. Available at: http://members.eb.com/bol/topic?eu=28350&sctn=1&pm=1. Accessed March 27, 2000.

Cross of Lorraine. Symbols.com [online]. Available at: http://www/symbols.com/encyclopedia/03/036.html. Accessed April 22, 2000.

Cumming E, Kaplan W. *The Arts & Crafts Movement.* London: Thames & Hudson; 1991.

Dalby R. *The Golden Age of Children's Book Illustration.* London: Michael O'Mara Books; 1991.

Dale R. *Louis Wain: The Man Who Drew Cats.* London: Chris Beetles; 1991.

Davidson G. *A Dictionary of Angels Including the Fallen Angels.* New York, NY: Macmillan; 1967.

Davis S, Davis J. About Samuel L. Schmucker [online]. 2001. Available at: http://www.samuellschmucker.com/schmucker.html. Accessed May 27, 2002.

Dr. John Harvey Kellogg. Battle Creek Historical Society [online]. Available at: http://www.geocities.com/Athens/Oracle/9840/kellogg.html. Accessed February 26, 2002.

The Dionne settlement: justice at last. *News in Review* [online]. 1998; April. Available at: http://www.tv.cbc.ca/newsinreview/apr98/dione/present.htm. Accessed July 10, 2002.

Donahue MP. *Nursing: The Finest Art: An Illustrated History.* St. Louis: Mosby; 1985.

Donahue MP. *Nursing: The Finest Art: An Illustrated History.* 2nd ed. St. Louis: Mosby; 1996.

Dell'Aquila A, Dell'Aquila P. *Raphael Kirchner and His Postcards.* Bari, Italy: Mario Adda; 1996.

Doherty K. Issues in professional nursing lecture notes [online]. 1998. Available at: http://ntmain.utb.edu/kdougherty/4311/lecture_notes.html. Accessed March 4, 2002.

Douglas A. (2001). Comedian Charlie Chaplin. *Time Magazine* [online]. Available at: http://www.time.com/time/time100/artists/profile/chaplin.html. Accessed July 18, 2002.

Dunant, Jean Henri. The Nobel foundation [online]. Available at: http://www.nobel.se/laureates/peace-1901-bio.html. Accessed February 4, 2002.

Duncan A. *Art Deco.* London: Thames & Hudson; 1998.

Edward VIII. *Britannia.com* [online]. 2000. Available at: http://www.britannia.com/history/monarchs/mon61.html. Accessed July 28, 2002.

Edwards N. Angel of Mons [e-mail to Michael Zwerdling]. January 6, 1999.

Eichenberg S. Biography of Bebe Daniels. Internet Movie Database [online]. 2001. Available at: http://us.imdb.com/Bio? Daniels, +Bebe. Accessed July 18, 2002.

Ellen Church. Iowa Division of Tourism [online]. 2002. Available at: http://www.crescoia.com/ellenchurch.html. Accessed August 5, 2002.

Ellis R. On cauterisation by electric heat in the treatment of certain diseases of women. London: *British Medical Journal (London).* 1862; January 4:20–21.

Emerson A. 1918: the great influenza pandemic. *The Bostonian Society News.* 2002; Winter. Boston: Boston Historical Society and Museum.

Emuang K. *The world at war series: the Boer War* [online]. 1999. Available at: http://content.miw.com.sg/LifeStyle/Military/ls_military01_20020920.asp. Accessed September 20, 2002.

Era of Development. Virtual museum of Virginia Tech [online]. Available at: http://www.ee.vt.edu/~museum/time/time3.html. Accessed January 3, 2000.

Fanelli G, Godoli E. *Art Nouveau Postcards.* New York, NY: Rizzoli; 1987.

Farella C. Doormats, devils and divas: nurses in the movies. *Nursing Spectrum.* 2001; 13(1):28–28

Farella, C. Group strives to polish nursing's image. *Nursing Spectrum.* 2000;10(4):10.

Farley S. Queen Victoria. *World of royalty* [online]. 2002. Available at: http://www.royalty.nu/Europe/England/Victoria.html. Accessed July 15, 2002.

Farley T. Private line's telephone history part 1—to 1870 [online]. Available at: http://www.privateline.com. Accessed February 23, 2000.

Fenkl H. *Caduceus.* [online]. Available at: http://www.endicott-studio.com/forcaduc.html. Accessed January 21, 2000.

Frankl V. *Man's Search for Meaning.* New York, NY: Simon & Schuster; 1963.

Freeman B. Sonoma County Tribune (October 13, 1892) [online]. 2001. Available at: http://www.newspaperabstracts.com/CA/Sonoma/1892/oct.html. Accessed March 16, 2002.

Fussell P. *The Great War and Modern Memory.* London: Oxford University; 1975.

Gallagher H. *By Trust Betrayed: Patients, Physicians, and the License to Kill in the Third Reich.* New York, NY: H. Holt; 1990.

Gallen Kellela Museum [online]. Available at: http://www.gallen-kallela.fi/akseli/1_tradition.html. Accessed April 24, 2002.

Genocide Research. (2001). *Armenian National Institute*[online]. Available at: http://www.armenian-genocide.org/research.htm. Accessed August 20–September 3, 2002.

Gibbs G. *The Topographical Locator for Picture Post Card Collectors.* Syracuse, NY: Gibbs; 1987.

Go-Card postcard advertising [online]. Available at: http://www.gocard.com/index2.html. Accessed March 14, 2002.

Goldsack B. *Remembering Benson's Wild Animal Farm.* Nashua, NH: Midway Museum Publications; 1998.

Gott T. *Don't Leave Me This Way: Art in the Age of AIDS.* Brisbane: National Gallery of Australia; 1994.

Graves R. *The Greek Myths.* New York, NY: Penguin; 1960.

Gravesites of prominent nurses. American Association for the History of Nursing [online]. Available at: http://www.aahn.org/gravesites/robb.html. Accessed March 1, 2002.

Great Depression. Encyclopedia Britannica [online]. Available at: http://www.britannica.com/eb/article?eu=38610&tocid=0&query=%22great%20depression%2. Accessed April 16, 2002.

Great Ormond Street Hospital. *Great Ormond Street Hospital* [online]. 2002. Available at: http://www.gosh.org/history/index.htm. Accessed November 21, 2002.

Green L. Stereotypes: negative racial stereotypes and their effect on attitudes toward African-Americans. *Perspectives on multiculturalism and cultural diversity.* 1998;10:1. Virginia Commonwealth University [online]. Available at: http://www.vcu.edu/safweb/counsel/MC/stereo.html. Accessed January 14, 2000.

Guinness Collectors Club [online]. Available at: http://www.guinnesscollectorsclub.co.uk/labels/bottlers.asp. Accessed February 27, 2000.

HDS. (1916). With the American Ambulance Field Service in France: personal letters of a driver at the front. Printed only for private distribution, January 1916 [online]. Available at: http://www.ku.edu/~libsite/wwi-www/Buswell/AAFS1.htm. Accessed August 15, 2002.

Hageman P, Kosanovich J. Allied Powers. Propaganda postcards of the Great War [online]. 2002. Available at: http://www.ww1-propaganda-cards.com/allied_powers.html. Accessed August 9, 2002.

Hall J. *Dictionary of Subjects and Symbols in Art.* New York, NY: Harper & Row; 1979.

Hapag-Lloyd [online]. Available at: http://www.hapaglloyd.com/pages/i_index.html. Accessed March 13, 2002.

Helfand W. *Medicine and Pharmacy: 100 Years of Poster Art.* New York, NY: New York State Museum; 1981.

Helfand W. *The Nightingale's Song: Nurses and Nursing in the Ars Medica Collection of the Philadelphia Museum of Art.* Philadelphia, Pa: Philadelphia Museum of Art; 2000.

Henry Street Settlement. National Park Service [online]. 1998. Available at: http://www.cr.nps.gov/nr/travel/pwwmh/ny31.htm. Accessed July 29, 2002.

Hepner Z. Circumcision. Mazel Tov [online]. 2001. Available at: http://imohel.com/. Accessed January 3, 2001.

Herzog P, Vazzana G. *Brigitte Helm, from Metropolis to Gold: Portrait of a Goddess.* New York, NY: Corvin; 1994.

Herzog P, McThomas R. Obituary of Brigitte Helm. *New York Times*. June 14, 1996.

Hill R. The history of the British iron lung 1832–1995 [online]. 1995. Available at: http://www.geocities.com/ironlungmuseum/ironlung.htm. March 18, 2002.

History of the American Lung Association. American Lung Association [online]. Available at: http://www.lungusa.org/history/history.html. Accessed May 1, 2000.

History of the Maltese Cross [online]. Available at: http://www.cvc.net/cvcmem/ods/histmalt.htm. Accessed April 22, 2000.

History of National Nurses Week. Nursing World [online]. Available at: http://www.nursingworld.org/pressrel/nnw/nnwhist.htm. Accessed April 15, 2002.

The history of a picture's worth [online]. Available at: http://fas.sfu.ca/~dhepting/personal/research/words/history.html. Accessed July 9, 2001.

History of St. John Ambulance [online]. Available at: http://www.cam.ac.uk/societies/cufas/bge/sjhist.htm. Accessed February 17, 2000.

History of tuberculosis. Lupin Group [online]. Available at: http://www.lupingroup.com/phtml/tball.htm. Accessed May 3, 2000.

Hodgin G. The history, synthesis, metabolism and uses of artificial sweeteners [online]. Available at: http://www.ecit.emory.edu/ECIT/chem_ram/synth/Hodgin.htm#Introduction. Accessed March 15, 2002.

Hoehling A. *A Whisper of Eternity: The Mystery of Edith Cavell*. New York, NY: Thomas Yoseloff; 1957.

Holy Bible. King James Version. New York, NY: Meridian; 1974.

Holt T, Holt V. Till the Boys Come Home: The Picture Postcards of the First World War. Newtown Square, Pa: Deltiologists of America; 1977.

Howe L. Florence Nightingale. An international forum for the discussion of nursing history [online]. 2002. Available at: E-mailing list. Accessed October 23, 2002.

Hubartt K. "Bird-Boy" Art Smith. *The News@Sentinel* [online]. 1999. Available at: http://www.news-sentinel.com/ns/projects/2000/1910/ind0.htm. Accessed April 13, 2000.

Hutchinson J. *Champions of Charity: War and the Rise of the Red Cross*. Boulder, Col: Westview Press; 1996.

Hygieia. Encyclopaedia Britannica [online]. Available at: http://www.britannica.com/bcom/eb/article/0/0,5716,42705+1,00.html. Accessed May 26, 2000.

Ice, T. *The Boer War: South Africa, 1899–1902*. [online]. 1995. Available at: http://www.geocities.com/Athens/Acropolis/8141/boerwar.html. Accessed September 23, 2002.

ICRC: answers to your questions. International Committee of the Red Cross [online]. Available at: http://www.irc.org/icrceng.nsf/8ec4e051a8. . . 1e8107617dffb412562b20032e6a? OpenDocument. Accessed May 2, 2000.

In Harm's Way: A History of Women with America's Armed Forces. Rohnert Park, Calif: Pomegranate; 2002.

Internal combustion history. Denner Power Co. [online]. Available at: http://www.dennerpower.com/InternalCombustionHistory.html. Accessed March 3, 2000.

International Council of Nurses (ICN) [online]. Available at: http://www.icn.ch/. Accessed March 3, 2002.

Isabel Adams Hampton Robb. American Nurses Association [online]. Available at: http://www.nursingworld.org/hof/robbia.htm. Accessed March 16, 2000.

James Montgomery Flagg. Spartacus educational [online]. Available at: http://www.spartacus.schoolnet.co.uk/. Accessed March 11, 2002.

Japan Tobacco International. (2001). State Academic Bolshoi Theatre press service [online]. Available at: http://www.bolshoi.ru/eng/projects/jt.shtml. Accessed July 28, 2002.

Jewison G, Steiner J. Austro-Hungarian land forces 1848–1918 [online]. 2000. Available at: http://www.austro-hungarian-army.co.uk/biog/erzfried.htm. Accessed July 30, 2002.

John F. Hutchinson. Royal Society of Canada [online]. Available at: http://www.rsc.ca/english/awards_hannah_1991–2000.html. Accessed March 18, 2002.

Judnick B. Mastroianni [online]. Available at: http://www.judnick.com/ArtistsM.htm. Accessed April 19, 2002.

Juliet Ann Opie Hopkins. Arlington National Cemetery Web site [online]. 1999. Available at: http://www.arlington cemetery.com/jhopkins.htm. Accessed September 20, 2002.

Juliet Opie Hopkins. Alabama Department of Archives & History [online]. 2001. Available at: http://www.archives.state. al.us/teacher/civilwar/civ2.html. Accessed September 20, 2002.

Kalmien V. *Art History of Photography.* New York, NY: Viking; 1974.

Kalevala. Encyclopedia Britannica [online]. Available at: http://www.britannica.com/ eb/article? eu=45423. Accessed April 22, 2002.

Kalisch P, Kalisch B. *The Advance of American Nursing.* 3rd ed. Philadelphia: Lippincott; 1995.

Karl Friedrich Benz. Camelot International [online]. Available at: http://www.camelotintl.com/world/ 02karl_friedrich_banz.html. Accessed March 3, 2000.

Kery P. *Great Magazine Covers of the World.* New York, NY: Abbeville; 1982.

Key W. *The Age of Manipulation: The Con in Confidence, the Sin in Sincere.* Lanham, Md: Madison Books; 1993.

Keiger D. Why metaphor matters. *Johns Hopkins Magazine* [online]. 1998. Available at: http://www.jhu.edu/ ~jhumag/0298web/metaphor.html. Accessed May 5, 2000.

Kerensky, Aleksandr Feodorovich. Infoplease Encyclopedia [online]. Available at: http://www.infoplease.com/ ce6/people/A0827440. html. Accessed May 14, 2002.

Knights, chivalry and orders [online]. Available at: http://www.thelema.net/ ramsey/knighthood.html. Accessed February 21, 2000.

Koehler L. *Saint Elisabeth the New Martyr.* New York, NY: Orthodox Palestine Society; 1988.

Kovacs R. *Electrotherapy and Light Therapy.* Philadelphia, Pa: Lea & Febiger; 1938.

Kole T, Abbondondolo T. Princess Marie of Greece [online]. 1999. Available at: http://www.katoufs.com/marie.html. Accessed July 28, 2002.

Kolata, G. *Flu.* New York, NY: Touchstone; 1999.

Kricfalusi J. *The Ren and Stimpy Show: Postcards Over the Edge.* New York, NY: Grosset & Dunlap; 1992.

Kukryniksy. *Bol'shaya sovetskaya entsiklope-diya [Big Soviet Encyclopedia].* Vol 23. Moscow; October, 1953:634–635.

Kurth P. *Tsar: The Lost World of Nicholas and Alexandra.* Boston: Little Brown; 1995.

Lacey R. *Majesty: Elizabeth II and the House of Windsor.* New York, NY: Harcourt Brace; 1977.

Landon B. Hamburg America Line [online]. 1997. Available at: http://www.uiowa. edu/~english/profpage/blandon/tlucht/ bthal.html. Accessed March 12, 2002.

Larson R. *White Roses: Stories of Civil War Nurses.* Gettysburg, Pa: Thomas; 1997.

Levi P. *The Drowned and the Saved.* New York, NY: Random House; 1989.

Liberty Theater. International Broadway Database [online]. 2002. Available at: http://www.ibdb.com/venue. asp?ID=1235. Accessed August 19, 2002.

Lieberman H. (2001). Incubator baby shows: a medical and social frontier [online]. Available at: http://www.historycooperative.org/ journals/ht/35.1/lieberman.html. Accessed July 5, 2002.

Lifton R. *The Nazi Doctors: Medical Killing and the Psychology of Genocide.* New York, NY: Perseus; 2000.

Lisa's postcard page [online]. Available at: http://www.geocities.com/Heartland/ Meadows/2487. Accessed March 30, 2002.

Lister, Joseph, Baron Lister, of Lyme Regis. Encyclopedia Britannica [online]. Available at: http://members.eb.com/bol/ topic? eu=49648&sctn=1&pm=1. Accessed March 15, 2002.

Lithography. Encyclopedia Britannica [online]. Available at: http://members.eb. com/bol/topic?artl=48518&seq_nbr=1& page=n&isctn=2&pm. Accessed March 6, 2000.

Louis Wain: A true cat lover. National Cat Club [online]. 1999. Available at: http://www.nationalcatclub.co.uk/ general/louisewain.htm. Accessed June 1, 2002.

Louis Wain's world—the history of the cat fancy. Wainsworld [online]. Available at: http://www.geocities.com/Heartland/ Estates/2313/wain1.htm. Accessed May 31, 2002.

Lowe J. *Deltiology.* 1970;11:1.

Macdonald G. *Camera, Victoria Eyewitness: A History of Photography 1826–1913.* New York, NY: Viking; 1980.

MacDonald L. *The Roses of No Man's Land.* New York, NY: Macmillan; 1989.

Madison B. The Russo-Japanese War. The Russo Japanese War Research Society [online]. 2002. Available at: http://www.russojapanesewar.com/. Accessed September 21, 2002.

The Maltese Cross [online]. Available at: http://home.keyworld.net/sanandrea/cyberfair/attractions/mcross.html. Accessed February 12, 2000.

Maltin L. Bebe Daniels. Internet movie database [online]. 1994. Available at: http://us.imdb.com/Bio?Daniels,+Bebe. Accessed July 18, 2002.

Manheimer M. Theresienstadt-Auschwitz-Warsaw-Dachau: recollections. *Dachau review.* Brussels: Comité International de Dachau; 1989:1, 55–92.

Marie Curie. Penn State University Department of Medicine [online]. 2001. Available at: http://www.xray.hmc.psu.edu/rci/ss7/ss7_2.html. Accessed September 15, 2002.

Marinetti FT. The founding and manifesto of Futurism. Paris: Le Figaro, (February 20, 1909). Niuean pop cultural archive [online]. Available at: http://www.unknown.nu/futurism/. Accessed March 12, 2002.

Martin L. Oxygen therapy: the first 150 years [online]. 1999. Available at: http://www.mtsinai.org/pulmonary/papers/ox-hist/ox-hist-intro.html. Accessed March 16, 2002.

Martin R, Martin C. *Vintage Illustration: Discovering America's Calendar Artists, 1900–1960.* Portland, Ore: Collectors Press; 1997.

Mashburn J. *The Postcard Price Guide.* Enka, NC: Colonial House; 1997.

Mason B. TB on the rise in Britain [World Socialist Web site]. 1999. Available at: http://www.wsws.org/articles/1999/jul1999/tb-j22.shtml. Accessed March 18, 2002.

McBryde B. *A Nurse's War.* Essex, Great Britain: Cakebread; 1993.

McCafferty L. Year of the nurse. *Advance for Nurses.* 2002; Jan. 21. King of Prussia, Pa: Merion Publications; 2002.

McCoy B. Dr. John Harvey Kellogg. The museum of questionable medical devices [online]. 2002. Available at: http://www.mtn.org/quack/amquacks/kellogg.htm. Accessed March 23, 2002.

McCoy B. *Quack: Tales of Medical Fraud from the Museum of Questionable Medical Devices.* Santa Monica, Calif: Santa Monica Press; 2000.

McDonald J. *Country Joe McDonald's tribute to Florence Nightingale* [online]. 2000. Available at: http://www.countryjoe.com/nightingale/index.html. Accessed May 23, 2000.

McGuinness M. Civil War wounded. *The Evangelist* [online]. 2002. Available at: http://www.evangelist.org/archive/htm/1126civl.htm. Accessed September 20, 2002.

McSherry P. Spanish American War Centennial Web site [online]. 1996. Available at: http://www.spanamwar.com/timeline.htm. Accessed September 21, 2002.

McThomas R, Herzog P. Obituary of Brigitte Helm. *New York Times.* June 14, 1996.

Meglaughlin J. *British Nursing Badges.* London: Vade-Mecum; 1990.

Methodist Hospital of Dallas [online]. Available at: http://www.mhd.com/. Accessed March 18, 2002.

Metropolis [videotape]. Quebec: Madacy Entertainment.

Michael Faraday. Bradley Department of Electrical and Computer Engineering, Virginia Polytechnic Institute and State University [online]. Available at: http://www.ee.vt.edu/~museum/time/Faraday.html. Accessed March 2, 2000.

Millar L. *Grand Duchess Elizabeth of Russia.* Redding, Calif: Nikodemos Orthodox Publication Society; 1991.

Million Dollar Babies [videotape]. Cinar Films. Ontario: Sony Entertainment.

Mirriam P. Littoriali [e-mail to Michael Zwerdling]. March 27, 2002. Available at e-mail: zna@nursepostcard.com.

Militia's 40-hour killing rampage. *Guardian International* [online]. 2001. Available at: http://www.guardian.co.uk/international/story/0,3604,638927,00.html. Accessed January 25, 2002.

Mizuki K. Dear candy's friends of the world. [online]. 1999. Available at: http://members.fortunecity.com/domesticviolence1/e_from_mizuki.htm. Accessed March 5, 2001.

Moon W. Biography of Majel Barrett Roddenberry [online]. 1999. Available at: http://www.roddenberry.com/. Accessed July 21, 2002.

Morgan H, Brown A. *Prairie Fires and Paper Moons: The American Photographic Postcard 1910–1920.* Boston: Godine; 1981.

Morgenthau H. Ambassador Morgenthau's story. University of Kansas [online]. 1918. Available at: http://www.ku.edu/~libsite/wwi-www/morgenthau/Morgen25.htm. Accessed July 28, 2002.

MVP Heritage. Advocate Health Care [online]. 2002. Available at: http://www.advocatehealth.com/. Accessed October 8, 2002.

Narbaez Jr, R. The star and the crescent. Mission Islam [online]. Available at: http://www.missionislam.com/islam/conissue/crescent.htm. Accessed June 1, 2000.

The National Trust and the National Gardens Scheme. National Trust [online]. 2002. Available at: http://www.nationaltrust.org.uk/environment/html/. Accessed July 28, 2002.

Neis S. A brief history of postcard types [online]. 1996. Available at: http://www.geocities.com/Heartland/Meadows/2487/pchistory.htm. Accessed March 3, 2002.

Neubecker O. A Guide to Heraldry. NewYork, NY: McGraw Hill; 1979.

Neudin G. Les meilleurs cartes postales d'illustrateurs. St. Hillaire, France: Neudin; 1991.

New Piper aircraft [online]. Available at: http://www.newpiper.com/history.htm. Accessed March 14, 2002.

Newhall B. The History of Photography from 1839 to the Present. Boston: Little, Brown; 1982.

Nichols D. The symbols of medicine. [online]. 1999. Available at: http://www.ualberta.ca/~msauofa/iatros/hermes.html. Accessed May 10, 2000.

Nicholson S. The Encyclopedia of Antique Postcards. Radnor, Pa: Wallace-Homestead; 1994.

Nicholson S. Milestones in postcard history. Postcard Collector Annual 2000. Iola, WI: Krause Publications; 2000:12–16.

Nursing Sister Georgina Fane Pope. Canadian War Museum [online]. 2000. Available at: http://www.civilization.ca/cwm/saw/person/pope_e.html. Accessed September 21, 2002.

NYK Line [online]. Available at: http://www.nykline.co.jp/english/about/history/index.htm. Accessed March 14, 2002.

Old Brewster Hospital. Soul of America [online]. 2002. Available at: http://www.soulofamerica.com/cityfldr/jksnvil1.html. Accessed October 10, 2002.

O'Neill C. A Picture of Health: Hospitals and Nursing on Old Picture Postcards. Oxford: Meadow Books; 1990.

O'Neill C. More Pictures of Health: Hospitals and Nursing on Old Picture Postcards. Oxford: Meadow Books; 1991.

Ortakales D. Mabel Lucie Attwell [online]. 2001. Available at: http://www.ortakales.com/Illustrators/index.html. Accessed May 28, 2002.

Our History. Shaare Zedek Medical Center, Jerusalem [online]. 2002. Available at: http://www.szmc.org.il/main.asp?top=2&id=43. Accessed October 11, 2002.

Owings, A. Frauen: German Women Recall the Third Reich. New Brunswick, NJ: Rutgers; 1995.

P. Buckley Moss: the people's artist [online]. Available at: http://www.p-buckley-moss.com/. Accessed March 7, 2002.

Pennok M, ed. Makers of Nursing History: Portraits and Pen Sketches of One Hundred and Nine Prominent Women. New York, NY: Lakeside; 1940.

Pierce K. The Yellow Kid [online]. Available at: http://www.kenpiercebooks.com/yelo-kid.htm. Accessed March 6, 2000.

Pimbley's Dictionary of Heraldry [online]. Available at: http://www.coatsofarms.addr.com/pimb_c.htm. Accessed May 14, 2000.

Poison Gases. Spartacus Educational [online]. 2002. Available at: http://www.spartacus.schoolnet.co.uk/FWWgas.htm. Accessed August 20, 2002.

Poller W. Medical Block 36. New York, NY: Lyle Stuart Books; 1960.

Postcards. Portobello.com [online]. Available at: http://www.portobello.com.au/reading/printed_postcards.htm. March 3, 2002.

Poster. Encyclopedia Britannica [online]. Available at: http://members.eb.com/bol/topic?eu=62591&sctn=1&pm=1. Accessed March 21, 2000.

Powers S. American Red Cross posters [online]. 2000. Available at: http://www.collectarc.com/postermain.html. Accessed March 3, 2002.

Preziosi D. Coffee? Tea? A Registered Nurse? The origin of the airline stewardess. Postcard Collector 2002;208:20–21. Iola, WI: Antique Trader Publications.

Processional cross. The Catholic Encyclopedia [online]. Available at: http://www.adveent.org/cathen/12488a.htm. Accessed May 18, 2000.

Publication Manual of the American Psychological Association. 4th ed. Washington, DC: American Psychological Association; 1994.

The Queens Nursing Institute [e-mail to Michael Zwerdling]. July 23, 2002. Available at: e-mail: zna@nursepostcard.com.

Raigmore Hospital. North of Scotland Institute of Postgraduate Medical Education [online]. 2002. Available at: http://www.inverness-pgmc.demon.co.uk/. Accessed September 14, 2002.

Randolph Caldecott. Randolph Caldecott Society [online]. Available at: http://www.randolphcaldecott.org.uk/. Accessed May 28, 2002.

Red Cross. The Nobel Foundation [online]. Available at: http://www.nobel.se/laureates/peace-1917-history.html. Accessed February 4, 2000.

Red Cross and Red Crescent. Encyclopedia Britannica [online]. Available at: http://members.eb.com/bol/topic?eu=64537&sctn= 1&pm=1. Accessed March 27, 2000.

Red Cross double standard. *Washington Post.* May 6, 2000;B6.

Reed W. Harrison Fisher. Illustration House [online]. 1999. Available at: http://www.illustration-house.com/. Accessed August 30, 2002.

Rempel G. The Crimean War [online]. 2001. Available at: http://mars.acnet.wnec.edu/~grempel/courses/russia/lectures/19crimeanwar.html. Accessed October 28, 2002.

Rempel G. The Russian Civil War [online]. 1998. Available at: http://mars.acnet.wnec.edu/~grempel/courses/russia/lectures/28civilwar.html. Accessed September 23, 2002.

Rempel G. The Crimean War [online]. 1999. Available at: http://mars.acnet.wnec.edu/~grempel/courses/russia/lectures/19crimeanwar.html. Accessed September 21, 2002.

Renou A. The telephone [online]. Available at: http://messel.emse.fr/~arenou/telephone.html. Accessed February 13, 2000.

Revolution by design: the soviet poster. International Poster Gallery [online]. Available at: http://www.internationalposter.com/ru-text.cfm#NEP. Accessed March 3, 2002.

Rhodes A. Histore mondiale de la propagande de 1933 à 1945. Paris: Elsevier Séquoia; 1980.

Richards E. *The Knife and Gun Club: Scenes From an Emergency Room.* New York, NY: Atlantic Monthly; 1989.

Riggs H. *Days of Tragedy in Armenia: Personal Experiences in Harpoot, 1915–1917.* Ann Arbor, Mich: Gomidas Institute; 1997.

Ringle K. Ferreting out the elusive enemy. *Washington Post.* December 29, 2001; C1, C4.

Roberts R. The smash-up kid: Fort Wayne aviator Art Smith. *Traces.* Fort Wayne: Indiana Historical Society; 1998.

Rock Island Railroad [online]. Available at: http://www.rock-island.org/. Accessed February 27, 2002.

Rossi A. *Posters.* London: Paul Hamlyn; 1966.

Royal Warrants. Official Web site of the British Monarchy [online]. Available at: http://www.royal.gov.uk. Accessed July 24, 2002.

Rubin C, Williams M. Larger than life: the American tall-tale postcard, 1905–1915. New York, NY: Abbeville; 1990.

Russian Civil War. (2000). Spartacus [online]. Available at: http://www.spartacus.schoolnet.co.uk/RUScivilwar.htm. Accessed September 23, 2002.

Russo-Turkish Wars. *Columbia Encyclopedia.* [online]. 6th ed. 2000. Available at: http://www.bartleby.com/65/ru/RussoTur.html. Accessed May 25, 2000.

Ryder R. *Edith Cavell.* New York, NY: Stein and Day; 1975.

SS Amerkia. Maritimes Matters [online]. Available at: http://www.maritimematters.com/amerika.html. Accessed March 13, 2002.

SS Nobska historical notes [online]. Available at: http://www.nobska.org/bgnd/a2.htm. Accessed February 21, 2002.

Santos C. RE: 1977 ICN in Tokyo [e-mail to Michael Zwerdling]. March 14, 2002. Available at: e-mail: zna@nursepostcard.com.

Schriver G. *A History of the Illinois Training School for Nurses 1880–1929.* Chicago: Board of Directors of the Illinois Training School for Nurses; 1930.

Schwertfeger R. *Women of Theresienstadt.* New York, NY: Berg; 1989.

Shackelford M. Medals of Finland [online]. 1997. Available at: http://www.ku.edu/~kansite/ww_one/medals/finmedl/finland.html. Accessed April 22, 2002.

Sigel R. The cultivation of medicinal herbs in the concentration camp. *Dachau Review*. 1990;2:78–86. Brussels: Comité International de Dachau.

Smith A. *Art Smith, His Own Story of His Thrilling Career*. Ft. Wayne: News-Sentinel; 1915.

Smith E. *Visual Arts in the Twentieth Century*. New York, NY: Abrams; 1996.

Smith J. Baby incubators. Neonatology on the web [online]. 1999. Available at: http://www.neonatology.org/classics/smith/smith.html. Accessed July 16, 2002.

Smith J. *Royal postcards*. Lombard, IL: Wallace-Homestead; 1987.

Sobieszek R. *The Art of Persuasion: A History of Advertising Photography*. New York, NY: Abrams; 1988.

Sovereign Grand Lodge Independent Order of Odd Fellows [online]. Available at: http://norm28.hsc.usc.edu/IOOF.shtml. Accessed February 21, 2002.

Spanish Civil War. *Encyclopedia Britannica* [online]. 2002. Available at: http://www.britannica.com/eb/article?eu=70775. Accessed September 22, 2002.

Staff F. *The Picture Postcard and Its Origins*. London: Lutterworth; 1979.

Stangos N, ed. *Concepts of Modern Art from Fauvism to Postmodernism*. 3rd ed. London: Thames & Hudson; 1994.

SS Nobska historical notes [online]. Available at: http://www.nobska.org/bgnd/a2.htm. Accessed February 21, 2002.

Steam engine. *Compton's encyclopedia* [online]. Available at: http://www.optonline.com/comptons/ceo/02400_A.html. Accessed March 3, 2000.

Stern G. Packaging: container as context [online]. 1999. Available at: http://www.balchinstitute.org/advert/package.html. Accessed September 24, 2000.

Story of the laws behind the labels. Food and Drug Administration [online]. Available at: http://vm.cfsan.fda.gov/~lrd/history1.html. Accessed February 26, 2002.

Stout S. Story of the great Cherry Coal Mine disaster [online]. 1979. Available at: http://www.kentlaw.edu/ilhs/cherrymi.html. Accessed June 6, 2000.

Stuart D. *Dear Duchess: Millicent Duchess of Sutherland, 1867–1955*. London: David & Charles; 1982.

Sturani E. *Curarsi con le cartoline*. Rome: Rinaldo Cutini; 1983.

Suburban Hospital Healthcare System [online]. Available at: http://www.openseason.com/suburban/welcome/about.html. Accessed March 8, 2000.

Taylor T. The doctors trial—the medical case of the subsequent Nuremberg proceedings: the indictment [online]. 1946. Available at: http://www.ushmm.org/research/doctors/indiptx.htm. Accessed January 6, 2001.

Terning J. The Dionne Quintuplets [online]. 1999. Available at: http://schwinger.harvard.edu/~terning/bios/Dionne.html. Accessed July 13, 2002.

Teutonia Society. San Francisco history: societies [online]. 2002. Available at: http://www.zpub.com/sf50/sf/hgsoc.htm. Accessed August 22, 2002.

Theofiles J. *American Posters of World War I*. New York, NY: Dafran House; 1984.

Timeline: Lebanon. BBC News [online]. Available at: http://news.bbc.co.uk/hi/english/world/middle_east/newsid_819000/819200.stm. Accessed February 8, 2002.

Tipper H, Hollingwood H, Hotchkiss G, Parsons F. *Advertising, Its Principles and Practice*. New York, NY: Ronald Press; 1919.

Toland J. *Hitler: The Pictorial Documentary of his Life*. New York, NY: Doubleday; 1978.

Toledo's Attic [online]. Available at: http://www.attic.utoledo.edu/att/time/t1908.html. Accessed February 27, 2002.

Tony awards. American Theatre Wing [online]. Available at: http://www.tonys.org/news/features/7773ea0590bae20085256a5f006acd70.html. Accessed March 2, 2002.

Tryon N. Royalty and its influence on photographic images. *Postcard Collector*; April 1958.

Turner E. *The Shocking History of Advertising*. New York, NY: Ballantine; 1953.

Ukraine. Flick, Inc. [online]. Available at: http://www.flick.com/onomastikon/Former-Soviet-Union/Europe&Caucasus/Ukraine.htm. Accessed March 3, 2002.

Unger A. Edith Cavell: No hatred or bitterness for anyone. *British Heritage Magazine*. 1997; May. Women's history [online]. Available at: http://womenshistory.about.com/library/prm/bledith_cavell1.htm. Accessed November 26, 2002.

United Kingdom National AIDS Trust [online]. Available at: http://www.nat.org.uk/. Accessed March 15, 2002.

United States Census Bureau National Population Estimates [online]. Available at: http://www.census.gov:80/population/estimates/nation/popclockest.txt. Accessed February 24, 2000.

Vanderwood P, Samponaro F. *Border Fury: A Picture Postcard Record of Mexico's Revolution and U.S. War Preparedness, 1910–1917*. Albuquerque: University of New Mexico; 1988.

Vassiltchikov M. *Berlin Diaries 1940–1945*. New York, NY: Random House; 1998.

Vorres I. The art of the last Romanov Grand Duchess of Russia [online]. 2002. Available at: http://www.si.edu/oahp/olga/. Accessed August 22, 2002.

Waco UIC. Smithsonian national air and space museum [online]. Available at: http://www.nasm.si.edu/nasm/aero/aircraft/wacouic.htm. Accessed March 14, 2002.

Wagner C, Weidner D. Belgian Royalty: Queen Elizabeth. Historical boys' royal costume [online]. 2002. Available at: http://histclo.hispeed.com/royal/gers/bav/eliz.htm. Accessed July 30, 2002.

Wagner C, Weidner D. British Royalty: Prince Albert Victor. Historical boys' royal costume [online]. 1999. Available at: http://histclo.hispeed.com/royal/eng/royal-ukav.htm. Accessed July 31, 2002.

Wagner C, Weidner D. European Royalty: Italy. Historical boys' royal costume [online]. 1998. Available at: http://histclo.hispeed.com/royal/ita/royal-it.htm. Accessed July 30, 2002.

Wagner C, Weidner D. European Royalty: Thurn and Taxis. Historical boys' royal costume [online]. 1999. Available at: http://histclo.hispeed.com/royal/gers/royal-thurn. htm. Accessed July 31, 2002.

Wald, Lillian D. Encyclopedia Britannica [online]. 2002. Available at: http://www.britannica.com/eb/article?eu=77909. Accessed July 29, 2002.

Ward R. *Investment Guide to North American Real Photo Postcards*. Bellevue, Wash: Antique Paper Guild; 1991.

Ward R. *Real Photo Postcards: The Life-Size Edition*. Bellevue, Wash: Antique Paper Guild; 1994.

Wells D. A history of ships named Enterprise [online]. 2001. Available at: http://www.cs.umanitoba.ca/~djc/startrek/SNE.html. Accessed July 27, 2002.

Wells W, Burnett J, Moriarty S. *Advertising Principles and Practice*. 3rd ed. Englewood Cliffs, NJ: Prentice Hall; 1995.

Wenborn N, et al. *Pictorial History of the Twentieth Century*. North Dighton, MAA: JG Press; 1995.

What is The Lorraine-Cross? Danish Lung Association [online]. Available at: http://www.lunge.dk/eng-Lorraine.htm. Accessed May 8, 2000.

Winthrop University Hospital [online]. Available at: http://www.winthrop.org/. Accessed March 7, 2002.

World AIDS Day Organization [online]. Available at: http://www.worldaidsday.org/. Accessed March 14, 2002.

World War I. *Encyclopedia Britannica* [online]. 2002. Available at: http://www.britannica.com/eb/article?eu=118861. Accessed September 23, 2002.

Zeepvat C. *Queen Victoria's Family: A Century of Photographs*. Gloucestershire: Sutton; 2001.

Zodin S. Army nurses. *Caducean*. February 12, 1996;4–5. Honolulu: Tripler Army Medical Center.

Zodin S. Dr. Kildare [e-mail to Michael Zwerdling]. February 11, 2002. Available at: zna@nurspostard.com.

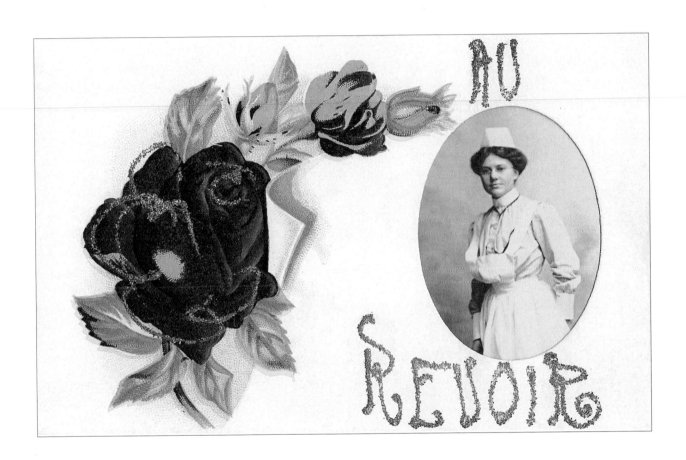

Index

Boer War, 266f, 282, 289
Bohemian Heart Charity, 143f
Bompard, Luigi, 103
Bonazzi, E., 154f
Bophuthatswana, 315f, 337
Boris, King, 219
Boulanger, G., 92f
Bovie Corporation, 133f, 164
Bowdle, Marie, 136f
Bowes-Lyon, Elizabeth, 217
Brazil, 316f
Brenton, Ray, 180f
Brewster, Mary M., 219
Brewster Hospital, 306f, 310
Bristol Visiting Nurse Association, 112f, 160
British Expeditionary Force (BEF), 286
British West Africa, 316f
Brown, Trevor, 68f–69f, 103, 159f, 167
Brownfield, Elizabeth, 173f
Buhl, Marthe, 48f–49f, 102
Bulgaria, 316f
Byzantine Emperor, 7

C

Caduceus, 4
Caldecott, Randolph, 88f, 105
Caldecott Medal, 105
California House, 17f, 32
Campbell, Blendon, 108f, 160
Camp Fire Girls, 296f, 309
Canada, 316f–317f
Canadian nurses, 190f–191f
Canadian Nursing Service, 290
Canadian Red Cross Memorial Hospital (CRCMH), 218
Candy Candy, 67f, 103
Capping ceremony, 27f, 33
Cato Street Conspiracy, 105
Cavell, Edith Louise, 248f, 253f, 256f, 287, 288
Challenger (railroad), 163
Chamberlain, Neville, 291
Chaplin, Charles Spencer, 183f, 213
Chesterton, Cecil, 106
Chicago, Rock Island, and Pacific Railroad, 161
Chieko, Sanjo, 221
Child hatchery, 215
China, 317f
Chiron, 4
Chlorine gas, 284
Christie, Mary B., 173f
Church, Ellen (Marshall), 163
Circumcision, 304f, 309
Collyer, June, 188f, 214
Compassion in nurses, 4–5
Coney Island, 215

Congo Free State, 315f, 337
Constructivism, 150f, 165
Cook County Hospital, 161
Coronis, 3–4
Couney, Martin, 215
Cox, Howard, 122f
Crimean War, 9, 283
Croatia, 317f
Crobella, Tito, 249f, 250f–252f, 288
Cross of Lorraine, 6–8
Cross of St. George, 8
Cross of St. John, 8
Cunningham, Alison, 332f, 337
Curie, Marie Sklodowska, 288
Czechoslovakia, 317f

D

Dahomey, 318f
Day, Larraine, 214
Day of Liberation, 291
de Boullion, Godefroy, 7
De Croy, Prince, 287
De Croy, Princess, 287
Delano, Jane A., 231f, 283
Denmark, 318f
Depage, Antoine, 287
Depage, Marie, 256f
Detroit Publishing Company, 104
Diana (Roman goddess), 32
Dionne quintuplets, 214
Doctor in the House (movie), 287
Dogali (town), 32
Dr. Kildare (film series), 189f, 214
Drayton, W. Heyward, 104
Drinker, Philip, 163
DRK (Deutsche Rotes Kreutz), 276f, 291
Duchess of Connaught Red Cross Hospital, 218
Duchess of Sutherland, 195f
Duchess of York, 195f
Dudovich, Marcello, 41f, 60f, 102
Dupuy, Father, 327f, 337

E

E & J Burke Bottling Company, 160
Easter, 62f, 103
Eaton, Seymour, 104
Edith Cavell Hospital School, 257f
Edward, Prince, 195f, 218
Edward III, King, 216
Edwards, Alice, 213
Edwards, Tom, 213
Edward VII, King, 216
Edward VIII, King, 217
Egypt, 318f
Élan and patriotism, 289
Electrostatic therapy, 161
Electrotherapies, 120f, 161
Elena, Princess (Montenegro), 220